LANGUAGES AND LINGUISTICS SERIES

SPEECH DISORDERS: CAUSES, TREATMENT AND SOCIAL EFFECTS

LANGUAGES AND LINGUISTICS SERIES

Critical Discourse Analysis: An Interdisciplinary Perspective
Thao Le, Quynh Le and Megan Short (Editors)
2009. ISBN: 978-1-60741-320-2

Critical Discourse Analysis: An Interdisciplinary Perspective
Thao Le, Quynh Le and Megan Short (Editors)
2009. ISBN: 978-1-60876-772-4 (Online Book)

Building Language Skills and Cultural Competencies in the Military
Edgar D. Swain (Editor)
2009. ISBN: 978-1-60741-126-0

Building Language Skills and Cultural Competencies in the Military
Edgar D. Swain (Editor)
2009. ISBN: 978-1-60876-597-3 (Online Book)

Second Languages: Teaching, Learning and Assessment
Ryan L. Jikal and Samantha A. Raner (Editors)
2009. ISBN: 978-1-60692-661-1

Aphasia: Symptoms, Diagnosis and Treatment
Grigore Ibanescu and Serafim Pescariu (Editors)
2009. ISBN: 978-1-60741-288-5

Building Strategic Language Ability Programs
Joshua R. Weston (Editor)
2010. ISBN: 978-1-60741-127-7

Speech Disorders: Causes, Treatment and Social Effects
Alan E. Harrison (Editor)
2010. ISBN: 978-1-60876-213-2

LANGUAGES AND LINGUISTICS SERIES

SPEECH DISORDERS: CAUSES, TREATMENT AND SOCIAL EFFECTS

ALAN E. HARRISON
EDITOR

Nova Science Publishers, Inc.
New York

LIBRARY OF CONGRESS CATALOGING-IN-PUBLICATION DATA

Speech disorders : causes, treatment and social effects / editor, Alan E. Harrison.
p. cm.
Includes bibliographical references and index.
ISBN 978-1-60876-213-2 (hardcover : alk. paper)
1. Speech disorders. 2. Language disorders. 3. Communicative disorders. I. Harrison, Alan E.
RC423.S63827 2009
616.85'5--dc22

2009031120

Published by Nova Science Publishers, Inc. ✢ New York

CONTENTS

PREFACE

Speech disorders or speech impediments, as they are also called, are a type of communication disorder where 'normal' speech is disrupted. This can mean stuttering, lisps, etc. Someone who is totally unable to speak due to a speech disorder is considered mute. Speech disorders refer to problems in producing the sounds of speech or with the quality of voice. In many cases the cause is unknown. However, there are various known causes of speech impediments, such as "hearing loss, neurological disorders, brain injury, mental retardation, drug abuse, physical impairments such as cleft lip and palate, and vocal abuse or misuse. This new and important book gathers the latest research from around the globe in the study of speech disorders with a focus on such topics as: speech and voice disorders in Parkinson's Disease, genetic causes, stuttering therapy for adolescents and adults, prosody and autism spectrum disorder, speech rehabilitation after oropharyngeal cancer, mutism, dyslexia and others.

Chapter 1 – This chapter starts with a description of the different aspects of speech disturbance in Parkinson's disease, considering previous findings based upon perceptual and acoustical analysis and kinematic studies. In the second section, there is an overview of different therapeutic approaches in the treatment of dysarthria. The third section deals with methodological issues which are relevant for the interpretation and weighting of study data on speech. Finally, all these different aspects of dysarthria are integrated into a preliminary pathophysiological concept of Parkinsonian dysarthria illustrated in the last section of this review.

Chapter 2 - Both speech production and literacy skills are of significant concern to educators and early interventionists. Longitudinal research has shown that children with speech and/or literacy problems remain at significant risk for limited academic, social, and occupational achievement. While these two behavioral domains have often been studied separately (as speech-language disorders and as reading disabilities), the co-occurrence of speech and literacy problems is well-documented, with deficits in one domain often accompanied by (sometimes subtle) deficits in the other. The theoretical link between speech and literacy-related skills in children is reviewed in this chapter, with emphasis on the phonological components of reading. Research is summarized on two main topics: the identification of individuals who are at risk for literacy problems through speech assessment, and the literacy-related skills of children with speech sound disorders. Data are then presented that demonstrate how short-term phonological memory may play an important connecting role between speech and literacy in children with speech sound disorders. Finally, the implications for assessment and intervention for children with speech sound disorders are summarized in an effort to provide a more comprehensive framework for translating research on the speech-literacy link into clinical practice.

Literacy skills, which must be explicitly taught, have their foundations in speech-related skills, which are often learned quite naturally. Alphabetic writing systems take advantage of the fact that there are discernable categories of speech sounds (phonemes) that are produced by speakers of the language. Thus, proficient literacy skills, particularly in an alphabetic orthography, are aided by one's facility with the phonology of the language. That is, successful reading of an alphabetic system involves mapping print to the speech signal, while spelling requires mapping speech to print. The goals of this chapter are to briefly review the well-established connection between speech and literacy, discuss the theoretical and empirical link (based primarily in phonological processing), and extend the discussion of speech and literacy skills to shed light on two clinical populations: children who do not have facility with literacy skills, and children who do not have facility with the productive phonology of their language. It will become apparent that children with literacy problems have been found to have subtle problems with productive phonological skills, and children with speech sound disorders often have problems with literacy-related skills. The implications for clinical research will be addressed throughout the chapter to highlight why the speech-literacy connection is of importance. Phonological short-term memory will be discussed as an important skill in literacy development, and data will be presented to demonstrate how this skill could be assessed in children with poor intelligibility.

The term *speech sound disorder (SSD)* will be used to refer to those children who have difficulty producing or using the sounds of their language, but for whom there is no obvious cause (such as hearing impairment, cleft palate, developmental disorder, etc.); other terminology, such as articulation impairment, phonological disorder, or expressive phonological impairment, have been used in the literature. The terms *dyslexia* or *reading difficulties* will be used to refer to children who demonstrate low performance on reading and/or spelling tasks in the absence of an obvious cause (cognitive problems, developmental disabilities, etc.). It should be noted that nearly every study reviewed here uses its own criteria for determining these categories (SSD or dyslexia), and many studies use different terms to refer to the same populations. In addition, both speech production and literacy skills are immensely complex and cannot be thoroughly reviewed here. Both rely on cognitive-behavioral skills that include attention, memory, perception, etc., all of which are the byproduct of genetic and environmental influences; thus, the relationships that will be discussed exist within the context of many other complex neural, psychological, and biological relationships. Accurately measuring the essential parameters of speech and reading is still a challenge even to the most experienced researchers and clinicians

Approximately 50-75% of children with SSD have been found to have long-term academic problems, and approximately 28% of children identified as "at-risk" for literacy problems are referred for speech therapy. Thus, the overlap among speech and reading problems is not negligible.

Reading educators often lack sufficient knowledge of phonology, and some speech-language pathologists judge that they lack sufficient knowledge of reading (e.g., a series of editorials in the *ASHA Leader* 2007-2008). Although this may be a limitation in our professional training programs, research demonstrates a robust relationship between phonological and literacy skills that should be of concern to both professions. Ultimately, we wish to understand speech and reading at the level both of the individual (a particular client or student, etc.) and in populations (persons with SSD, dyslexia, etc.). Thus, beginning with the simple notion that speech skills are a foundation for literacy, it is important to discuss how and why these skills should be considered together.

From a systems-based perspective, both SSD and reading problems have been discussed as arising from weaknesses in the auditory processing or perception of speech, skill automization, and timing mechanisms. For example, individuals with SSD as well as those with reading problems have been reported to show below-average identification of synthesized speech, and difficulty encoding the temporal order of perceived speech sounds. Both clinical populations have been shown to struggle with speech- and non-speech rhythmic tasks and motor coordination tasks. Given that reading skills rely heavily on oral language, it is not surprising that many of the same neural regions needed for speech perception and production are also required for reading and spelling.

From an etiological perspective, similar causes have been put forth as contributing to both speech and reading problems. Genetic influences and family histories of the respective disorders likely contribute to the manifestation of both speech and reading problems in children. Additionally, impoverished language environments, often associated with low socioeconomic status or low parental education, likely plays a role in some cases of speech and reading difficulty.

Chapter 3 - Positron Emission Tomography (PET) is at present the only method affording three-dimensional regional quantitation of various physiological, functional and molecular variables in man. Making use of tracers labelled with short lived positron emitting radio-nuclides and coincidence detection of annihilation radiation state of the art technology and advanced computing systems permit quantitative imaging of voluminous organs within one session. By 3-D data acquisition the distribution of small tracer amounts in the brain can be measured with a spatial resolution of down to 2 mm and values of various metabolic, functional and molecular parameters can be calculated applying kinetic and parametric analysis. Over the last 30 years PET has gained importance as a clinical diagnostic procedure yielding information on pathophysiologic mechanisms in various brain diseases. This method has also been used extensively as a tool of functional neuroanatomy when changes of metabolic or perfusional patterns were studied during various stimulations or task performances in healthy subjects or patients with localized brain lesions.

This approach was especially successful in the study of language, which as a complex brain function is based on the interplay of a distributed network in which partial functions are executed in various centres, which are hierarchically organized and lateralized into the dominant hemisphere. Following local brain lesions different language domains are impaired causing the various types of aphasia. Changes in the interactions within the functional network of language are important for the type of aphasia and for the capacity for recovery, e.g. after stroke. In this context, studies of activation patterns during speech tasks in the course after stroke could be used to predict extent of recovery, could demonstrate effects of supportive therapy and may be helpful in the development of procedures, e.g. cortical stimulation, for suppression of interfering or for enhancing compensatory effects in rehabilitation.

Chapter 4 - This study reports the first five years of a school readiness intervention called 'HABLA' (Home Based Activities Building Language Acquisition), It was designed to increase and enrich speech and literacy activities in the homes of economically and educationally disadvantaged Latino families with children between the age of 2 and 4. A team of trained home visitors provided two years of a 23-week program of visitation in which they met with parent(s) and child twice weekly. Both years presented a Spanish language adaptation of the Parent Child Home Program model; home visitors provide intensive modeling and coaching of non-directive Spanish language use, conversation, and literacy activities. Administration of the PLS-3 in Spanish at the onset and culmination of each year of the program indicates significant increases in receptive and expressive language for each year of visitation (7.8 standard points for the first year, 4.4 for the second) with effect size r ranging from .24 to .41. Participants had significantly improved their levels of oral Spanish skill and scored much higher than a comparison group of untreated peers. A subset of graduates of the two-year program was tested as kindergarteners; they showed a continued advantage over a comparison group of 18 peers who had not received the intervention. For the graduates, both their Spanish PLS-3 scores and English PLS-4 scores were significantly higher, and their parents reported a continued effort to provide literacy experiences at home. The HABLA participants also showed a clear advantage for an English language test of phonological awareness, one of the strongest predictors of school success.

During the early years of their lives, children in affluent and poor families experience a dramatic difference in exposure to speech. On average, those living in poverty hear 300 fewer words per hour and this culminates in a 30 million-word deficit by the time children enter kindergarten. Tied to this deficiency in spoken language exposure is a commensurate deficiency in children's speech that directly relates to the style, quality and diversity of their parent's language. As speech skills are key ingredients in school success, early deficiencies in the speech environment, if left unheeded, may cascade into educational disadvantages and a tragic loss of social capital.

Because the difference in the speech environment between advantaged and disadvantaged children begins so early in their lives, effective intervention must also begin early. An ideal intervention should increase the quality and quantity of parent to child language and should involve shared activities that can become self-sustaining after treatment ceases. The intervention should be home-based, and even if the children are to be English language learners once they begin school, the intervention should target the language of the home since that is the language the parent is most capable of delivering with appropriately rich vocabulary and grammar. Prompted by these considerations, we have developed a home-based intervention program to enrich the Spanish home language and literacy environments of poor Latino children. It is based on the highly successful Parent Child Home Program (PCHP).

Chapter 5 - The nature of speech sound disorder (SSD) is not yet well understood. Some view it as a single clinical entity, while others propose distinct subtypes, defined variously by criteria such as error types and suspected cause. A universally accepted disorder classification, based on relevant behavioral observations, does not yet exist. An account of genetic substrates would greatly enhance current understanding of SSD, but such an account is not yet available. This chapter reviews the history of genetic research in SSD from the first studies of familial clustering of SSD to the most recent studies in molecular genetics and points to new frontiers in the quest to characterize the biological causes of SSD.

Chapter 6 - Stuttering is a multifaceted communication disorder that not only affects the individual's speech fluency, but also impacts how he or she feels and thinks about themselves and communication. Thus, coping effectively with stuttering during adulthood often requires a multifaceted approach. The purpose of this chapter is to describe an intensive therapy program, the Intensive Stuttering Therapy for Adolescents and Adults, which utilizes such an approach. This proposed chapter is broken into three parts. First, the complex nature of stuttering and the rationale for a multifaceted approach will be discussed. Next, the author will describe the approach and the initial outcome data from this clinic. Finally, future directions for this clinical program will be explained, including the rationale and need for using telepractice as an adjunct to the intensive clinic.

Chapter 7 - Atypicalities in prosody are a prominent characteristic of all autism spectrum disorders. Despite the centrality of prosody to the behavioral presentation of the disorder, our knowledge of the nature of these deficits is limited. In this chapter, current research on prosody production and comprehension in autism spectrum disorders is examined. Particular attention will be given to the utility of prosody as an early diagnostic marker, as a behavioral indicator of subtypes of the disorder, and as a bellwether for strengths and weaknesses in an individual's cognitive profile. Future directions of prosody research will also be discussed, including the importance of acoustic analysis of speech and other psycholinguistic paradigms. Finally, the clinical implications research on prosodic deficits in autism spectrum disorders will be addressed, including the value of prosody for identifying individual differences and the promise of computerized instant feedback technology for treatment.

Chapter 8 - The Multi Dimensional Voice Program (MDVP) is a powerful software tool for quantitative acoustic assessment of voice quality; it is capable of calculating 33 parameters and provides flexible routines for graphical representation of the results.

Also a user-upgradeable voice database allows automatic comparison of the current results with different nosological groups. In our experience fundamental frequency (Fo), Jitter percent, Shimmer, noise to harmonics ratio (NHR), voice turbulence index (VTI), soft phonation index (SPI), degree of voiceless (DUV), degree of voice breaks (DVB) and peak amplitude variation (vAm) are the parameters which give the most objective information about the presence of vocal modification. A multiple regression analysis of these nine acoustic measures may provide a quick and relatively sensitive method that may be clinically useful in measuring change of vocal quality and articulation. These data provide a more complete analysis in conjunction with other tests: the mirror-fogging test from Glatzel and the Gutzmann test (for testing nasality); the voice handicap index (a validated questionnaire measuring psychosocial handicapping effects of voice disorders); Van Borsel's study (to evaluate articulation).

The authors have applied this protocol in the analysis of speech and voice before and one month after different surgical techniques (tonsillectomy, adenotonsillectomy, uvulopalatoplasty, septoplasty, microlaryngoscopy, etc).

Our protocol of voice and speech analysis provide objective, documentable and measurable data of vocal function, and these measurements are clinically helpful for the comparison of the patients' voice with those of healthy speakers. These measures maybe very useful to evaluate the patient affected by pathology and to provide a more secure diagnosis. For these reasons, otorhinolaryngologist should evaluate patients also using the MDVP, in conjunction with other test, at the beginning of their "diagnostic challenge".

Chapter 9 - During the second half of the 20th century the proportion of the United Kingdom population attending higher education increased from around 5% to more than 40%. It should not be surprising that the Higher Education learning environment has become more diverse as we move towards the government target of 50% of the population.

There is a growing awareness of the numbers of students who are diagnosed as dyslexic and perhaps to a lesser extent, students who may be dyscalculic.

Dyslexia is essentially a deficit in working memory. In the same way that sight impairment or hearing impairment may be mild or severe, dyslexia may also be mild or severe.

Sight, hearing, and working memory are clearly factors which affect learning, but consideration of a single factor cannot give a reliable assessment of a person's ability, intelligence or potential.

The term 'constructive alignment' is used to describe the desired harmony between the student and all of the elements which make up the learning environment. The assertion is that greater harmony will facilitate greater learning.

Disciplines such as psychology, sciences and social sciences, have significant mathematical and/or statistical concepts embedded in them. It is common for students to find themselves undertaking projects which involve the collection and analysis of data. Individual students might have returned to full time education after a number of years; they might not have a formal mathematics qualification and be a little surprised and daunted by the mathematics involved. In such situations any learning disability compounds the principal problem that the student is attempting to apply relatively complex statistical/mathematical analysis without having a good understanding of the necessary underpinning concepts, such as ratio, proportion and probability.

The study of mathematics requires assimilation of a hierarchy of concepts. Without an understanding of lower concepts on which the higher concepts are built, study of the higher concepts can be frustrating and unproductive.

Our student support facilities need to be developed so that students can be shown the necessary hierarchy of mathematical concepts and can assimilate them at their own pace. This will be of benefit to students with and without learning difficulties.

Chapter 10 - The intra-oral structures are essential for the chewing, swallowing, speech and vocal production functions, effects in these functions, as well as the aesthetic, social and emotional aspects related to oral cancers, do affect these patients. These effects are caused both by the tumor, and by its treatment (surgery, radiotherapy and/or chemotherapy). There are few studies with the use of objective or subjective instruments to evaluate the resulting speech and voice, still scarcer are the studies that discuss the speech-therapy strategies and their results for these oncology patients. Objective: Review and present both the voice and speech evaluation instruments, and the therapy strategies used for the improvement of the oral communication of oral cavity and oropharynx cancer patients. Method: Perform a literature review between 1967 and 2009 with the Medline describer (speech OR voice OR therapy) AND (oral cancer OR oropharynx cancer), with the exclusion of the papers that present results without formal evaluation instruments and case studies. Results: Eighty four studies were found meeting the criteria established. Thirty-four studies used quality of life protocols for functional evaluation and in 50 studies there was the citation of the utilization of some type of voice or speech evaluation clinical observations to describe function. Speech therapy procedures and their strategies/results concerning speech and voice were found in only 5 studies. Conclusions: Perceptive-auditory evaluation was the most used, with speech intelligibility as the most analyzed parameter. But studies concerning the speech-therapy treatment of these patients are still scarce, and their results seem to be influenced by the size of the samples, by the number of speech-therapy sessions, and by the eventual effects of the variety of the exercises performed.

Chapter 11 - This case report investigated audience/no-audience effects on stuttering, speech rate, and fundamental frequency (F_0) by analyzing the oral reading performance of an adult Japanese male stutterer in an A_1-B_1-A_2-B_2 paradigm, where A represents an audience phase and B a no-audience phase. The subject read a passage five times in each phase. The audience/no-audience effects on the three variables were found significant. The plausibility of higher F_0 as an indicator and 'precursor' of stuttering, in conjunction with the relation of anxiety to stuttering and F_0, is discussed. The possibility is also suggested that oral reading practice in a no-audience condition may be used as treatment for stuttering.

Chapter 12 - Selective mutism is a poorly understood condition at the interface between speech-language disorders and psychiatric disorders of childhood. Affected children fail to speak in one or more specific situations, impairing their social and academic development, often for years. Previous underestimates of its prevalence may account for the limited research attention it has received. Social anxiety, second language acquisition, developmental delays, auditory processing problems, and subtle language impairments may contribute to selective mutism, but a clear understanding of its etiology remains elusive. Key aspects of assessment include evaluating anxiety, cognition, and language using nonverbal methods and collateral information from parents and schools; obtaining a detailed baseline of communication attempts in various situations; and ruling out the presence of impaired hearing, pervasive developmental disorder, other communication disorders, normal second language acquisition, and mutism secondary to a traumatic event. Intervention has focused largely on behavioral methods to encourage social speech, but adding serotonin-specific medications is often helpful in severe cases, despite some concerns about using these in young children. Teamwork between clinicians, families, and school personnel is essential for treatment success. Further studies to elucidate the etiology of selective mutism and its optimal treatment are needed.

Chapter 13 – The tongue of the human being is the muscular mass which takes a seat in the mandibular bone and occupies the oral floor. The musculature of the human tongue is consisted of both four extrinsic lingual muscles and four intrinsic tongue muscles. The extrinsic lingual muscles are attached to the structures outside of the tongue including the jaw, the styloid process, and the hyoid bone, and end in the tongue. The intrinsic lingual muscles are contained entirely within the tongue. It had been considered that the gross position of the tongue body might be accomplished by the contraction of the extrinsic lingual muscles, while the intrinsic lingual muscles might determine the shape of the surface of the tongue. In practice, the extrinsic lingual muscles or the intrinsic muscles work not only respectively, but also together to accomplish more fine and efficiently movement of the tongue, i.e., articulatory movement and masticatiory movement. Before considering the musculature of the human tongue, let us see the history and origins the tongue muscles.

Chapter 14 - The effectiveness of using speech rate-conversion software by artificially decreasing sound waveforms without changing the pitch was studied in 62 individuals with dysarthria. Besides having patients read a standard common passage entitled "The North Wind and the Sun" aloud, they had casual conversations on a different occasion. Both reading and conversations were recorded on a digital audiocassette recorder in a sound-treated studio. Using speech rate-conversion software, the two types of speech samples (reading and speaking) were played back under 5 rate-delay conditions (100, 150, 200, 250, and 300%

slower than the original recording) for evaluation of intelligibility and naturalness by 3 speech and language pathologists. With regard to both intelligibility and naturalness, a significant difference was observed among the 5 rate-delay conditions regardless of the type and severity of dysarthria. A 200% delay in rate delivered the greatest improvement in intelligibility; conversely, any rate-delay less or more than 200% resulted in slight deterioration. In addition, a 150% rate-delay in speech yielded the greatest improvement in naturalness, while any delay less or more than 150% resulted in a significant deteriorating tendency. These findings suggest that reducing verbal speed within the range of 150 - 200% may be useful in the clinical management of dysarthria.

Chapter 15 - The persistent reading difficulties of developmental dyslexics are often accompanied by a host of speech processing deficits. Dyslexics typically have inordinate difficulties in processing noise-degraded speech as opposed to non-speech stimuli despite exhibiting normal audiometric profiles. Furthermore, dyslexics often show relatively poor categorization of phonetically similar but phonologically contrastive speech sounds. However, some speech contrasts such as /d/-/g/ provoke more discriminative difficulty than others such as /b/-/s/ or /b/-/w/. If speech and speech disorders are modular, the dyslexic pattern of speech problems may not be limited to the auditory domain. Less often reported in the literature is a reduced influence of visual articulatory gestures on dyslexic perception of auditory cues. The question posed by the current study is whether or not dyslexic speech processing in the auditory channel is similarly nuanced in the visual channel. To this end, an auditory-visual twist on the standard categorical perception experiment was used to assess dyslexics' and controls' categorization of synthetic speech sounds along /ada/-/aga/ and /aba/-/awa/ continua. Presentation of each acoustic continuum involved a 3-factor design: 1) noise masked vs. clear presentation, 2) with and without a simultaneous video of a speaker, 3) articulating either endpoint of the respective continua. Results show that the dyslexics exhibited less precise, flatter categorical functions for acoustic /ada/ vs. /aga/ in noise; their responses were also less influenced by the introduction of visual cues to /d/ or /g/ than were those of the controls. In contrast, the dyslexics showed more control-like categorization of acoustic /aba/-/awa/ stimuli, as well as greater influences of the corresponding visual cues than controls. This parallel between the visual and auditory speech perception of dyslexics can be described phonologically: dyslexics may find place of articulation contrasts more problematic than manner contrasts. It is possible that poor apprehension or representation of key phonological features may imperil the categorical labeling of minimally contrastive speech stimuli. Discussion considers this account as compared to auditory temporal accounts, general magnocellular dysfunctions, and integrative failures.

In: Speech Disorders: Causes, Treatment and Social Effects ISBN: 978-1-60876-213-2
Editor: Alan E. Harrison, pp. 1-41

Chapter 1

SPEECH AND VOICE DISORDERS IN PARKINSON'S DISEASE

Sabine Skodda
Department of Neurology, Ruhr-University of Bochum, Bochum, Germany

INTRODUCTION

Parkinson´s disease (PD) is a neurodegenerative disorder characterized by progressive loss of dopaminergic neurons, primarily in the substantia nigra pars compacta, and affects 1-2% of people age over 60 years [179]. According to the Braak staging, PD begins as a synucleopathy in non-dopaminergic structures of the lower brainstem or in the olfactory bulb with subsequent rostral progression and affection of the substantia nigra [33, 34]. The progressive dopaminergic loss is associated with a variety of motor and non-motor deficits in PD patients. In addition to the most ostensible symptoms as muscular rigidity, tremor, bradykinesia and postural instability, many patients develop a distinctive alteration of speech characterized as hypokinetic dysarthria. In a survey, the prevalence of dysarthria in PD was about 70% [110]. Affected patients may complain about a quiet or weak voice and about difficulties to get speech started. Further, they often report that they are asked to repeat their words because listeners have difficulties to understand although patients themselves may self-estimate their speech as loud and sufficiently articulated [74]. Dysarthria can emerge at any stage of the disease and worsen in the later stages [192, 244], causing a progressive loss of communication and leading to social isolation. Already James Parkinson noted in his "essay on the shaking palsy" that PD patients often became "scarcely intelligible" in the course of the disease [201].

Dysarthria is a collective name for impairments of speech-organ motor control resulting from dysfunction of structures on the supralaryngeal (jaw, lips, tongue, velum, pharynx), laryngeal (larynx) or infralaryngeal (trachea, lungs, diaphragma) level. Hypokinetic dysarthria in PD is interpreted as manifestation of rigor and hypokinesia on the speech effector organs, leading to a multidimensional motor speech impairment including alterations of speech respiration, phonation, articulation and prosody. Thus, based upon global clinical impression,

PD dysarthria is characterized by monotony of pitch and loudness, reduced stress, variable speech rate, imprecise articulation and a breathy and harsh voice [47, 49, 57, 58].

Since dysarthric speech is the end product of the pathological dynamics of the speech effector organs, perceptual analysis of speech may be useful for a qualitative evaluation of speech impairment and for estimation of overall intelligibility as the superordinate parameter of successful verbal communication. This approach can be supplemented by quantitative measurement of different speech variables by the means of acoustical analysis and assessment of articulatory movements by kinematic techniques. Understanding the disturbed motor patterns is the assumption for an insight in the underlying pathophysiology in Parkinsonian dysarthria.

Therefore, the actual review starts with a description of the different aspects of speech disturbance in PD considering previous findings based upon perceptual and acoustical analysis and kinematic studies. In the second section, there is an overview of different therapeutic approaches in the treatment of dysarthria. The third section deals with methodological issues which are relevant for the interpretation and weighting of study data on speech. Finally, all these different aspects of dysarthria are integrated into a preliminary pathophysiological concept of Parkinsonian dysarthria illustrated in the last section of this review.

I. Description of Parkinsonian Dysarthria

Based upon the perceptual analysis of a large sample of dysarthric speakers, Darley, Aronson and Brown primarily defined a salient cluster of deviant speech dimensions in Parkinsonian dysarthria including a harsh breathy voice quality, reduced variability of pitch and loudness, reduced stress, imprecise consonant articulation and short rushes of speech interrupted by inappropriate periods of silence [57, 58]. Together, these features give hypokinetic dysarthria its distinctive gestalt of a flat, attenuated and sometimes accelerated quality which has been attributed to a reduced range of articulatory movement [57, 58]. Logeman and colleagues established a general profile of hypokinetic dysarthria in a group of 200 PD patients, where almost 90% had voice disorders characterized by hoarseness, roughness, tremulousness and breathiness [169]. About half of the speakers featured articulatory problems, and 20% had speech rate abnormalities characterized by syllable repetitions, irregularities of syllable length and excessive speech pauses. According to this study, the authors supposed voice abnormalities to be the prominent attribute of hypokinetic dysarthria with the assumption of further subgroups including articulatory and speech rate deviations. These suggestions were consolidated by the findings of Zwirner and Barnes who confirmed the higher frequency of laryngeal than articulatory impairment in PD, maybe as an evidence that hypokinetic dysarthria tends to begin with laryngeal manifestation [279].

I.1. Speech Respiration

The rigidity associated with PD can include respiratory muscles and therefore lead to an increased resistance of the respiratory system mirrored by a reduced vital capacity and tidal volume as well as by reduced amplitude of chest wall muscles during breathing, reduced respiratory muscle strength and endurance and irregular breathing patterns [28, 126, 127, 250, 265, 270]. Respiratory insufficiency in PD has been attributed to a variety of abnormal speech findings as reduced maximum vowel duration, reduced airflow volume during vowel prolongation, fewer syllable production per breath group, use of greater than average percentage of vital capacity per syllable and increased breath groups during reading [32, 48, 49, 127, 189]. Solomon and Hixon found abnormally small rib cage volumes and compensatory large abdominal volumes at the initiation of speech breath groups in PD speakers who produced fewer words and spoke for less time per breath group than healthy controls [250]. Respiratory support for speech may also be measured by vowel prolongation time which has been reported to be reduced in PD speakers as compared to healthy controls and to show further decline in the course of disease [47, 49, 148, 185]. However, there are further studies negating a decrease of maximum phonation time in PD [8, 243], perhaps because of different test methods and inherent variability within and across individuals. Murdoch and colleagues reported on abrupt and paradoxical movements of chest wall parts during vowel prolongation and syllable repetition tasks in a subgroup of PD speakers which have been interpreted as abnormal rigidity of respiratory muscles, but the interpretation had been questioned because of methodological concerns [191, 250].

Since most of the measures on speech breathing assess airstream after it has been acted upon by the larynx and upper-airway structures, there are methodological difficulties to parse out the contribution of the breathing subsystem. Furthermore, besides simple mechanical mechanisms of impaired speech breathing, there is experimental support for the presence of impaired respiratory control at least in some PD speakers, suggested by documentation of longer latencies before beginning exhalation following forceful inhalation, delayed initiation of phonation once exhalation begins, problems with altering automatic respiratory rhythms for speech and difficulty with tracking a sinusoidal target with respiratory movements [147, 181].

I.2. Phonation

Numerous acoustical and physiologic studies have examined laryngeal function which in general confirm perceptual impression of multifaceted changes of voice in Parkinsonian dysarthria and thus provide additional insight in the underlying mechanisms.

The majority of studies on average pitch of voice as obtained by measurement of fundamental frequency (F_0) report an elevation of F_0 in PD patients as compared to age-matched controls [47, 48, 49, 69, 114, 124, 131, 146, 236, 243] which, however, not always reaches statistical significance [146, 160, 185] and seems to be more consistent in male than in female PD patients [124]. These findings stand in contrast to the perceptual findings of Darley and colleagues who found that pitch was tended to be perceived as low [57, 58] which might be attributed to a distortion of subjective pitch estimation by further voice abnormalities as e.g. reduced loudness. The increased F_0 in PD patients is generally ascribed to rigidity of the laryngeal musculature resulting in increased stiffness of the vocal folds. While average F_0 has been found to be increased when examined during sustained vowel production, reading passages and monologues, several studies discovered an increase of F_0 range and variability during vowel prolongation in PD [69, 114, 137, 279]. Similarly, some examiners describe an increased jitter, which serves as a measure of F_0 micropertubation, in prolonged vowel production [114, 137], which, however, could not be reproduced in female PD patients [143]. Although not consistently reproducible by the different examiners, raised F_0 variability, jitter and shimmer, which gives information about short-time instability of speech intensity, serve as an indication for irregular vocal fold vibration and therefore are thought to reflect reduced short-term neuromuscular control of the laryngeal abductory or adductory mechanisms in PD [124, 159].

Voice tremor, although no prominent perceptual feature of Parkinsonian dysarthria, can be detected by acoustical analysis or videostroboscopy in a subgroup of PD speakers [84, 203, 236]. Voice tremor frequency was found to lie within the same 4 to 7 Hz range as the typical Parkinsonian rest tremor and was more often seen in late stages of the disease [124, 136].

Investigation on speech loudness unambiguously document a reduced vocal intensity during various speech tasks, vowel prolongation tasks and alternate motion rate tasks which can be assessed by perceptual analyses [57, 58] and acoustical analyses techniques as well [72, 81, 119, 124, 131, 146, 237]. In an electromyographic (EMG) study, Baker and colleagues documented a reduction in thyroarytenoid muscle EMG amplitudes in PD speakers which was correlated to reduced sound pressure levels interpreted as a possible manifestation of hypokinesia on laryngeal structures responsible for low voice in PD [17]. Ho and colleagues found a reduction of conversional loudness in PD speakers at various distances from their listeners, but the ability to increase speech volume when the interlocutor distance increased was found to be preserved indicating a dampened speech intensity level. Since PD patients tended to overestimate the loudness of speech, additional perceptual deficits may contribute to a dysfunctional self-monitoring and adjustment of speech intensity [120]. Finally, loudness problems in PD may be exacerbated under conditions of divided attention, such as speaking while performing a motor task [122].

A further phonatory measure that has been studied in PD is the voice onset time (VOT) which is defined as the duration of time from articulatory release of a consonant to the onset of voicing of the following vowel [166]. Therefore, in the description of speech, VOT is at the intersection of phonation and articulation. Forrest and colleagues found increased mean VOT in PD patients which they attributed to coordination deficits of the laryngeal tractus [79]. On the other hand, there are contradictory findings of reduced VOT in Parkinsonian speakers which have been explained by a primarily reduced vocal fold opening produced by laryngeal rigidity allowing a faster vocal fold closure evidenced in a shorter VOT [78, 271].

Since phonatory abnormalities in PD are caused by a dysfunctional co-operation of phonatory and laryngeal effector organs, dynamic measurements of laryngeal movements during phonation by means of laryngoscopy, electromyography and aerodynamic can give insight into the disturbed functions. Hanson and colleagues documented numerous visible abnormalities in a cinelaryngoscopic study of 32 PD patients [108]. The most characteristic finding, that later has been replicated by subsequent studies [84, 203, 236], was vocal fold bowing during phonation represented by a significant glottic gap but with tightly approximated vocal processes, which was observed in 30 of the patients and was correlated to breathiness of voice and reduced intensity. Besides vocal fold bowing, laryngeal structure irregularities were apparent in many of the patients with asymmetries of vocal fold length, degree of bowing and paradoxical approximation of the ventricular folds during phonation. Electromyographic and aerodynamic studies provide further information about restricted vocal fold movements which might reflect a loss of appropriate reciprocal activity between agonist and antagonist muscles rather than general muscle weakness [118]. In support, observations of vocal fold bowing and impairment of voice onset and offset control were associated with increased thyroarytenoid and cricothyroid activity increasing vocal fold tension and stiffness and leading to reduced subtle motor control of phonation [84]. Aerodynamic studies also suggested an increase of subglottic pressure and laryngeal resistance during speech in some speakers with hypokinetic dysarthria [135] which may contribute to the patients′ impression of higher speech effort, nevertheless producing a low intensity of voice.

In summary, acoustic and physiological studies of phonatory attributes in PD speakers provide evidence of reduced laryngeal efficiency, flexibility and control. Many of these abnormalities can be related to the underlying muscle rigidity, reduced range and slowness of movements in the laryngeal muscles.

I.3. Resonance

There is a scarceness of research examining the characteristics of resonance in PD speech, although Ludlow and Bassich reported that nasality was a strong perceptual feature in differentiating the speech of PD speakers from healthy controls [170], which has also been confirmed by acoustic analysis [74]. On the other hand, in the first extensive systematic description of different kinds of motor speech disorders performed by Darley and colleagues, resonatory disturbance was not found to be a salient perceptual feature of Parkinsonian dysarthria [57]. It was speculated that the perception of resonance might be masked by further phonatory problems because the nasal airflow measures performed by Hoodin and Gilbert did not correlate strongly with perceptual ratings of hypernasality [125]. Some further studies have demonstrated that nasalization may spread across several consecutive syllables and that the degree and velocity of velar movements during speech tasks can be reduced [116, 117, 142, 194]. Hirose noted that velar displacement as measured by x-ray microbeam became limited and irregular at faster speech rates and that the velum tended to stay in an elevated posture, probably due to a loss of reciprocal suppression between functionally antagonistic velar muscles [118]. Therefore, summarized, velopharyngeal dysfunction responsible for hypernasality found in some PD speakers mirrors a similar underlying pathology of slow and reduced range of movement as it was demonstrated to be present in other aspects of impaired speech function.

I.4. Articulation

A number of acoustic and physiologic studies on articulatory dynamics support the perceptual impression of imprecise articulation of consonants and vowels in PD speakers, which have in general been attributed to a reduction of range and velocity of the articulators (lips, tongue, jaw) caused by rigidity, weakness or fatigue [145].

Inaccurate articulation illustrated as failure to completely reach articulatory targets or sustain contact for sufficient durations can lead to the phenomenon of "spirantization" during stop consonant production. Spirantization, usually taken as evidence for articulatory "undershooting" is characterized acoustically by the replacement of a stop consonant gap with low-intensity frication and has been proven by a variety of studies [4, 48, 142, 243]. It is attributed to a failure of complete articulatory closure for stop consonant productions and perceived as aperiodic, fricative-like noise [271]. Another method of evaluating articulatory skills in PD speakers has been the use of oral diadochokinetic tasks which consist of the rapid production of syllables containing consonant-vowel combinations with bilabial, alveolar and velar places of articulation, such as /pα tα kα/ [77]. The diadochokinetic tasks are used to examine the speakers′ ability to produce rapidly alternating articulatory movements and have been found to show some irregularities in PD patients [5]. In an optoelectric movement study, Ackermann and colleagues found a tendency to keep speech rate on a normal level at the expense of amplitude of articulatory movements to compensate for bradykinesia of the articulator muscles [5]. However, the more severely affected PD patients were unable to fully compensate with this "articulatory undershooting" strategy [3, 4]. Several studies were able to confirm the rigidity, reduced range of movement and abnormal speed of articulator movements in PD. Findings include kinematic evidence of lip muscle stiffness, reduced range and velocity of lip and jaw movements [45, 79, 80, 118, 129, 194]. Electromyographic studies have also documented poor reciprocal patterns of activation between jaw opening and closing muscles during speech tasks [118]. It has been suggested that such persistent abnormal muscle contractions – reflecting difficulties with reciprocal adjustments of antagonistic muscles or a loss of reciprocal suppression between functionally antagonistic muscle pairs – may represent the physiological basis of hypokinesia and rigidity [118, 163]. Further studies in PD speakers, although with some inconsistencies, revealed reduced tongue strength and endurance and a faster decline of tongue pressure when instructed to keep a constant effort of the tongue, which has been interpreted as "fatigue" of articulator muscles in PD [251, 252, 253]. Supplementary research on articulatory structures revealed weakness in the lips and velum as well [194]. The presence of weakness and fatigue is not necessarily linearly related to abnormal perceptual speech characteristics. Solomon and colleagues found no significant relationship between tongue strength and articulatory precision and overall speech impairment. The authors noted that the operating range for speech muscles is approximately 10% to 25% of their maximum strength, so the threshold for articulator muscle weakness to result in perceptible speech deficits obviously is not exceeded during the routine speech tasks [252].

Evidence from acoustic studies also supports conclusions that the range of articulator movements is reduced in PD, leading to impaired vowel articulation caused by diminished "formant" transitions [79, 272]. Vowels are formed primarily by movements of the tongue, lips and jaw creating oropharyngeal resonating cavities which amplify certain frequency bands of the voice spectrum. These harmonics are called "formants". Formants define the single vowels by their typical distinct peaks of acoustic energy. The position of the articulators (tongue, lips and jaw) therefore defines the three dimensional characteristics of the vocal tractus and influences the formant frequencies, especially of the first (F1) and second (F2) formant. Vowel production may also be affected by deficits in articulator control and mobility as evidenced by differences in vocal tract resonances. As a consequence, limited movements of the articulators as suggested in PD lead to inadequate vowel formation by a restriction of formant production which should be characterized by a lowering of normally high frequency formants and by an elevation of normally low frequency formants. Connor and colleagues examined F1 and F2 transitions from syllable repetitions to infer information about articulator movement. Both F1 and F2 transition rates were flatter in PD compared to control speakers [51]. Similarly, Flint and colleagues found flatter F2 transition rates in PD speakers during sentence reading [78]. Acoustic vowel space (i.e., the space covered by the first and second formant values for the corner vowels /ɑ/, /i/ and /u/) was found to be restricted, suggestive of a smaller working space for vowels in PD [233, 246, 272].

In summary, PD patients generally demonstrate deficits in articulation which affect oral closure for stop consonant production and the ability to quickly move the articulators. Also, amplitude and velocity of lip and mandible movements have been shown to be defective, in addition to slowed articulator movement during vowel production. Rigor and hypokinesia manifestation on the articulator structures leading to inappropriate coactivation of antagonistic muscles are supposed to be responsible for what has been described "undershooting" of articulatory gestures in PD. Furthermore, there is evidence that at least some PD speakers suffer from reduced oromotor control, diminished steadiness in orofacial structures and varying instability of tongue, lips and jaw perhaps as a function of the degree of tremor in each of these structures [1, 279].

I.5. Prosody

Prosody is the term applied to the natural variations of pitch, intensity, articulatory rate and rhythm occurring during running speech and serves to transport emotional speech contents and meets further linguistical demands [2, 59]. A number of studies have found that PD speakers exhibit an impaired speech prosody, whereas monopitch speech mirrored by a reduction of fundamental frequency (F_0) range and variability seems to be the most conspicuous feature of Parkinsonian dysprosody [47, 48, 49, 229, 240]. Numerous studies on prosody indicate a significantly reduced F_0 range and variability in reading and sentence production in PD patients as compared to healthy controls [78, 85, 99, 185]. F_0 variability was also found to be decreased in untreated PD patients [137] and showed a further decline in the course of the disease [185, 224]. Reduced pitch variability has also been demonstrated based upon the analysis of question-answer pairs [160, 161]. Darkins and colleagues used a semantically governed paradigm and examined F_0 changes in noun phrases and similar sounding compound nouns; healthy speakers, but not PD patients, produced a significant F_0 declination in the second word of compound nouns, indicating a loss of linguistically demanded prosodic capacities in PD [56]. It has been hypothesized that the diminished F_0 variability in PD patients is caused by reduced laryngeal and vocal fold mobility as a result of hypokinesia manifestation in PD [96, 248].

Prosodic intensity changes have been shown to be reduced in PD speakers. Caekebeke and colleagues examined emotion-related intensity changes with subjects producing sentences containing emotional content (e.g. angry versus neutral) and found the PD speakers to produce smaller intensity changes than healthy controls [42]. Metter and Hanson reported reduced ability to use intensity changes during reading of a standard passage in PD [185]. In summary, PD speakers demonstrated reduced ability to use pitch and intensity changes to signify semantic or emotional differences during sentence and paragraph reading, thus leading to the perceptual impression of "monopitch" and "monoloudness" speech [234].

In previous studies, the findings concerning speech rate in PD patients remained inconclusive. Some of the discrepancies may be task-related, since the examination of speech rate based upon syllable repetition may rather indicate articulatory capacities, whereas speech rate and pause ratios calculated from meaningful sentences, standardized reading tasks or a free monologue are likely to reflect prosodic aspects instead. Some examiners documented slow syllable repetition rates in PD speakers [75, 171]; in contrast, there are further studies giving proof of accelerated alternate motion rates, sometimes with further evidence of reduced amplitude of articulator movements at least in some speakers [4, 116, 117, 194]. It has been suggested that abnormally fast syllable repetition rates in PD speakers indicate a mode of speech with a loss of voluntary control [194]. This hypothesis seems to be substantiated by the finding that there are at least some PD speakers who have difficulty altering speech rate when requested [171]. A similar phenomenon of heterogeneous speech rates in PD has been found when related to connected speech tasks [62, 78, 185, 243, 271]. Weismer stated that PD patients may produce speech at a faster rate because of articulatory difficulties, in which patients may "blur contrast" between different speech sound, causing an increased speech rate [271]. Impaired self-timing for motor movements has also been offered as an explanation for the increased rate of speech sometimes seen in PD [5]. On the other hand, Ludlow and colleagues found PD speakers to demonstrate slower speaking rates than control subjects, but this difference was not significant [171]. Still other research has revealed that there are no statistical significant group differences between speech rates of PD and healthy speakers, while some individual PD patients with more severe symptoms of the disease exhibited abnormally slow or fast rates [47, 185]. As these extreme rate disturbances were found in both directions (i.e., slower and faster), the mean rate differences between PD and control speakers were not found to be significant [185]. A recent study on speech rate based upon a standardized reading task found no differences in overall speech rate between PD and control subjects, but a significant acceleration in the course of reading in the PD speakers only. Furthermore, the PD speakers featured a characteristic speech-to-pause ratio pattern with less numerous but longer speech pauses which has been interpreted as an impaired speech rhythm and timing organization [243]. Summarized, the results of these studies indicate that speech rate is heterogeneous within the population of PD speakers. Because such variability is probably not simply a function of disease severity, this raises the possibility of the existence of subtypes of the disorder, especially in view of the fact that hypokinetic dysarthria is the only type of motor speech disorder in which speech rate is accelerated at least in some individuals. However, Weismer has suggested that the perception of fast speech rate could be an artefact of features such as articulatory imprecision and continuous voicing that "blur" discrete acoustic contrasts which may lead to the impression of increased rate [271].

Moreover, some additional factors, mostly related to speech pauses and between-syllable durational differences, round out the features of dysprosody in Parkinsonian speech. Although Canter found no differences between Parkinsonian and control subjects in number of pauses or mean pause duration during reading [47], several studies demonstrated such abnormalities. PD speakers have been shown to exhibit a higher percentage of pauses within speech samples [106, 185] with inconsistent findings concerning the number of pauses which have been found to occur slightly more [106] or less frequently [243]. Illes and colleagues found an increased frequency and duration of speech pauses exceeding 200 ms. These hesitations tended to be longer and occur more frequently at the beginning of sentences, which may be an evidence for impaired speech initiation. There was also an increase in number of words between silent intervals which perceptually are recognized as short "rushes" of speech in PD [131]. Moreover, the authors discovered that PD speakers exhibited fewer interjections and "modalizations" (comments that bear on verbal behaviour) during narrative speech, suggesting that silent speech pauses are displayed instead of fillers [131]. On the other hand, stuttering-like speech dysfluencies called "palilalia" have been observed in some people with PD [57, 232]. Palilalia, sometimes referred to as autoecholalia, is the compulsive repetition of utterances, often in a context of increasing speech rate and decreasing loudness and in general is considered of speech production impairment, probably reflecting damage to inhibitory motor circuits that help terminate action [23].

I.6. Sensory and Perceptual Deficits

Although the speech problems associated with PD are considered to be related to the motor dysfunctions of the disease, numerous studies have documented sensory problems including sensorimotor deficits in the orofacial system [44, 66, 235] and abnormal auditory, temporal and perceptual processing of voice and speech [3, 102, 119, 121, 235] which have been implicated as important etiological factors in Parkinsonian speech abnormalities [83]. Some insights into the sensory deficits affecting speech and voice in PD patients have been provided by studies on the regulation of speech loudness to increased levels of background noise and instantaneous auditory feedback in PD speakers and controls [119, 120]. The PD patients demonstrated an abnormal pattern of speech loudness modulation and failed to increase or decrease loudness in response to auditory feedback and background noises in the same manner as the healthy speakers.

II. Treatment

II.1. Pharmacological Treatment

The beneficial effect of l-dopa on motor impairment in PD, first introduced 1968 and acting to replenish the diminishing dopamine levels in the brain, has been well documented over the decades. Further drugs developed to ameliorate Parkinsonian symptoms are MAO-B inhibitors and COMT inhibitors which prolong the antiparkinsonian action of l-dopa by inhibiting its degradation, as well as dopaminergic agents realizing agonistic effects on the different striatal dopamine receptors, and anticholinergic agents which act by blocking the relatively predominant acetylcholine in the Parkinsonian basal ganglia.

Because of its undeniable positive effects on motor impairment, l-dopa is still appreciated as "gold standard" in the neuropharmacological treatment of PD. However, the impact of l-dopa treatment on speech and voice is highly variable across published reports. Findings appear to show mixed results in improvement of speech production through the use of l-dopa. Perceptual analyses of speech following l-dopa therapy have noted an amelioration of overall speech adequacy, clarity of articulation, normalcy of nasal resonance and temporal aspects of speech although these improvements were not found to be as convincing as the amelioration of limb symptoms [223]. Further studies based on perceptual analyses, reported improved overall intelligibility after l-dopa treatment, primarily as a result of improved loudness and more regular distribution of speech time and pauses [61, 180, 193]. Wolfe and colleagues examined the overall speech improvement after a steady-state of l-dopa treatment rated by independent speech pathologists who documented an amelioration of voice quality as well as improvements in pitch variation and articulation [275]. On the other hand, Quaglieri and colleagues found an amelioration in rating of global speech performance under l-dopa therapy only in 2 of 14 PD speakers [212]. Furthermore, there are case reports and studies dealing with PD patients in advanced stages of the disease demonstrating a worsening of global speech performance which had been attributed to dyskinesia related dysarthria and an increase of speech dysfluencies under l-dopa admission [12, 22, 53, 98, 178], supporting the hypothesis that speech disfluencies may be related to an increase or decrease of the dopamine concentration in the brain [98].

No systematic differences in rest breathing were found in PD patients before and after l-dopa admission, but significant changes were measured in 11 of 14 patients in a subset of speech breathing variables throughout the l-dopa drug cycle [250]. Another study indicated some improvement in the diaphragm component of breathing at rest, although some worsening seemed to be indicated for intercostal muscles after l-dopa administration [267].

Electrophysiological studies on l-dopa effects on articulation in PD speakers also produced contradictory findings. Some studies have found quantitative l-dopa related improvements in articulatory performance [43, 46, 162, 260]. By measuring labial rigidity using a transduction system, Caligiuri found a decrease of non-speech labial rigidity and an increase of labial movement amplitudes after l-dopa administration [46]. Leanderson and colleagues noted a l-dopa induced elimination of formally abnormal lip muscle activation patterns during rest and during movements in PD patients [162]. Moreover, mandibular movements during syllable repetition tasks were found to be improved under l-dopa [260]. Nakano and colleagues performed an electromyographic analysis of lip function during speech and found an elimination of abnormal tonic lip movements under l-dopa [193]. Labial pressures in speech and non-speech tasks also tended to improve following l-dopa therapy [87]. On the other hand, some further studies failed to confirm a positive l-dopa effect on the maximum force and contraction of laryngeal and articulatory muscles based upon measurements of lip and longue force [60, 84, 86]. The relationship between non-speech and speech-related oral movements has been a matter of debate; especially as a l-dopa induced reduction of rigidity of articulatory muscles does not automatically imply improvements in articulatory movements or function.

Some electrophysiological studies on phonation in PD speakers brought about an improvement of voice quality and an increase of sound pressure levels measured by coupled acoustic and glottographic recordings, whereas other phonatory variables remained unchanged under l-dopa [134, 275]. Electromyography of laryngeal muscles confirmed the assumption of l-dopa induced reduction of rigor and hypokinesia as producing an amelioration of some phonatory functions [84] which was partially confirmed by acoustic analysis of phonation [97, 230]. On the contrary, some other studies showed no change in phonatory factors after l-dopa administration [85, 123, 209]. There are also reports on some improvement of pitch variation under l-dopa as one important parameter of Parkinsonian dysprosody, whereas speech rate was unchanged [15, 62, 97, 123, 275].

Compared to the large amount of research on l-dopa effects on Parkinsonian speech, there are only a few studies examining the influence of dopamine agonists, anticholinergics or MAO-B inhibitors on dysarthria in PD speakers. One report showed no significant improvement in laryngeal and articulatory speech components after administration of apomorphine, a short acting dopaminergic receptor agonist [152]. It has been suggested that pramipexole may have positive effects on the oro-facial system and auditory system and thus may have a beneficial influence on speech [239]. As dopamine D2 receptors are located in the secondary auditory cortex and may play some role in higher order auditory processing, activation of D2 receptors may improve auditory feedback mechanisms which have shown to be dysfunctional in PD [101]. An investigation on voice and speech in 5 individuals with PD after fetal dopamine transplants showed a different influence of dopamine restorage on phonatory, articulatory and limb motor system without convincing improvement of Parkinsonian dysarthria [16]. When comparing trihexyphenidyl, an anticholinergic agent, to placebo, subjective improvement was noted in maximum intensity speech range and speaking rate, however, objectively, little significant effect on overall speech capacities was found [37, 54]. Selegiline, which inhibits the degradation of dopamine by inhibiting MAO-B, has been shown to improve rate and range of articulator movements in oral diadochokinetic tasks as well as in measures of vital capacity and words per exhalation during reading [241], but had no consistent effect on acoustic speech measures in the monotherapy in early stage PD [257]. Interestingly, low dose administration of clonazepam, a benzodiazepine without dopaminergic properties, has proved a beneficial effect on short speech rushes, imprecise consonants and inadequate silences in a placebo controlled study on 12 male PD speakers; only little improvement was reported in voice quality and pitch behaviour [25].

Hence, the effect of pharmacotherapy with special emphasis on l-dopa treatment seems to be limited and variable among PD patients – even if some small phonatory or articulatory improvements owing to dopaminergic pharmacotherapy can be seen in individual patients [97, 123]. Schulz emphasized that such variability in the findings may result from variation of dysarthria severity, stage of the disease, pre-existing drug treatment or the occurrence of motor fluctuations or dyskinesia [238]. Furthermore, the comparability of the aforementioned studies is limited because of methodological diversities, different outcome measures, small sample sizes and heterogeneity of disease specific parameters as disease duration or global motor impairment.

II.2. Surgical Treatment

Before the rise of dopamine therapy, functional neurosurgery procedures, such as thalamotomy and pallidotomy, were used to treat Parkinsonian symptoms. Some significant improvement after lesional surgical treatment has been observed for motor impairment of limb; however, the effect on Parkinsonian dysarthria has shown to be more deleterious than beneficial. Thalamotomy, generally performed in the ventrolateral and ventrointermediate nuclei of the thalamus, was mainly performed to improve Parkinsonian tremor, whereas rigor and hypokinesia show only inconsistent improvement. Unilateral thalatomy has been shown to worsen speech regardless if the lesion is in the dominant or non-dominant hemisphere [20, 204]. Bilateral thalamotomy has been associated with word blocking, slow speech and hypophonia and a persistent worsening of dysarthria, some of the patients developed palilalia [50, 258, 262]. Because of these serious adverse advents on Parkinsonian speech, thalamotomy has been abandoned for the treatment of PD.

Pallidotomy usually involves lesions of the posteroventral portion of the internal part of the globus pallidus and was used to alleviate Parkinsonian symptoms and reduce contralateral dyskinesias [156]. Reports on the effect of unilateral or bilateral pallidotomy on speech function are contradictory; whereas some studies describe no beneficial effect on Parkinsonian dysarthria [38, 93, 157, 239]; others report a worsening of speech function with development of transient dysarthria, facial weakness, swallowing problems and alterations in verbal fluency [264]. On the other hand, there are opposite descriptions of positive changes in phonatory and articulatory measurements in PD speakers after unilateral and bilateral pallidotomy [19, 236]. Barlow and colleagues reported that half of the patients involved in a study of labial force production and stability experienced improvement on this motor component of speech after bilateral posteroventral pallidotomy [19].

In the last years, much attention has been paid to the effects of functional stereotactic neurosurgical procedures on Parkinsonian speech, as high frequency deep brain stimulation has been proved to provide stable beneficial effects on motor functions especially in advanced PD [65]. The results of studies looking at postsurgery speech outcome are variable [207]. Deep brain stimulation of the ventral intermediate nucleus of the thalamus has been reported to have a worsening effect on perceptual assessment [200, 211, 261] and electrophysiological outcome parameters of speech [89]. According to Gross and colleagues, clinical dysarthria assessment based upon it 18 of the UPDRS III showed an improvement of speech relative to baseline in seven patients under deep brain stimulation of the globus pallidus internus (GPi) [104]. However, worsening of speech according to perceptual analysis has been observed in other studies [92, 154]. Lyons and colleagues estimated the decline of speech function as an adverse effect of GPi stimulation that can be resolved with adjustments of the stimulation parameters [173]. Perceptual assessment of dysarthria by the use of UPDRS III/item 18 showed a beneficial effect of nucleus subthalamicus (STN) stimulation on the speech of PD patients, although the improvement was much less pronounced than that on limb movements and tended to decrease in the long-term [153, 164, 228]. On the other hand, there are reports on a worsening of overall speech functions under STN stimulation as assessed by UPDRS or more subtle dysarthria sores [109, 187, 226]. There are further studies which combine perceptual assessment of overall speech function with acoustic analysis and electrophysiological measurements which suggested that STN stimulation can improve articulatory and phonatory components of Parkinsonian speech [71, 88, 89, 90, 206]. Pinto and colleagues found an improvement of speech function in the majority of 26 PD patients with STN stimulation using perceptual analysis and electrophysiological measurements [205]. They stated that STN stimulation had a beneficial long-term effect on the articulatory organs involved in speech production, and this indicated that Parkinsonian dysarthria is associated, at least in part, with an alteration in STN neuronal activity [205]. In a recent study performed by D´Alatri and colleagues, no negative speech effects of STN deep brain stimulation were seen in 12 PD patients; on the contrary, some aspects of speech, as vocal tremor, tended to improve but without effects on global speech intelligibility [55]. Klostermann and colleagues reported that STN stimulation worsened speech performance according to perceptual rating methods applied in 19 PD patients [149]. In contrast, technical measures showed stimulation-induced improvements of single speech dimensions affected by the PD-specific motor disorder. The authors stated that STN stimulation reduces designated disease-inherent dysarthrophonic symptoms, such as glottic tremor. However, these actions on speech have found to be predominantly outweighed by the general dysarthrogenic effects of STN stimulation, probably based on a decline of complex (e.g. prosodic) functions. They concluded that stimulation-induced speech impairment should be considered a likely problem in the course of this treatment [149]. Two other studies tried to asses some findings regarding the effects of unilateral STN stimulation on speech subcomponents. Santens and colleagues reported that selective left-sided stimulation had a profoundly negative effect on prosody, articulation, and hence, intelligibility [231], which has in general been confirmed by similar observations made by Wang and colleagues [269].

Most of the studies of the effects of deep brain stimulation on Parkinsonian dysarthria are uncontrolled with selected patients that may not be representative. A further bias may be added by the fact that presurgery selection of patients is needed to ensure the minimum risk for those patients in terms of the surgery itself. Since, for example, PD patients with severe cognitive impairment or predominant axial symptoms as gait disorders usually are excluded from stereotactic surgery, the effect of deep brain stimulation on postsurgery dysarthria may be underestimated due to the preoperative patients′ selection criteria. Moreover, pre-existing speech disturbance is less responsive to deep brain stimulation than global motor limb dysfunction. Stimulation of the target and probably of surrounding structures can induce specific speech impairment that differs from "pure" Parkinsonian dysarthria concerning severity and quality. Summarized, according to the available data, speech intelligibility which reflects the overall speech production understood by a listener, has a poor response to STN stimulation whereas motor subcomponents of speech, such as lip or laryngeal movements assessed separately, could show some improvement induced by deep brain stimulation.

II.3. Speech Therapy

For many years, speech and voice disorders in PD were considered resistant to traditional behavioral speech therapy [9, 13, 233]. Although changes in speech may be achieved in the treatment room, carryover and long-term treatment outcomes in general have been relatively poor [8]. Moreover, although there is a varied number of speech therapy approaches reported in literature, including training in control of speech rate, prosody, loudness, articulation and respiration sometimes assisted by special feedback or pacing devices [7, 68, 113, 277], only very few clinical trials have been performed. Delayed auditory feedback increased speech intelligibility in two of 11 PD patients [68]. Another report of two cases documented an increase in vocal loudness and pitch modulation and decrease of fast speech rate after delayed auditory feedback in a 3-month follow up [107]. In a case study of a microcomputer-based wearable biofeedback device, patients themselves were able to consciously modulate speech loudness, which led to an improvement of perceptual and acoustic assessments [103, 227]. Significant improvement of vocal loudness has been reported in ten patients by the application of masking noise forcing the users to increase their speech intensity [7].

The newest and generally perceived as state-of-the-art treatment for Parkinsonian dysarthria is the Lee Silverman Voice Treatment (LSVT®). LSVT® is an intensive, high effort speech treatment designed to rescale the amplitude of motor output of PD speakers based upon elements derived from neurology, physiology, motor learning, muscle training and neuropsychology [215]. The five essential concepts of the LSVT® include 1) focus on voice (increase amplitude of movement / increase vocal loudness), 2) improve sensory perception of effort, 3) administer treatment in a high effort style, 4) intensity (4 times a week for 16 sessions in one month), and 5) quantify treatment related changes. The LSVT® approach centers on the specific therapeutic target of increasing vocal loudness which acts as a "trigger" to increase effort and coordination across the speech production system. By incorporating sensory awareness training with motor speech exercises, LSVT® facilitates acceptance and comfort with increased loudness and the ability to self-monitor vocal loudness in PD speakers. Furthermore, a simple, redundant and intensive training may help to accommodate the processing speed, memory and executive function deficits observed in some individuals with PD and promote overlearning and internalization of the vocal effort required for normal loudness [83]. Findings from initial treatment studies on 45 PD patients documented a significant increase of post-treatment voice intensity after LSVT® compared to an alternative group which achieved a different kind of speech therapy (respiratory treatment) [214]. Follow-up studies documented maintenance of this effect out to one and two years after treatment [215, 217]. The data of these studies offer strong support for the short- and long-term efficacy of LSVT® for PD speakers [214, 215, 218]. After LSVT® treatment, PD speakers showed significant improvements in vocal fold closure, as measured by videostroboscopy as well as electroglottography [248], subglottic air pressure and maximum air flow rate [216] without any evidence of increased vocal hyperfunction defined as unwanted strain or excessive vocal fold closure [213, 248]. These studies have also provided important information about mechanisms underlying speech and voice disorders in PD and have identified fundamental elements of treatment-related change. Data have documented that successful speech treatment generates other important effects across the vocal tract, encompassing positive changes in articulation, swallowing and facial expression [70, 76, 232].

Evidence-based appraisal of the effect of speech therapy on Parkinsonian dysarthria has been the subject of recent reviews [63, 254, 278]. The review sponsored by the Movement Disorder Society was performed on four clinical studies on speech therapy [138, 214, 224, 238] and a further study on electrophysiological measures on participants of one of the antecedent examinations [248]. Although the effects of LSVT® study seemed to be the most convincing as compared to the other studies [214], the review concluded that there is not enough evidence for substantial improvement after any speech therapy because of insufficient study design (small sample sizes, lack of control group, only short time follow up etc.) [254]. Deane and colleagues reached the same conclusions when comparing randomized controlled trials of speech and language therapy with placebo or no intervention and different kinds of speech therapy concluding five trials all published before 2001 totaling 134 PD patients. Members of the Academy of Neurologic Communication Disorders and Sciences (ANCDS) reviewed the evidence for behavioral management of respiratory and phonatory dysfunction from dysarthria including studies of speech therapy for PD speakers [278]. These authors did not limit the review to randomized controlled trials, but rather included case, single subject and group designs. For speech therapy related to PD this review included three studies of biofeedback devices totaling 39 participants, five studies with other devices totaling 16 people, 14 studies of LSVT® totaling about 90 persons and 3 miscellaneous studies of group treatment. In summary, the review concluded that for LSVT®, most outcome measures were positive and interpretable with confidence [278].

Summarized, the majority of PD patients experience speech and voice disorders at some point during the course of disease and these deficits impair their quality of life. Medical and surgical treatment alone has not shown to sufficiently alleviate these speech disorders. Thus, a combination of behavioural speech therapy, specifically the LSVT® approach, in medically managed PD patients appears at present to be the most effective type of speech intervention, although more studies and clinical trials are necessary.

III. Methodological Issues

There are a number of methodological issues in the examination of voice and speech which are to be considered in the planning and conducting of studies on dysarthria and in the interpretation of data and comparison of results.

III.1. Normal Variations in Speech Production

Normal aging is associated with changes in speech that are physiologically, acoustically and perceptually detectable. They include at least changes in pitch, voice quality and stability, loudness, speech breathing patterns, speech rate and prosodic variations [18, 64, 190, 217, 247]. Baker and colleagues found a decrease of sound pressure levels and a reduction of laryngeal electromyographic signals in healthy elder adults as compared to the young individuals [18]. In another study, changes of chest wall compliance and pulmonary elastic recoil were held responsible for different speech breathing patterns in elderly adults as compared to younger ones [128]. A study on voice characteristics in 205 healthy elderly participants documented a convergence of male and female pitch of voice while range and variability both increased; furthermore, there was evidence for growing voice instability in the elder participants [64]. Using electromyographic recording techniques, Luschei and colleagues found changes in the discharge patterns of laryngeal muscles in healthy elderly men and male PD speakers, but not in female speakers. This was interpreted as different impact of aging on the male and female voice apparatus [172]. Formant frequency characteristics have been found to exhibit significant alterations in elderly men, while elderly female speakers generally maintained formant frequency integrity during vowel articulation [220]. Smith and colleagues found a reduction of speech rate and an increase of segment and syllable duration in elderly speakers [247]. Because many neurologic disorders such as PD are overlaid on an aging nervous system, and because some speech changes associated with aging are similar to those associated with dysarthria, the identification of a speech characteristic as "deviant" and possibly indicative of dysarthria often requires an awareness of what is "normal" for the participant's age and general physical condition. Furthermore, gender has some influence on speech characteristics, as male and female voice and speech are perceptually different. These differences can influence the detection of abnormalities, at least with some methods of analysis. For example, acoustic indices of laryngeal abnormalities may differ among men and women with the same underlying neurologic disease [143], and some of the acoustic heterogeneity within specific categories of dysarthria may be explained by gender [146]. A further aspect is that the qualitative character of speech varies as a function of normal differences in personality, emotional state and speaking roles. Such variations often and justifiably go unnoticed by clinicians′ and researchers′ intent upon recognizing abnormalities, but they sometimes must be identified explicitly for accurate differential diagnosis [74].

According to this condensed overview on physiological factors influencing certain aspects of speech and voice, studies on Parkinsonian dysarthria have to be performed with comparison to an age- and gender-matched control group.

III.2. Task Dependency

The task which has been chosen for examination of an underlying dysarthria may itself influence the results. Since speech is a highly complex, dynamic motor activity through which individuals express thoughts and emotions and respond to and control their environment, the setting of a "speech examination" in a scientific surrounding with technical equipment and recording devices guided by an examiner may create an artificial atmosphere that leads to a "non-natural" kind of speech. Therefore, the data obtained by such studies may not be representative for the speech abnormalities occurring in participants´ every-day life. For example, even in healthy individuals, external cues are known to influence certain prosodic parameters such as loudness, stress, speech rate and pitch variability [205] which has been found to be relevant in PD patients as well [47, 100, 185, 186]. Therefore, examiners have to bear in mind that certain aspects of speech, especially prosodic parameters, may differ significantly, depending on the respective task: e.g., if the participant is asked to perform a free monologue, a standardized reading task or if he is asked to execute the speech task in an accentuated emotional style. Moreover, some of the speech tasks usually applied to examine phonatory or articulatory aspects of speech, as for example maximum phonation time or diadochokinesis and syllable repetition tasks, deal with simplified and somewhat artificial aspects of vocalization under the hypothesis that complex speech is based upon the synthesis of such plain modules. However, abnormalities detected by those simple tasks may not necessarily be relevant for the integrity of much more complex speech functions.

III.3. Methodological Differences

Motor speech disorders can be studied in many ways, all of which contribute to their characterization and understanding. The methods can be categorized under two broad headings: perceptual and instrumental. Each method has strengths and shortcomings, each has varying sensitivity to abnormalities in different parts of the speech system, and each has varying relevance to the numerous clinical and theoretical questions that are relevant to the understanding of Parkinsonian dysarthria and motor speech disorders in general.

Perceptual methods are based primarily on the auditory-perceptual attributes of speech. At the same time, they are subject to unreliability of judgments among clinicians, they may be difficult to quantify, and they cannot directly test hypotheses about the pathophysiology underlying perceived speech abnormalities [144]. But, as the auditory-perceptual classification of disturbed speech is a valid and essential diagnostic tool in the hand of experienced examiners, it is unlikely that it will be completely replaced by other methods, because the evaluation of speech disorders always begins with a perceptual judgment that speech has changed or is abnormal or different in some way. Darley and colleagues pioneered the modern use of auditory perceptual assessment to characterize the dysarthrias and to identify the clusters of salient perceptual characteristics that are associated with lesions in different parts of the central and peripheral nervous system [57, 58, 59]. In fact, one result of their work was the generation of numerous hypotheses about the pathophysiological bases of the dysarthrias. Therefore, they helped to set the direction of acoustic and pathophysiological studies based upon acoustic and other instrumental methods that with high frequency have confirmed and further refined the perceptually based hypotheses generated from the work of Darley and colleagues.

In the last years, a variety of instrumental methods have demonstrated clinical value for the description and analysis of motor speech disorders, and they often contribute to the differential diagnosis of dysarthria. Instrumental methods can be roughly organized under three headings: acoustic, physiologic and visual imaging.

Acoustic methods can visually display and numerically quantify numerous aspects of the acoustic speech signal. They are tightly bound to auditory-perceptual judgments of speech, because they use the same data, the acoustic speech signal. They have provided refined, confirmatory and quantified support for perceptual judgments that e.g. speech rate is slow, voice is breathy or contains tremor or interruptions, pitch and loudness variability are reduced, and so on [213]. In addition, qualitative acoustic analyses can make important contributions to theoretical constructs in explaining components of motor speech disorders [167]. The capacity of acoustic analysis to make visible and quantify the speech signal can provide baseline data and serve as an index of stability, improvement or deterioration over time. However, its capacity to add to, modify or refine perceptually based clinical diagnoses has yet to be firmly established [144].

Auditory-perceptual and acoustic analyses, by definition, are focused on the sound emitted from the vocal tract. Physiologic methods move "upstream" toward the source of activity that generates the speech signal and therefore represent another level of explanation. They focus on the movements of speech structures and air, the muscle contractions that generate movement, the relationship among movements at different levels of the musculoskeletal speech mechanism, and the temporal parameters and relationships among central and peripheral neural and biomechanical activity. The most commonly employed physiologic methods used to study the movement of air and peripheral structures associated with dysarthrias include electromyographic, kinematic and aerodynamic measures. Physiologic analyses have increased the understanding of speech motor control and how it can break down. They have refined and sometimes challenged perceptually based explanations for the pathophysiology of certain motor speech disorders by clarifying whether various abnormal movements during speech reflect weakness, spasticity, incoordination, reduced range of movement and so on. In addition, they have provided insight into whether certain disorders reflect linguistic, motor planning or programming or neuromuscular deficits, distinctions that can be very difficult or impossible to be made on the basis of clinical perceptual assessment alone.

In addition to acoustic and physiologic methods, numerous instruments are available for visually imaging parts of the upper aerodigestive tractus during speech, a process that cannot be appreciated simply by watching people talk. The most common clinically used visual imaging methods include videofluoroscopy, nasoendoscopy, laryngoscopy and videostroboscopy, all of which can be videotaped, saved and analyzed. The instrumentally-provided visual image is usually interpreted by way of a non-quantified perceptual judgement by the clinician doing the examination.

Summarized, the insight into the value and restrictions of each of the aforementioned methods used for description and analysis of disturbed speech is essential for interpretation of study data. Since none of the methods, alone or in combination, is able to comprehensively explain all the aspects of a certain motor speech disorder, results and conclusions have to be interpreted regarding the limitations implicated by the chosen method. Furthermore, until now there are no standardized study protocols neither related to the used speech tasks nor related to the methods. Therefore, further research and cooperation are necessary to establish valuable and standardized study designs and convincing surrogate parameters for the examination of disturbed speech to guarantee validity and comparability as the basis for a better pathophysiological understanding of the underlying mechanisms.

III.4. Heterogeneity of PD Patients

The interpretation of findings derived from research on dysarthria in PD speakers is restricted by the broad variability concerning kind and degree of speech disturbance in this disease. Although the work of Darley and colleagues based upon a large sample of PD speakers has lead to a widely accepted characterization of a typical pattern of Parkinsonian dysarthria described as "monopitch, monoloudness" with "harsh and breathy voice quality" [57, 58, 59], this prototypic speech style can vary significantly in the individual PD patient. Furthermore, there are some distinctive phenomena such as palilalia that only occur in a small subgroup of PD patients. Some other aspects of speech, such as articulatory velocity, show no significant difference in PD speakers as compared to healthy controls when related to the average values of the accordant study group, but can be atypically slow or accelerated in subgroups of PD speakers which raise the possibility of distinctive subtypes of speech disturbance which may be overlooked because of lacking statistical significance in large sample sizes. Moreover, some speech parameters as articulatory velocity, mean fundamental frequency or pitch variability, have been shown to be correlated not only to speakers´ age but also to disease duration or general motor impairment [124, 243, 259]. Therefore, these disease related variables have to be taken into account for the data interpretation. A further factor which may influence kind and degree of speech disturbance in PD can be the antiparkinsonian treatment. Although the findings concerning the general effect of l-dopa and other antiparkinsonian drugs on the specific speech parameters are contradictory, there are at least individual PD patients that show a benefit from dopaminergic therapy concerning their speech deficits. On the other hand, many PD patients in advanced stages of the disease suffer from l-dopa related so called "response fluctuations" which itself can have some influence on speech performance. Response fluctuations experienced by PD patients include changes in motor performance that may or may not co-vary with l-dopa dosage or schedule. There are a number of causes of response fluctuations, but as a whole, motor fluctuations are related to both chronic treatment with dopaminergic agents, especially l-dopa, and the degenerative process of the continuing progression of PD [67, 158]. Besides the hypokinetic or "off-state" response fluctuations that are characterized by unexpected periods of intensification of motor symptoms, there are also "on-state" dyskinesias which are thought to be caused by short-term excessive central dopamine levels [67]. These dyskinesias include hyperkinetic choreiform movements which can occur in all parts of the body and can include facial, oromandibular and thoracoabdominal muscles [130] and therefore may lead to a further deterioration of speech in some individual PD patients [53]. Since there were reasonable ethical concerns to perform studies on dysarthria in advanced stage PD patients completely off-medication to examine the kind and degree of speech disturbance in the course of the disease undisturbed by drug effects, the majority of such studies have a pre- and after-treatment design with taking speech measurements before and after morning medication [45, 134, 140, 209, 230, 267]. However, since the nightly withdrawal of medication is not able to completely washout the antiparkinsonian drugs, the performance of speech tasks in the morning before the first drug intake is not able to give a representative clinical picture of the underlying impairment uninfluenced of medication effects. Furthermore, the time period of full medication effect after drug administration may vary between the PD participants as well as the extent of motor response to a single drug admission, both exemplary aspects which are capable to distort the study results.

Summarized, as demonstrated by these few examples, the drug regimen and possible side effects of antiparkinsonian medication may have an important influence on kind and extent of speech disturbance at least in individual PD speakers and should therefore ideally be controlled in clinical studies on Parkinsonian dysarthria. Therefore, studies on speech disturbance in PD either demand the inclusion of a representatively large number of participants to allow subsequent subgroup formation, or the careful control of a broad variety of participants′ characteristics as disease duration, general motor impairment, stage of the disease, presence and kind of motor fluctuations and so on.

IV. Pathophysiology of Speech Impairment in PD

Despite the multitudinous studies dealing with numerous different aspects of the speech disturbance in PD, until now research on Parkinsonian dysarthria has not been able to generate one global pathophysiological theory being able to comprehensively integrate all the single findings. The fundamental basis for an insight into the pathophysiology of motor speech disorders is an understanding of the neurology of speech under physiological conditions, which requires the integrity and integration of numerous neurocognitive, neuromuscular and musculoskeletal activities that can be summarized as follows:

1). The "cognitive-linguistic processes" implicate the organization of thoughts, feelings and emotions generating an intention to communicate and the conversion of these intentions into verbal symbols in a manner that abides by the rules of language.
2). The activity of "motor speech planning and programming" implicates the organization of the intended verbal message for neuromuscular execution; this activity comprehends the selection and sequencing of sensorimotor programs that activate the speech muscles at appropriate coarticulated times, durations and intensities.
3). The activity of "neuromuscular execution" implies the "translation" of the motor speech program into the adequate innervation of respiratory, phonatory, resonatory and articulatory muscles in a manner that generates an acoustic signal that faithfully reflects the goals of the program and can be controlled and modified by feedback mechanisms.

However, although sufficient for a basic understanding of the physiology of speech, this level-based paradigm is high-grade simplified, because the different systems of neural function rather cooperate in widespread networks than in hierarchically organized sections and the disorder of single neural components can induce dysfunctions of different "levels" (e.g. basal ganglia disorders can affects motor speech planning as well as neuromuscular execution). Regardless of these constrictions, adhering to the "level"-model, the complex features of Parkinsonian dysarthria result from a multidimensional impairment affecting all the aforementioned aspects of motor speech production albeit with varying degree and focus in the individual patients.

A variety of studies deal with the organs of neuromuscular execution of speech namely the functional systems of speech respiration, phonation, resonance and articulation which for the most part have been analyzed by physiologic measures. Spirometric and kinematic assessment of speech breathing revealing abnormalities chest wall movements in a subgroup of PD speakers had been interpreted as rigor manifestation [191], whereas other examiners have rather suggested altered compliance of rib cage and abdomen to be responsible for impaired speech breathing patterns in PD [250]. A recent examination of lung volume use during extemporaneous speaking in PD revealed a dysfunctional utilization of the tidal volume for speaking which was not to be attributed to rigor or hypokinesia of the respiratory system, but rather to disturbed motor execution [40]. Some studies provide electromyographic evidence for reduced activity of laryngeal muscles in PD speakers accompanied by low sound pressure levels which has been interpreted as manifestation of hypokinesia on the phonatory system [17, 172]. On the contrary, an abnormal contraction of the laryngeal muscles leading to particular vocal fold bowing has been documented in untreated PD speakers with impaired voice onset and offset, which partially was reversible by l-dopa administration explained as rigor manifestation on the vocal folds [84]. In the same vein, restricted vocal fold movements measured by electromyographic and aerodynamic studies have been attributed to a loss of appropriate reciprocal activity between agonist and antagonist phonatory muscles [118]. An analogue pattern of impaired reciprocal activation and abnormal co-contractions of functional antagonistic muscles has been documented in lip and jaw muscles leading to a reduced range of articulator movements, which again has been interpreted as manifestation of rigor as a cause of imprecise vowel and consonant articulation in PD [46, 79, 80, 118, 129, 163, 194]. In summary, although research on neuromuscular performance in Parkinsonian dysarthria also has produced some inconsistencies, the dysfunctional motor patterns of the executive speech organs have been attributed to rigor and hypokinesia manifestation resulting from dopamine depletion in PD, as at least some of the abnormal findings were found to be l-dopa responsive [43, 45, 86, 162, 193, 260]. The finding of improved force of the articulatory organs under bilateral deep brain stimulation has been taken as an evidence for altered STN neuronal activity being at least partially responsible for Parkinsonian dysarthria [206, 208].

According to the "level model" of speech performance introduced in the section above, albeit the supposedly beneficial effect of dopaminergic or deep brain stimulation on some aspects of neuromuscular execution in Parkinsonian speech, the superordinate capabilities of cognitive-linguistic processes as well as of motor speech planning and programming (which include e.g. some aspects of prosody, speech timing and overall speech adequacy) have been rather found to be refractory to dopaminergic therapy. Therefore, the aggravation of Parkinsonian dysarthria which often accompanies the overall progression of the disease, suggests a link to the increasing severity of non-dopaminergic lesions in PD [30]. Since the cognitive-linguistic processes can be compromised by the development of cognitive decline and dementia developing in the later stages of PD, the aspect of motor speech planning and programming has have been attributed to a motor-cortex-basal ganglia-cortex loop which has been shown to be tightly connected to cortex-basal ganglia-cerebellum circuits [6, 274].

More recent research has led to a reinterpretation of the functional organization of the basal ganglia and the impact of dopaminergic depletion which might – although primarily referred to the limb motor system – establish explanations for some clinical features of Parkinsonian dysarthria as well [199]. According to this theory, the motor circuit of the basal ganglia has two entry points, the striatum and the subthalamic nucleus (STN), and one output, the globus pallidus pars interna (GPi), which connects to the cortex via the motor thalamus. Neuronal afferents coding for a given movement or task project to the basal ganglia by two different systems, called the "direct circuit" (projections to the GPi via the striatum and STN, which are primarily inhibited by corticostriatal afferents) and the "indirect circuit" (projections to the GPi via the globus pallidus pars externa (GPe), which are facilitated by corticostriatal afferents). Dopaminergic depletion in PD disrupts the corticostriatal balance leading to increased activity the indirect circuit and reduced activity in the direct circuit. Therefore, the Parkinsonian state is thought to be characterized by the disruption of the internal balance of the basal ganglia leading to hyperactivity in the two main entry points of the network (striatum and STN) and excessive inhibitory output from the GPi. Replacement therapy with standard l-dopa creates a further imbalance, producing an abnormal pattern of neuronal discharge and synchronization of neuronal firing that sustain the "off" and "on with dyskinesia" states. The effect of l-dopa is robust but short-lasting and converts the Parkinsonian basal ganglia into a highly unstable system, where pharmacological and compensatory effects act in opposing directions. This creates a scenario that substantially departs from the normal physiological state of the basal ganglia and might be responsible not only for motor fluctuations but also for some of the dopamine refractory aspects of speech impairment in PD [198, 199].

According to a PET study on 12 healthy individuals conducted by Wise and colleagues based upon a word repetition task, the formulation of an articulatory plan is a function of the left anterior insula and lateral premotor cortex, whereas the left basal ganglia seemed to be dominant for speech, although the axial phonatory muscles involved reached their output from both cerebral hemispheres [274]. In general, speech production under physiological conditions, has particularly been attributed to the supplementary motor area (SMA) and anterior cingular cortex for the generation of speech [174], whereas the left insula has been shown to be essential for planning of speech articulatory movements [73, 274]; the speech movements themselves have been found to be initiated in the primary motor cortex corresponding to the trunk and orofacial somatotopic areas [36, 274]. Furthermore, the language components of speech are known to involve the participation of prefrontal, frontal and temporal cortices, such as Broca´s and Wernicke´s areas [115]. Supplementary to these general hypotheses of speech production, there is further research emphasizing the aspect of speech motor performance mostly based upon syllable repetition tasks using functional magnetic imaging (fMRI) techniques. Riecker and colleagues identified different cerebral structures of speech motor control including SMA, primary sensorimotor regions, dorsolateral prefrontal cortex, anterior insula, thalamus, putamen/pallidum and cerebellar hemispheres which were found to diversify dependent from repetition frequency and were organized into two separated networks, most presumably to motor preparation (SMA, dorsolateral frontal cortex, anterior insula, superior cerebellum) and motor execution processes (sensorimotor cortex, basal ganglia, thalamus, inferior cerebellum) [221, 222]. These findings were widely substantiated by the study of Bohland and Guenther with further evidence for an increased engagement of the basic speech network (including primary and sensorimotor cortices, SMA, anterior insula, portions of basal ganglia, thalamus and cerebellum) and recruitment of additional areas dependent from the complexity of the speech task [29]. In the same vein, Bookheimer and colleagues were able to demonstrate different patterns of neural activation in a speech task when based upon automatic repetition of nonsense syllables in comparison to a complex linguistic speech task [31]. These findings underline the methodological difficulties to locate distinct neural networks involved in speech performance even in healthy speakers as cognitive-linguistic activities and activities of motor speech planning and programming are supposed to be connected and superimposed to each other and therefore, the artificial task-related disjunction of hypothetic subunits of speech performance may lead to a significant bias.

While the wealth of studies on speech has generated valuable hypotheses about speech physiology and has provided a sketchy insight into some aspects of motor speech planning and programming in healthy speakers, the pathophysiological mechanisms of dysfunctional motor speech control in Parkinsonian dysarthria are poorly understood. Liotti and colleagues examined Parkinsonian speakers before and after Lee Silverman Voice Treatment (LSVT®) based upon PET imaging and found an overactivation of orofacial primary motor cortex, inferior lateral premotor cortex and SMA in the pre-treatment state. After LSVT®, the clinical improvement of dysarthria in the PD speakers was accompanied by a reduction of cortical motor-premotor activations, resembling the functional pattern observed in healthy speakers [165]. Moreover, an additional recruitment of right anterior insula, caudate head, putamen and dorsolateral prefrontal cortex have suggested a treatment-induced functional reorganization from an abnormally effortful to a more automatic implementation of speech motor actions [165]. On the contrary, Pinto and colleagues found a lack of activation in the right orofacial primary motor cortex when performing a PET study on speech performance in PD speakers in the "off" and "on" state of STN deep brain stimulation. Furthermore, there was a decreased activation of the bilateral cerebellar hemispheres and an overactivation in the right superior premotor cortex and the bilateral dorsolateral prefrontal cortex and – confirming the findings of Liotti and colleagues – of the SMA [208]. These abnormal activations have been interpreted as compensatory mechanisms, but might also arise directly as part of the pathophysiology of PD. According to these PET studies, the basal ganglia only seem to hold a subordinate role in the intricate neuronal networks required for speech performance, but this might be a methodological artifact, since other investigators have accented the particular relevancy of the basal ganglia for some aspects of motor speech programming [255].

Based upon studies on limb movements, PD patients have been found to feature a reduced ability to rapidly switch from one movement or motor program to another [21, 52, 273] which has been interpreted as difficulty with modifying or inhibiting an ongoing response or with activating new motor programs [132, 155]. Furthermore, limb reaction time studies have supported the premise that PD patients have difficulties maintaining programmed information prior to movement initiation which has gained empirical support from numerous kinematic investigations leading to the speculation that programmed representations of movements might decay prior to and during movement initiation [24, 91, 225]. These phenomena of limb movement motor programming seem to parallel some aspects of Parkinsonian dysarthria, as abnormally placed speech pauses, problems with progression through an utterance, impaired initiation of articulation or decrease of pitch variability in the course of speaking [105, 245, 260] could result from difficulties in maintaining the speech motor program. Exemplarily, Moreau and colleagues were able to detect correlations between articulatory hastening and festination of gait in PD patients which suggests a shared pathophysiological mechanism of dysfunctional stability of repetitive movements over time [187]. Furthermore, reduced ability to switch between speech motor programs would be consistent with speech behavior such as difficulty stopping an ongoing response and marked hesitation between movement segments [8, 74]. However, the few pioneering studies on speech motor programming in PD speakers failed to support a disruption of speech motor planning or programming so far, which might be attributed to methodological or theoretical concerns, as most of the examinations focused on different potential manifestations of programming deficits such as impaired relative timing [52, 171, 242]. For example, Connor and colleagues examined production of isolated syllables compared to more complex polysyllabic words produced as quickly as possible under the presumption that speech planning in PD should be more impaired for longer and more complex speech tasks. Though the authors found no significant acoustic differences between speech production of PD patients and healthy controls, it is to be speculated that the complexity of the task was insufficient to adequately engage speech motor programming operations [51].

Further parallels between limb movement and motor speech impairment of Parkinsonian dysarthria refer to the aspect of time processing, which itself is thought to be a component of motor programming. Dysfunctional time processing in PD has exemplarily been found to be reflected in increased reaction and movement time [27], impaired ability to maintain a fixed rhythm in tapping tasks [197, 256] and increased speech production time [268]. Timing deficits in the non-motor domain have been shown to include impaired temporal discrimination of pairs of stimuli in the somatosensoric, visual and auditory modalities and impaired time estimation [14, 202]. Since PD patients have been shown to feature deficits both in production and perception tasks that involve time-related decisions one should suggest a common timekeeping mechanism involving basal ganglia circuits which are dysfunctional in PD. In fact, a wealth of experimental evidence suggests the existence of a common timing mechanism for motor and perceptual tasks in healthy individuals [111]. For instance, significant correlations between interval tapping and interval discrimination tasks have been documented [41, 141]. Variability on both production and perception tasks have been found to increase linearly as a function of the target interval, following the scalar property [94, 183] of interval timing. One explanation for the scalar property is based upon an internal clock model [263], implying a comparison of the current subjective time interval to internal representations stored in the reference memory [95]. This paradigm implicates the dissociation between memory, which can be affected by anticholinergic manipulations, and the internal clock, which is related to dopaminergic basal ganglia circuits [95]. In the same vein, functional magnetic resonance imaging (fMRI) studies on healthy individuals have demonstrated that the basal ganglia-thalamocortical pathway is activated during both perceptual and motor timing tasks [184, 210] implicating this network as part of the neural substrate of the "internal clock" [39]. Given that the basal ganglia receive dopaminergic input from the substantia nigra, it is not surprising that, for example, dopaminergic antagonists produce a deceleration of the subjective internal clock speed in proportion to their dopamine D2 receptor affinity [177, 182]. Therefore, interval timing had been attributed to the integrity of cortico-striatal pathways which seemed to be substantiated by the finding of an impairment of interval estimation and reproduction in unmedicated Parkinsonian patients, which was reversible under dopaminergic therapy and deep brain stimulation of the subthalamic nucleus [14, 175, 176, 219]. Contrariwise, further studies on interval discrimination and estimation in PD failed to demonstrate an impairment of time processing related to intervals within the hundreds of milliseconds range [112, 150]. On the other hand, it has been shown that cerebellar pathways are likewise essential for correct millisecond timing [133, 151], as one of the capacities required for speech performance and perception [39].

Some further understanding of the basal ganglia function has been achieved by research on developmental stuttering which bears resemblance the accidental involuntary repetition of utterances in some individual PD speakers called "palilalia" [10]. Because of the clinical similarities of palilalia and stuttering including situational exacerbation of symptoms [11, 26], alleviating effects of external sensory cues [168], facilitory effects of focused attention [266] and sensitivity to fluctuating dopamine levels [276], stuttering has been etiologically attributed to a dysfunction of the basal ganglia and its associated cortico-striato-thalamo-cortical connections [139]. Brain imaging studies were able to demonstrate dysfunctional activation in different neuronal structures in stutterers similar to the patterns found in PD speakers including left superior and posterior temporal lobes, circumscribed areas of the left frontal and prefrontal cortex, the left primary motor cortex and the left SMA [35, 82, 195, 196]. Moreover, there was evidence for deficits in motor sequence skill learning and development of automaticity in persons with developmental stuttering [249] clinically similar to some motor features in PD patients, which has been assigned to dysfunctional basal ganglia circuits. Although a direct comparison of stutterers and PD patients on limb and speech motor skill learning has not been performed until now, both syndromes seem to go along with the transition of sequential motor skills to increasing automaticity [249]. In PD speakers, repetitive speech phenomena resembling stuttering have been found to emerge predominantly in a subgroup of patients with advanced disease and to occur more often in effort demanding speech tasks than in semiautomatic forms of speech and therefore have been interpreted as an evidence of deficient motor speech control [22].

Summarized, the multidimensional alterations of speech related to neuromuscular performance, motor planning and programming as well as cognitive-linguistic functions cannot be explained by dopaminergic deficits alone, but rather represent a polymorphic dysfunction of task-dependent interconnected neuronal networks which have to be further investigated in future research.

References

[1] Abbs, JH; Hunker, CJ; Barlow, SM. Differential speech motor subsystem impairments with suprabulbar lesions: neurophysiologic framework and supporting data. In: Berry, WR, ed. *Clinical Dysarthria.*, San Diego: College-Hill Press, 1984.

[2] Ackermann, H; Ziegler, W. Die Dysarthrophonie des Parkinson-Syndroms. *Fortschritte der Neurologie - Psychiatrie*, 1989, 57, 149-160.

[3] Ackermann, H; Ziegler, W. Articulatory deficits in Parkinsonian dysarthria. Journal of *Neurology, Neurosurgery, and Psychiatry,* 1991, 54, 1093-1098.

[4] Ackermann, H; Hertrich, I; Hehr, T. Oral diadochokinesis in neurological dysarthias. *Folia Phoniatrica et Logopaedia* 1995, 47, 15-23.

[5] Ackermann, H; Konczak, J; Hertrich, I. The temporal control of repetitive articulatory movements in Parkinson's disease. *Brain and Language* 1997, 57, 312-319.

[6] Ackermann, H; Wildgruber, D; Daum, I; Grodd, W. Does the cerebellum contribute to cognitive aspects of speech production? A functional magnetic resonance imaging (fMRI) study in humans. *Neuroscience Letters,* 1998, 247, 187-190.

[7] Adams, SG; Lang, AE. Can the Lombard effect be used to improve low voice intensity in Parkinson's disease? *European Journal of Communication Disorders,* 1992, 27, 121-127.

[8] Adams, SG. Hypokinetic dysarthria in Parkinson's disease. In: McNeil MR, ed. *Clinical management of sensorimotor speech disorders*. New York: Thieme, 1997.

[9] Allan, CM. Treatment of non-fluent speech resulting from neurological disease: Treatment of dysarthria. *British Journal of Disorders of Communication* 1970, 5, 3-5.

[10] Alm, PA. Stuttering and the basal ganglia circuits: a critical review of possible relations. *Journal of Communication Disorders,* 2004, 37, 325-369.

[11] Alsobrook, J; Pauls, D. Molecular approaches to child psychopathology. *Human Biology*, 1998, 70, 413-432.

[12] Anderson, JM; Hughes, JD; Rothi, LJ; Crucian, GP; Heilman, KM. Developmental stuttering and Parkinson's disease: the effects of levodopa treatment. *Journal of Neurology, Neurosurgery, and Psychiatry,* 1999, 66, 776-778.

[13] Aronson, AE. *Clinical voice disorders*. New York: Thieme-Stratton, 1990

[14] Artieda, J; Pastor, MA; Lacruz, F; Obeso, JA. Temporal discrimination is abnormal in Parkinson's disease. *Brain,* 1992, 115, 199-210.

[15] Azevedo, LL; Cardoso, F; Reis, C. Acoustic analysis of prosody in females with Parkinson's disease: effect of l-dopa. *Arquivos de Neuro-Psiquiatria,* 2003 , 61 , 995-998.

[16] Baker, KK; Ramig, LO; Johnson, AB; Freed, CR. Preliminary voice and speech analysis following fetal dopamine transplants in 5 individuals with Parkinson Disease. *Journal of Speech, Language, and Hearing Research,* 1997, 615-626.

[17] Baker, KK; Ramig, LO; Luschei, ES; Smith, ME. Thyroarytenoid muscle activity associated with hypophonia in Parkinson's disease and aging. *Neurology,* 1998, 51, 1592-1598.

[18] Baker, KK; Ramig, LO; Sapir, S; Luschei, ES; Smith, ME. Control of vocal loudness in young and old adults. *Journal of Speech, Language, and Hearing Research,* 2001, 44, 297-305.

[19] Barlow, SM; Iacono, RP; Paseman, LA; Biswas, A; D'Antonio, L. The effects of posteroventral pallidotomy on force and speech aerodynamics in Parkinson's disease. In: Cannito, M; Yorston, KM; Beukelman, DR; eds. *Neuromotor speech disorders: nature assessment and management.* Baltimore: Brooks, 1998, 117-155.

[20] Bell, DS. Speech functions of the thalamus inferred from the effects of thalamotomy. *Brain,* 1968, 91, 619-638.

[21] Benecke, R; Rothwell, JC; Dick JPR; Day, BL; Marsden, CD. Disturbance of sequential movements in patients with Parkinson's disease. *Brain,* 1987, 110, 361-379.

[22] Benke, T; Hohenstein, C; Poewe, W; Butterworth, B. Repetitive speech phenomena in Parkinson´s disease. *Journal of Neurology, Neurosurgery, and Psychiatry,* 2000, 69, 319-324.

[23] Benke, T; Butterworth, B. Palilalia and repetitive speech: two case studies. *Brain and Language,* 2001, 78, 62-81.

[24] Berardelli, A; Rothwell, JC; Thompson, PD; Hallett, M. Pathophysiology of bradykinesia in Parkinson´s disease. *Brain,* 2001, 124, 2131-2146.

[25] Biary, N; Pimental, PA; Langenberg, PW. A double-blind trial of clonazepam in the treatment of parkinsonian dysarthria. *Neurology,* 1988, 38, 255-258.

[26] Bloodstein, O. *A handbook of stuttering.* Chicago: Easter Seals Society, 1995.

[27] Bloxham, CA; Dick, DJ; Moore, M. Reaction times and attention in Parkinson´s disease. *Journal of Neurology, Neurosurgery, and Psychiatry,* 1987, 50, 1178-1185.

[28] Bogaard, JM; Hovestadt, A; Meerwaldt, J; van der Meche, FG; Stigt, J. Maximal exspiratory and inspiratory flow-volume curves in Parkisnon´s disease. *American Review of Respiratory Disease,* 1989, 139, 610-614.

[29] Bohland, JW; Guenther, FH. An fMRI investigation of syllable sequence production. *Neuroimage,* 2006, 32, 821-841.

[30] Bonnet, AM; Loria, Y; Saint-Hilaire, MH; Lhermitte, F; Agid, Y. Does long-term aggravation of Parkinson´s disease result from non-dopaminergic lesions? *Neurology* 1987, 37, 1539-1542.

[31] Bookheimer, FY; Zeffiro, TA; Blaxton, TA; Gaillard, PW; Theodore, WH. Activation of language cortex with automatic speech tasks. *Neurology,* 2000, 55, 1151-1157.

[32] Boshes, B. Voice changes in parkinsonism. *Journal of Neurosurgery*, 1966, 24, 286-291.

[33] Braak, H; Del Tredici, K; Rüb, U; de Vos, RA; Jansen Steur, EN; Braak, E. Staging of brain pathology related to sporadic Parkinson´s disease. *Neurobiology of Aging,* 2003, 24, 197-211.

[34] Braak, H; Bohl, JR; Müller, CM; Rüb, O; de Vos, RA; del Tredici, K. Stanley Fahn Lecture 2005, The staging procedure for the inclusion body pathology associated with sporadic Parkinson´s disease reconsidered. *Movement Disorders,* 2006, 21, 2042-2051.

[35] Braun, AR; Varga, M; Stager, SV; Schulz, GM; Selbie, S; Maisog, JM; Carson, RE; Ludlow, CL. Altered patterns of cerebral activity during speech and language production in developmental stuttering: An H2(15)O positron emission tomography study. *Brain,* 1997, 120, 761-784.

[36] Brown, S; Laird, AR; Pfordresher, PQ; Thelen, SM; Turkeltaub, P; Liotti, M. The somatotopy of speech: Phonation and articulation in the human motor cortex. *Brain and Cognition,* 2009 (in press).

[37] Brumlik, J; Canter, G; De La Torre, R; Mier, M; Petrovick, M; Boshes, B. A critical analysis of the effects of trihexyphenidyl (artane) on the components of the Parkinsonian syndrome. *Journal of Nervous and Mental Disease,* 1964, 138, 424-431.

[38] Buck, JF; Cooper, IS. Speech problems in parkinsonian patients undergoing anterior choroidal artery occlusion or chemopallidotomy. *Journal of the American Geriatric Society,* 1956, 4, 1285-1290.

[39] Buhushi, CV; Meck, WH. What makes us tick? Functional and neural mechanisms of interval timing. *Nature Reviews Neuroscience,* 2005, 14, 1-6.

[40] Bunton, K. Patterns of lung volume use during an extemporaneous speech task in persons with Parkinson's disease. *Journal of Communication Disorders,* 2005, 38, 331-348.

[41] Buonomano, DV; Karmarkar, UR. How do we tell time? *Neuroscientist,* 2002, 8, 42-51

[42] Caekebeke, J; Jennekens-Schinkel, A; van der Linden, A; Buruma, I; Roos, R. The interpretation of dysprosody in patients with Parkinson's disease. *Journal of Neurology, Neurosurgery, and Psychiatry,* 1991, 54, 145-148.

[43] Cahill, LM; Murdoch, BE; Theodoros, DG; Triggs, EJ; Charles, BG; Yao, AA. Effect of oral levodopa treatment on articulatory function in Parkinson's disease: preliminary results. *Motor Control,* 1998, 2, 161-172.

[44] Caligiuri, MP; Abbs, JH. Response properties of the perioral reflex in Parkinson's disease. *Experimental Neurology,* 1987, 98, 563-572.

[45] Caligiuri, MP. Short-term fluctuations in orofacial motor control in Parkinson's disease. In: Yorkston, K; Beukelman, D, eds. *Recent advances in clinical dysarthria.* Boston: College-Hill Press, 1989a, 199-212.

[46] Caligiuri, MP. The influence of speaking rate on articulatory hypokinesia in parkinsonian dysarthria. *Brain and Language,* 1989b, 36, 493-502.

[47] Canter, GJ. Speech characteristics of patients with Parkinson's disease. I: Intensity, pitch, and duration. *Journal of Speech and Hearing Disorders,* 1963, 28, 221-229.

[48] Canter, GJ. Speech characteristics of patients with Parkinson's disease: II. Physiological support for speech. *Journal of Speech and Hearing Disorders,* 1965a, 30, 44-49.

[49] Canter, GJ. Speech characteristics of patients with Parkinson's disease. III. Articulation, diadochokinesis, and overall speech adequacy. *Journal of Speech and Hearing Disorders,* 1965b, 30, 217-224.

[50] Canter, GJ; van Lancker, DR. Disturbances of the temporal organization of speech following bilateral thalamic surgery in a patient with Parkinson's disease. *Journal of Communication Disorders,* 1985, 18, 329-349.

[51] Connor, N; Ludlow, C; Schulz, G. Stop consonant production in isolated and repeated syllables in Parkinson's disease. *Neuropsychologia,* 1989, 27, 829-838.

[52] Contreraz-Vidal, JL; Stelmach, GE. Effects of Parkinsonism in motor control. *Life Sciences,* 1996, 58, 165-176.

[53] Critchley, EM. Peak-dose dysphonia in parkinsonism. *Lancet,* 1976, I, 544.

[54] Critchley, EM. Speech disorders of Parkinsonism : a review. *Journal of Neurology, Neurosurgery, and Psychiatry,* 1981, 44, 751-758.

[55] D'Alatri, L; Paludetti, G; Contarino, MF; Galla, F; Marchese, MR; Bentivoglio, AR. Effects of bilateral subthalamic stimulation and medication on parkinsonian speech impairment. *Journal of Voice,* 2008, 22, 365-372.

[56] Darkins, A; Fromkin, V; Benson, D. A characterization of the prosodic loss in Parkinson's disease. *Brain and Language* 1988, 44, 751-758.

[57] Darley, FL; Aronson, AE; Brown, JR. Clusters of deviant speech dimensions In the dysarthrias. *Journal of Speech and Hearing Research,* 1969a, 12, 462-496.

[58] Darley, FL; Aronson, AE; Brown, JR. Differential diagnostic patterns of dysarthria. *Journal of Speech and Hearing Research* 1969b, 12, 246-269.

[59] Darley, FL; Aronson, AE; Brown, JR. *Motor Speech Disorders.,* Philadelphia: Saunders, 1975.

[60] De Letter, M; Santens, M; van Borsel, J. The effect of levodopa on tongue strength and endurance in patients with Parkinson´s disease. *Acta Neurologica Belgica,* 2003, 103, 35-38

[61] De Letter, M; Santens, P; van Borsel, J. The effect of levodopa on word intelligibility in Parkinson´s disease. *Journal of Communication Disorders* 2005, 38,187-196

[62] De Letter, M; Santens, P; De Bodt, M; Boon, P; Van Borsel, J. Levodopa-induced alterations in speech rate in advanced Parkinson`s disease. *Acta Neurologica Belgica,* 2006, 106, 19-22

[63] Deane, KHO; Whurr, R; Playford, ED; Ben-Shlomo, Y; Clarke, CE. Speech and language therapy versus placebo or no intervention for dysarthria in Parkinson´s disease. (Cochrane Review). In: *The Cochrane Library (Issue 2),* Chichester: John Wiley & Sons Ltd, 2004.

[64] Decoster, W; Debruyne, F. The ageing voice: changes in fundamental frequency, waveform stability and spectrum. *Acta Otorhinolaryngologica Belgica,* 1997, 51, 105-112.

[65] Deuschl, G; Schade-Brittinger, C; Krack, P; Volkmann, J; Schäfer, H; Bötzel, K; Daniels, C; Deutschländer, A; et al for the German Parkinson Study Group, Neurostimulation Section. A randomized trial of deep-brain stimulation for Parkinson´s disease. *New England Journal of Medicine,* 2006, 31, 896-898.

[66] Diamond, SG; Schneider, JS; Markham, CH. Oral sensorimotor defects in people with Parkinson´s disease. *Advances in Neurology,* 1987, 45, 335-338.

[67] Djaldetti, R; Melamed, E. Management of response fluctuations: practical guidelines. *Neurology,* 1998, 51(Suppl.2), S36-40.

[68] Downie, AW; Low, JM; Lindsay, DD. Speech disorders in parkinsonism: usefulness of delayed auditory feedback in selected cases. *British Journal of Disorders of Communication,* 1981, 16, 133-139.

[69] Doyle, P; Raade, A; St Pierre, A; Desai, S. Fundamental frequency and acoustic variability associated with production of sustained vowels by speakers with hypokinetic dysarthria. *Journal of Medical Speech-Language Pathology,* 1995, 3, 41-50.

[70] Dromey, C; Ramig, LO; Johnson, A. Phonatory and articulatory changes associated with increased vocal intensity in Parkinson disease: A case study. *Journal of Speech and Hearing Research,* 1995, 38, 751-763.

[71] Dromey, C; Kumar, R; Lang, AE; Lozano, AM. An investigation of the effects of subthalamic nucleus stimulation on acoustic measures of voice. *Movement Disorders,* 2000, 15, 1132-1138.

[72] Dromey, C. Spectral measures and perceptual ratings of hypokinetic dysarthria. *Journal of Medical Speech-Language Pathology,* 2003, 11, 85-91.

[73] Dronkers, NF. A new brain region for coordinating speech articulation. *Nature,* 1996, 384, 159-161.

[74] Duffy, JR. Hypokinetic Dysarthria. In: *Motor Speech Disorders*, Duffy JR, ed. St. Louis: Elsevier, 1995, 187-215.

[75] Dworkin, JP; Aronson, AE. Tongue strength and alternate motion rates in normal and dysarthric speakers. *Journal of Communication Disorders,* 1986, 19, 115-132.

[76] El Sharkawi, A; Ramig, LO; Logemann, JA; Pauloski, BR; Rademaker, AW; Smith, CH; Pawlas, A; Baum, S; Werner, C. Swallowing and voice effects of Lee Silverman

Voice Treatment (LSVT®): A pilot study. *Journal of Neurology, Neurosurgery, and Psychiatry,* 2002, 71, 31-36.

[77] Fletcher, S. Time-by-count measurement of diadochokinetic syllable rate. *Journal of Speech and Hearing Research,* 1972, 15, 757-762.

[78] Flint, A; Black, S; Campbell-Taylor, I; Gailey, G; Levinton, C. Acoustic analysis in the differentiation between Parkinson's Disease and major depression. *Journal of Psycholinguistic Research,* 1992, 21, 383-399.

[79] Forrest, K; Weismer, G; Turner, GS. Kinematic acoustic and perceptual analyses of connected speech produced by parkinsonian and normal geriatric adults. *Journal of the Acoustical Society of America,* 1989, 85, 2608-2622.

[80] Forrest, K; Weismer, G. Dynamic aspects of lower lip movement in parkinsonian and neurologically normal geriatric speakers' production of stress. *Journal of Speech and Hearing Research,* 1995, 38, 260-272.

[81] Fox, CM; Ramig, LO. Vocal sound pressure level and self-perception of speech and voice of men and women with idiopathic Parkinson's disease. *American Journal of Speech-Language Pathology,* 1997, 6, 85-93.

[82] Fox, PT; Ingham, RJ; Ingham, JC; Zamarripa, F; Xiong, JH; Lancaster, JL. Brain correlates of stuttering and syllable production: A PET performance-correlation analysis. *Brain,* 2000, 123, 1985-2004.

[83] Fox, CM; Morrison, CE; Ramig, LO; Sapir, S. Current perspectives on the Lee Silverman Voice Treatment (LSVT®) for people with idiopathic Parkinson's disease. *American Journal of Speech-Language Pathology,* 2002, 11, 111-123.

[84] Gallena, S; Smith, PJ; Zeffiro, T; Ludlow, CL. Effects of levodopa on laryngeal muscle activity for voice onset and offset in Parkinson's disease. *Journal of Speech, Language, and Hearing Research,* 2001, 44, 1284-1299.

[85] Gamboa, J; Jimenez-Jimenez, FJ; Nieto, A. Acoustic voice analysis in patients with Parkinson's disease treated with dopaminergic drugs. *Journal of Voice,* 1997, 11, 314-320.

[86] Gentil, M; Tournier, CL; Perrin, S. Pollak, P. Effects of levodopa on finger and orofacial movements in Parkinson's disease. *Progress in Neuro-Psychopharmacology and Biological Psychiatry,* 1998, 22, 1261-1274

[87] Gentil, M; Garcia-Ruiz, P; Pollak, P; Benabid, AL. Effect of stimulation of the subthalamic nucleus on oral control in patients with Parkinson's disease. *Journal of Neurology, Neurosurgery, and Psychiatry,* 1999a, 67, 329-333.

[88] Gentil, M; Tournier, CL; Pollak, P; Benabid, AL. Effect of bilateral subthalamic nucleus stimulation and dopatherapy on oral control in Parkinson's disease. *European Neurology,* 1999b, 42, 136-140.

[89] Gentil, M; Garcia-Ruiz, P; Pollak, P; Benabid, AL. Effect of bilateral deep-brain stimulation on oral control of patients with parkinsonism. *European Neurology,* 2000, 44, 147-152.

[90] Gentil, M; Chauvin, P; Pinto, S; Pollak, P; Benabid, AL. Effect of bilateral stimulation of the subthalamic nucleus on parkinsonian voice. *Brain and Language,* 2001, 78, 233-240.

[91] Gentilucci, M; Negrotti, A. Planning and executing an action in Parkinson's disease. *Movement Disorders,* 1999, 14, 69-79.

[92] Ghika, J; Villemure, JG; Fankhauser, H; Favre, J; Assal, G; Ghika-Schmid, F. Efficiency and safety of bilateral contemporaneous stimulation (deep brain stimulation) in levodopa-responsive patients with Parkinson´s disease with severe motor fluctuations: a 2-year follow-up review. *Journal of Neurosurgery,* 1998, 89, 713-718.
[93] Ghika, J; Ghika-Schmid, F; Frankhauser, H; Assal, G; Vingerhoets, F; Albanese, A; Bogousslavsky, J; Favre, J. Bilateral contemporaneous posteroventral pallidotomy for the treatment of Parkinson´s disease: neuropsychological and neurological side effects. Report of four cases and review of the literature. *Journal of Neurosurgery,* 1999, 91,313-321.
[94] Gibbon, J. Scalar expectancy theory and Weber´s law in animal timing. *Psychological Review*, 1977, 84, 279-325.
[95] Gibbon, J; Church, RM; Meck, WH. *Timing and Time Perception Vol 423* The New New York: York Academy of Sciences, 1984, 52-77.
[96] Goberman, AM; Coelho, C. Acoustic analysis of parkinsonian speech I: Speech characteristics and L-dopa therapy. *NeuroRehabilitation,* 2002a, 17, 237-246.
[97] Goberman, A; Coelho, C; Robb, M. Phonatory characteristics of parkinsonian speech before and after morning medication: the ON and OFF states. *Journal of Communication Disorders,* 2002b, 35, 217-239.
[98] Goberman, AM; Blomgren, M. Parkinsonian speech disfluencies: effects of L-dopa related fluctuations. *Journal of Fluency Disorders,* 2003, 28, 55-70.
[99] Goberman, AK. Correlation between acoustic speech characteristics and non-speech motor performance in Parkinson Disease. *Medical Science Monitor* 2005, 11 (3), pp. 109 – 116.
[100] Goberman, AM; Elmer, WE. Acoustic analysis of clear versus conversional speech in individuals with Parkinson´s disease. *Journal of Communication Disorders,* 2005, 38, 215-230.
[101] Goldsmith, SK; Joyce, JN. Dopamine D2 receptors are organized in bands in normal human temporal cortex. *Neuroscience,* 1996, 74, 435-451.
[102] Graber, S; Hertrich, I; Daum I; Spieker, S; Ackermann, H. Speech perception deficits in Parkinson´s disease: underestimation of time intervals compromises identification of durational phonetic contrasts. *Brain and Language,* 2002, 82, 65-74.
[103] Greene, MC; Watson, BW. The value of speech amplification in Parkinson´s disease patients. *Folia Phoniatrica (Basel),* 1968, 20, 250-257.
[104] Gross, C; Rougier, A; Guehl, D; Boraud, T; Jlien, J; Bioulac, B. High-frequency stimulation of the globus pallidus internalis in Parkinson´s disease: a study of seven cases. *Journal of Neurosurgery,* 1997, 87, 491-498.
[105] Gurd, JM; Bessel, N; Watson, I; Coleman, J. Motor speech versus digit control in Parkinson´s disease: A cognitive neuropsychology investigation. *Clinical Linguistics & Phonetics,* 1998, 12, 357-378.
[106] Hammen, VL; Yorkston, KM; Beukelman, DR. Pausal and speech duration characteristics as a function of speaking rate in normal and dysarthric individuals. In: Yorkston KM, Beukelman DR, eds. *Recent advances in clinical dysarthria*. Austin, Texas: Pro-Ed, 1989.
[107] Hanson, WR; Metter, EJ. DAF speech rate modification in Parkinson´s disease: a report of two cases. In: Berry W, ed., *Clinical dysarthria*. San Diego: College-Hill, 1981, 250-57.

[108] Hanson, DG; Gerrat, BR; Ward, PH. Cinegraphic observations of laryngeal function in Parkinson′s disease. *Laryngoscope,* 1984, 94, 348-353.

[109] Hariz, MI; Johansson, F; Shamsgovara, P; Johansson, E; Hariz, GM; Fagerlund, M. Bilateral subthalamic nucleus stimulation in a parkinsonian patient with preoperative deficits in speech and cognition: persistent improvement in mobility but increased dependency: a case study. *Movement Disorders,* 2000, 15, 136-139.

[110] Hartelius, L; Svensson, P. Speech and swallowing symptoms associated with Parkinson′s disease and multiple sclerosis: a survey. *Folia Phoniatrica et Logopaedica,* 1994, 46, 9-17.

[111] Hazeltine, E; Helmuth, LL; Ivry, RB. Neural mechanisms of timing. *Trends in Cognitive Sciences* 1997, 1, 163-169.

[112] Hellström, A; Lang, H; Portin, R; Rinne, J. Tone duration discrimination in Parkinson′s disease. *Neuropsychologia,* 1997, 35, 737-740.

[113] Helm, N. Management of palilalia with a pacing board. *Journal of Speech and Hearing Disorders,* 1979, 44, 350-353.

[114] Hertrich, I; Ackermann, H. Gender-specific vocal dysfunction in Parkisnon′s disease: Electroglottographic and acoustical analyses. *Annals of Otology, Rhinology, and Laryngology,* 1995, 104, 197-202.

[115] Hickok, G; Erhard, P; Kassubek, J; et al. A functional magnetic resonnace imaging study of the role of left posterior superior temporal gyrus in speech production: Implications fort he explanation of conduction aphasia. *Neuroscience Letters,* 2000, 287, 156-160.

[116] Hirose, H; Kiritani, S; Ushijima, T; Yoshioka, H; Sawashima, M. Patterns of dysarthric movements in patients with parkinsonism. *Folia Phoniatrica et Logopaedica,* 1981, 33, 204-215.

[117] Hirose, H; Kiritani, S; Sawashima, M. Velocity of articulatory movements in normal and dysarthric subjects. *Folia Phoniatrica et Logopaedica,* 1982, 34, 210-215

[118] Hirose, H. Pathophysiology of motor speech disorders (dysarthrias). *Folia Phoniatrica et Logopaedica* 1986, 38, 61-88.

[119] Ho, AK; Bradshaw, JL; Iansek, R; Alfredson, R. Speech volume regulation in Parkinson′s disease: Effects of implicit cues and explicit instructions. *Neuropsychologia* 1999a, 37, 1453-1460.

[120] Ho, AK; Iansek, R; Bradshaw, JL. Regulation of parkinsonian speech volume: the effect of interlocutor distance. *Journal of Neurology, Neurosurgery, and Psychiatry* 1999b, 67, 199-202.

[121] Ho, AK; Bradshaw, JL; Iansek, R. Volume perception in parkinsonian speech. *Movement Disorders,* 2000, 15, 1125-1131.

[122] Ho, AK; Iansek, R; Bradshaw, JL. The effect of a concurrent task on parkinsonian speech. *Journal of Clinical and Experimental Neuropsychology,* 2002, 24, 36-47.

[123] Ho, AK; Bradshaw, JL; Iansek, R. For better or worse: The effect of levodopa on speech in Parkinson′s disease. *Movement Disorders,* 2008, 23 (4), 575-580.

[124] Holmes, RJ; Oates, J; Phyland, D; Hughes, A. Voice characteristics in the progression of Parkinson′s disease. *International Journal of Language & Communication Disorders* 2000, 35, 417-418.

[125] Hoodin, R; Gilbert, H. Parkinsonian dysarthria: An aerodynamic and perceptual description of velopharyngeal closure for speech. *Folia Phoniatrica et Logopaedica,* 1989, 41, 249-258.

[126] Hovestadt, A; Bogaard, JM; Meerwaldt, J; van der Meche, FG; Stigt, J. Pulmonary function in Parkinson´s disease. *Journal of Neurology, Neurosurgery, and Psychiatry,* 1989, 52, 329-333.

[127] Huber, JE; Spruill, J. Respiratory function and variability in individuals with Parkinson´s disease: pre- and post-Lee Silverman Voice Treatment. *Journal of Medical Speech-Language Pathology,* 2003, 11, 185-192.

[128] Huber, JE; Spruill, J. Age-related changes to speech breathing with increased vocal loudness. *Journal of Speech, Language, and Hearing Research,* 2008, 51, 351-368

[129] Hunker, C; Abbs, J; Barlow, S. The relationship between parkinsonain rigidity and hypokinesia in the orofacial system: a quantitative analysis. *Neurology,* 1982, 32, 749-754.

[130] Hurtig, H. Problems with current pharmacologic treatment of Parkinson´s disease. *Experimental Neurololy,* 1997, 144, 10-16.

[131] Illes, J; Metter, EJ; Hanson, WR; Iritani, S. Parkinson´s disease: acoustic and linguistic considerations. *Brain and Language,* 1988, 33,146-160.

[132] Inzelberg, R; Plotnik, M; Flash, T; Schechtman, E; Shahar, I; Korczyn, AD. Mental and motor switching in Parkinson´s disease. *Journal of Motor Behavior,* 2001, 33, 377-385

[133] Ivry, RB; Spencer, RM. The neuronal representation of time. *Current Opinion in Neurobiology,* 2004, 14, 225-232.

[134] Jiang, J; Lin, E; Wang, J; Hanson, D. Glottographic measures before and after levodopa treatment in Parkinsons´disease. *Laryngoscope,* 1999a, 109, 1287-1294.

[135] Jiang, J; O`Mara, T; Chen, HJ; Stern, JI; Vlagos, D; Hanson, D. Aerodynamic measurements of patients with Parkinson´s disease. *Journal of Voice,* 1999b, 13, 583-591.

[136] Jiang, J; Lie, E; Hanson, DG. Acoustic and airflow spectral analysis of voice tremor. *Journal of Speech, Language, and Hearing Research,* 2000, 43, 191-204.

[137] Jimenez-Jimenez, F; Gamboa, J; Nieto, A; Guerrero, M; Orti-Pareja, M; Molina, J; Garcia-Albea, E. Cobeta, I. Acoustic voice analysis in untreated patients with Parkinson´s disease. *Parkinsonism and Related Disorders,* 1997, 3, 111-116.

[138] Johnson, JA; Pring, TR. Speech therapy and Parkinson´s disease: a review and further data. *British Journal of Disorders of Communication,* 1990, 25, 183-184.

[139] Jones, RD; White, AJ; Lawson, KHC; Anderson, TJ. Visuoperceptual and visuomotor deficits in developmental stutterers: An exploratory study. *Human Movement Science* 2002, 21, 603-619.

[140] Karlsson, S; Persson, M; Johnels, B. Levodopa-induced ON-OFF motor fluctuations in Parkinson´s disease related to rhythmical masticatory jaw movements. *Journal of Neurology, Neurosurgery, and Psychiatry,* 1992, 55, 304-307.

[141] Keele, S; Nicoletti, R; Ivry, RB; Pokorny, R. Do perception and motor production share common timing mechanisms: a correlation analysis. *Acta Psychologica,* 1985, 60, 173-191.

[142] Kent, RD; Rosenbek, JC. Prosodic disturbance and neurologic lesion. *Brain and Language,* 1982, 15, 259-291.

[143] Kent, R; Kim, H; Weismer, G; Kent, J; Rosenbek, J; Brooks, B; Workinger, M. Laryngeal dysfunction in neurological disease: Amyotrophic lateral sclerosis, Parkinson's disease, and stroke. *Journal of Medical Speech-Language Pathology,* 1994, 6, 157-175.

[144] Kent, RD. Hearing and believing: some limits to the auditory-perceptual assessment of speech and voice disorders. *American Journal of Speech-Language Pathology,* 1996, 5, 7-23.

[145] Kent, RD; Weismer, G; Kent, J; Rosenbek, J. The dysarthrias: speech-voice profiles, related dysfunctions, and neuropathology. *Journal of Medical Speech-Language Pathology,* 1998, 6, 165-187.

[146] Kent, RD; Vorperian, AK; Kent, JF; Duffy, JR. Voice dysfunction in dysarthria: application of the Multi-Dimensional Voice Program. *Journal of Communication Disorders,* 2003, 36, 281-306.

[147] Kim, R. The chronic residual respiratory disorder in post-encephalitic parkinsonism. *Journal of Neurology, Neurosurgery, and Psychiatry,* 1968, 31, 393-398.

[148] King, J; Ramig, L; Lemke, J; Horii, Y. Parkinson's disease: Longitudinal changes in acoustic parameters of phonation. *Journal of Medical Speech-Language Pathology,* 1994, 2, 29-42.

[149] Klostermann, F; Ehlen, F; Vesper, J; Nubel, K; Gross, M; Marzinzik, F; Curio, G; Sappok, T. Effects of subthalamic deep brain stimulation on dysarthrophonia in Parkinson's disease. *Journal of Neurology, Neurosurgery, and Psychiatry,* 2008, 79, 522-529.

[150] Koch, G; Costa, A; Brusa, L; Peppe, A; Gatto, I; Torriero, S; Gerfo, EL; Salerno, S; Oliveri, M; Carlesimo, GA; Caltagirone, C. Impaired reproduction of second but not millisecond time intervals in Parkinson's disease. *Neuropsychologia,* 2008, 46, 1305-1313.

[151] Koekkoek, SKE; Hulscher, HC; Dortland, BR; Hensbroek, RA; Elgersma, Y; Ruigrok, TJ; De Zeeuw, CI. Cerebellar, LTD and learning – dependent timing of conditioned eyelid responses. *Science,* 2003, 301, 1736-1739.

[152] Kompoliti, K; Wang, QE; Goetz, CG; Leurgans, S; Raman, R. Effects of central dopaminergic stimulation by apomorphine on speech in Parkinson's disease. *Neurology,* 2000, 5, 458-462 .

[153] Krack, P; Batir, A; Van Blercom, N; Charbades, S; Fraix, V; Ardouin, C; Koudsie, A; Limousin, PD; Benazzouz, A; LeBas, JF; Benabid, AL; Pollak, P. Five-year follow-up of bilateral stimulation of the subthalamic nucleus in advanced Parkinson's disease. *New England Journal of Medicine,* 2003, 349, 1925-1934.

[154] Krause, M; Fogel, W; Heck, A; Hacke, W; Bonsanto, M; Trenkwalder, C; Tronnier, V. Deep brain stimulation for the treatment of Parkinson's disease: subthalamic nucleus versus globus pallidus internus. *Journal of Neurology, Neurosurgery, and Psychiatry,* 2001, 70, 464-470.

[155] Kropotov, JD; Etlinger, SC. Selection of actions in the basal ganglia-thalamocortical circuits: Review and model. *International Journal of Psychophysiology,* 1999, 31, 197-217.

[156] Laitinen, LV; Bergenheim, AT; Hariz, MI. Ventroposterolateral pallidotomy can abolish all parkinsonian symptoms. *Stereotactic and Functional Neurosurgery,* 1992, 58, 14-21.

[157] Lang, AE; Lozano, AM; Montgomery, E; Duff, I; Tasker, R; Hutchinson, W. Posteroventral medial pallidotomy in advanced Parkinson´s disease. *New England Journal of Medicine,* 1997, 337, 1036-1042.

[158] Lang, AE; Lozano, A. Parkinson´s disease: second of two parts. *New England Journal of Medicine,* 1998, 339, 1130-1143.

[159] Larson, KK; Ramig, LO; Scherer, RC. Acoustic and glottographic voice analysis during drug-related fluctuations in Parkinson´s disease. *Journal of Medical Speech-Language Pathology,* 1994, 2, 227-252.

[160] Le Dorze, G; Ouellet, L; Ryalls, J. Intonation and speech rate in dysarthric speech. *Journal of Communication Disorders,* 1994, 27, 1-17.

[161] Le Dorze, G; Ryalls, J; Brassard, C; Boulanger, N; Ratte, D. A comparison of the prosodic characteristics of the speech of people with Parkinson´s disease and Friedreich´s ataxia with neurologically normal speakers. *Folia Phoniatrica et Logopaedica,* 1998, 50, 1-9.

[162] Leanderson, R; Meyerson, B; Persson, A. Effect of l-dopa on speech in parkinsonism: An EMG study of labial articulatory function. *Journal of Neurology, Neurosurgery, and Psychiatry,* 1971, 34, 679-681.

[163] Leanderson, R; Meyerson, BA; Persson, A. Lip muscle function in parkinsonian dysarthria. *Acta Oto-Laryngologica,* 1972, 74, 350-357.

[164] Limousin, P; Krack, P; Pollak, P; Benazzouz, A; Ardouin, C; Hoffmann, D; Benabid, AL. Electrical stimulation of the subthalamic nucleus in advanced Parkinson´s disease. *New England Journal of Medicine,* 1998, 339, 1105-1111.

[165] Liotti, M; Ramig, LO; Vogel, D; New, P; Cook, CI; Ingham, RJ; Ingam, JC; Fox, PT. Hypophonia in Parkinson´s disease: neural correlates of voice treatment revealed by PET. *Neurology,* 2003, 60, 432-440.

[166] Lisker, L; Abramson, A. A cross-language study of voicing in initial stops: Acoustical measurements. *Word,* 1964, 20, 384-422.

[167] Liss, JM; Weismer, G. Qualitative acoustic analysis in the study of motor speech disorders (letter). *Journal of the Acoustical Society of America,* 1992, 92, 2984.

[168] Liu, X; Tubbesing, S; Aziz, T; Miall, R; Stein, J. Effects of visual feedback on manual tracking and action tremor in Parkinson´s disease. *Experimental Brain Research,* 1999, 129, 477-481.

[169] Logemann, JA; Fisher, HB; Boshes, B; Blonsky, ER. Frequency and cooccurrence of vocal tract dysfunctions in the speech of a large sample of Parkinsonian patients. *Journal of Speech and Hearing Disorders,* 1978, 43, 47-57.

[170] Ludlow, C; Bassich, C. The results of acoustic and perceptual assessment of two types of dysarthria. In: Berry W, ed. *Clinical Dysarthria*. San Diego: College-Hill Press, 1983, 121-153.

[171] Ludlow, CL; Connor, NP; Bassich, CJ. Speech timing in Parkinson´s and Huntington´s disease. *Brain and Language,* 1987, 32, 195-214.

[172] Luschei, ES; Ramig, LO; Baker, KL; Smith, ME. Discharge characteristics of laryngeal single motor units during phonation in young and older adults and in persons with Parkinson´s disease. *Journal of Neurophysiology,* 1999, 81, 2131-2139

[173] Lyons, K; Wilkinson, S; Troster, AI; Pahwa, R. Long-term efficacy of globus pallidus stimulation for the treatment of Parkinson´s disease. *Stereotactic and Functional Neurosurgery,* 2002, 79, 214-220.

[174] MacNeilage, PF; Davis, BL. Motor mechanisms in speech ontogeny: phylogenetic, neurobiological and linguistic implications. *Current Opinion in Neurobiology,* 2001, 11, 696-700.

[175] Malapani, C; Rakitin, B; Lewy, R; Meck, WH; Deweer, B; Dubois, B; Gibbon, J. Coupled temporal memories in Parkinson's disease: a dopamine-related dysfunction. *Journal of Cognitive Neuroscience,* 1998, 10, 316-331.

[176] Malapani, C; Deweer, B; Gibbon, J. Seperating storage from retrieval dysfunction of temporal memory in Parkinson's disease. *Journal of Cognitive Neuroscience,* 2002, 14, 311-322.

[177] Marico, AV; Church, RM. The differential effects of haloperidol and methamphetamine on time estimation in the rat. *Psychopharmacology (Berl.),* 1983, 79, 10-15.

[178] Marsden, CD; Parkes, JD. "on-off" effects in patients with Parkinson's disease on chronic levodopa therapy. *Lancet,* 1976, I: 292-296.

[179] Marsden, CD. Parkinson's disease. *Journal of Neurology, Neurosurgery, and Psychiatry,* 1994, 57, 672-681.

[180] Mawdsley, C; Gamsu, CV. Periodicity of speech in parkinsonism. *Nature,* 1971, 231: 315-316.

[181] McClean, MD; Beukelman, DR; Yorkston, KM. Speech-muscle visuomotor tracking in dysarthric and nonimpaired speakers. *Journal of Speech and Hearing Research,* 1987, 30, 276-282.

[182] Meck, WH. Selective adjustment of the speed of an internal clock and memory processes. *Journal of Experimental Psychology: Animal Behavior Processes,* 1983, 9, 171-201.

[183] Meck, WH; Benson, AM. Dissecting the brain's internal clock: how fronto-striatal circuitry keeps time and shifts attention. *Brain and Cognition,* 2002, 48, 195-211.

[184] Meck, WH; Malapani, C. Neuroimaging of interval timing. *Brain Research. Cognitive Brain Research,* 2004 , 21 , 133-137.

[185] Metter, J; Hanson, W. Clinical and acoustical variability in hypokinetic dysarthria. *Journal of Communication Disorders,* 1986, 19, 347-366.

[186] Möbes, J; Joppich, G; Stiebritz, F; Dengler, R; Schröder, C. Emotional speech in Parkinson's disease. *Movement Disorders,* 2008, 23, 824-829.

[187] Moreau, C; Ozsancak, C; Blatt, JL; Derambure, P; Destee, A; Defebvre, L. Oral festination in Parkinson's disease: Biomechanical analysis and correlation with festination and freezing of gait. *Movement Disorders,* 2007, 22, 1503-1506.

[188] Moretti, R; Tore, P; Antonello, RM; Campus, L; Gioulis, M; Zambito Marsala, S; Cazzato, G; Bava, A. "Speech initiation hesitation" following subthalamic nucleus stimulation in a patient with Parkinson's disease. *European Neurology,* 2003, 49, 251-253.

[189] Mueller, PB. Parkinson's disease: Motor speech behaviour in a selected group of patients. *Folia Phoniatrica et Logopaedica,* 1971, 23, 333-346.

[190] Mueller, PB. The ageing voice. *Seminars in Speech and Language,* 1997, 18, 159-168.

[191] Murdoch, BE; Chenery, HJ; Bowler, S; Ingram, JCL. Respiratory function in Parkinson's subjects exhibiting a perceptible speech deficit: A kinematic and spirometric analysis. *Journal of Speech and Hearing Disorders,* 1989, 54, 610-626.

[192] Mutch, WJ; Strudwick, A; Roy, SK; Downie, AW. Parkinson's disease: disability, review, and management. *British Medical Journal,* 1986, 293, 675-677.

[193] Nakano, K; Zubick, H; Tyler, H. Speech defects of parkinsonian patients: Effects of levodopa therapy on speech intelligibility. *Neurology,* 1973, 23, 865-870.

[194] Netsell, R; Daniel, B; Celesia, GG. Acceleration and weakness in parkinsonian dysarthria. *Journal of Speech and Hearing Disorders,* 1975, 40, 170-178.

[195] Neumann, K; Euler, HA; von Gudenberg, AW; Giraud, AL; Heinrich, L; Lanfermann, H; Gall, V; Preibisch, C. The narure and treatment of stuttering as revealed by fMRI: A within- and between-group comparison. *Journal of Fluency Disorders,* 2003, 28, 381-410.

[196] Neumann, K; Preibisch, C; Euler, HA; von Gudenberg AW; Lanfermann, H; Gall, V; Giraud, AL. Cortical plasticity associated with stuttering therapy. *Journal of Fluency Disorders,* 2005, 30, 23-39.

[197] O´Boyle, DJ; Freeman, JS; Cody, FWJ. The accuracy and precision of timing of self-paced repetition movements in subjects with Parkinson´s disease. *Brain,* 1996, 119, 51-70.

[198] Obeso, JA; Marin, C; Rodriguez-Oroz, MC; Blesa, FJ; Benitez-Temino, B; Mena-Segovia, J; Rodriguez, M; Olanow, CW. The basal ganglia in Parkinson´s disease: current concepts and unexplained observations. *Annals of Neurology,* 2008, 64 (Suppl.2), S30-46.

[199] Obeso, JA; Rodriguez-Oroz, MC; Benitez-Temino, B; Blesa, FJ; Guridi, J; Marin, C; Rodriguez, M. Functional organization of the basal ganglia: therapeutic implications for Parkinson´s disease. *Movement Disorders,* 2008, 23 (Suppl.3), S548-559.

[200] Obwegeser, AA; Uitti, RJ; Witte, RJ; Lucas, JA; Turk, MF; Wharen, RE; Jr; Quantitative and qualitative outcome measures after thalamic deep brain stimulation to treat disabling tremors. *Neurosurgery,* 2001, 48, 274-81.

[201] Parkinson, J. An essay on the shaking palsy. In: Critchley M; ed. *James Parkinson, 1755-1824.*, New York: Macmillan and Co, 1955, 145-218.

[202] Pastor, MA; Artieda, J; Jahanshahi, M; Obeso JA. Time estimation and reproduction is abnormal in Parkinson´s disease. *Brain,* 1992, 115, 211-225.

[203] Perez, KS; Ramig, LO; Smith, ME; Dromey, C. The parkinson larynx: tremor and videoscopic findings. *Journal of Voice,* 1996, 10, 354-361.

[204] Petrovici, JN. Speech disturbances following stereotaxic surgery in ventrolateral thalamus. *Neurosurgical Review,* 1980, 3, 189-195.

[205] Picheny, M.; Durlach, N.; Braida, L. Speaking clearly for the hard of hearing II: Acoustic characteristics of clear and conversional speech. *Journal of Speech and Hearing Research,* 1986, 29, 434-446.

[206] Pinto, S; Gentil, M; Fraix, V; Benabid, AL; Polak, P. Bilateral subthalamic stimulation effects on oral force control in Parkinson´s disease. *Journal of Neurology,* 2003, 250, 179-187.

[207] Pinto, S; Ozsancak, C; Tripoliti, E; Thobois, S; Limousin-Dowsey, P; Auzou, P. Treatments for dysarthria in Parkinson´s disease. *Lancet* 2004, 3, 547-556.

[208] Pinto, S; Thobois, S; Costes, N; Le Bars, D; Benabid, AL; Broussolle, E; Pollak, P; Gentil, M. Subthalamic nucleus stimulation and dysarthria in Parkinson´s disease: a PET study. *Brain,* 2004, 127, 602-615.

[209] Poluha, PC; Teulings, HL; Brookshire, RH. Handwriting and speech changes across the levodopa cycle in Parkinson´s disease. *Acta Psychologica (Amst.)* 1998, 35, 217-239.

[210] Pouthas, V; George, N; Poline, JB; Pfeuty, M; VandeMoorteele, PF; Hugueville, L; Ferrandez, AM; Lehericy, S; LeBihan, D; Renault, B. Neural network involved in time perception: an fMRI study comparing long and short interval estimation. *Human Brain Mapping,* 2005, 25, 433-441.

[211] Putzke, JD; Wharen, RE; Jr; Wszolek, ZK; Turk, MF; Strongosky, AJ; Uitti, RJ. Thalamic deep brain stimulation for tremor-predominant Parkinson´s disease. *Parkinsonism and Related Disorders,* 2003, 10, 81-88.

[212] Quaglieri, CE; Celesia, GG. Effect of thalamotomy and levodopa therapy on the speech of Parkinson patients. *European Neurology,* 1977, 15, 34-39.

[213] Rabinov, CR; Kreiman, J; Gerratt, BR; Bielamowicz, S. Comparing reliability of perceptual ratings of roughness and acoustic measures of jitter. *Journal of Speech and Hearing Research,* 1995, 38, 26-32.

[214] Ramig, LO; Countryman, L; Thompson, L; Horii, Y. Comparison of two forms of intensive speech treatment for Parkinson disease. *Journal of Speech and Hearing Research,* 1995, 38, 1232-1251.

[215] Ramig, LO; Countryman, S; O´Brien, C; Hoehn, M; Thompson, L. Intensive speech treatment for people with Parkinson´s disease: short and long term comparison of two techniques. *Neurology,* 1996a, 47, 1496-1504

[216] Ramig, LO; Dromey, C. Aerodynamic mechanisms underlying treatment-related changes in SPL in people with Parkinson disease. *Journal of Speech and Hearing Research,* 1996b, 39, 798-807.

[217] Ramig, LO; Gray, S; Baker, K; Corbin-Lewis, K; Buder, E; Luschei, E; Coon, H; Smith, M. The aging voice: a review, treatment data and familial and genetic perspectives. *Folia Phoniatrica et Logopaedica,* 2001, 53, 252-265.

[218] Ramig, LO; Sapir, S; Fox, CM; Countryman, S. Changes in vocal loudness following intensive voice treatment (LSVT) in individuals with Parkinson´s disease: a comparison with untreated patients a normal age-matched controls. *Movement Disorders,* 2001, 16, 79-83.

[219] Rammsayer, TH. Are there dissociable roles of the mesostriatal and mesolimbocortical dopamine systems on temporal information processing in humans? *Neuropsychobiology,* 1997, 35, 36-45.

[220] Rastatter, MP; McGuire, RA; Kalinowski, J; Stuart, A. Formant frequency characteristics of elderly speakers in contextual speech. *Folia Phoniatrica et Logopaedica,* 1997, 49, 1-8.

[221] Riecker, A; Mathiak, K; Wildgruber, D; Erb, M; Hertrich, I; Grodd, W; Ackermann, H. fMRI reveals two distinct cerebral networks subserving speech motor control. *Neurology,* 2005, 64, 700-06.

[222] Riecker, A; Kassubek, J; Gröschel, K; Grodd, W; Ackermann, H. The cerebral control of speech tempo: Opposite relationship between speaking rate and BOLD signal changes at striatal and cerebellar structures. *Neuroimage,* 2006, 29, 46-53.

[223] Rigrodsky, S; Morrison, EB. Speech changes in parkinsonism during l-dopa therapy: Preliminary findings. *Journal of the American Geriatric Society* 1970, 18, 142-151.

[224] Robertson, SJ; Thomson, F. Speech therapy in Parkinson´s disease: a study of the efficacy and long term effects of intensive treatment. *British Journal of Disordered Communication,* 1984, 19, 213-224.

[225] Romero, DH; Van Gemmert, AWA; Adler, CH; Bekkering, H; Stelmach, GE. Altered aiming movements in Parkinson´s disease patients and elderly adults as a function of delays in movement onset. *Experimental Brain Research,* 2003, 151, 249-261.

[226] Romito, LM; Scerrati, M; Contarino, MF; Iacoangeli, M; Bentivoglio, AR; Albanese, A. Bilateral high frequency subthalamic stimlation in Parkinson´s disease: long-term neurological follow-up. *Journal of Neurosurgical Sciences,* 2003, 47, 119-128.

[227] Rubow, R; Swift, E. A microcomputer-based wearable biofeedback device to improve transfer of treatment in parkinsonian dysarthria. *Journal of Speech and Hearing Disorders,* 1985, 50, 178-185.

[228] Rousseaux, M; Krystkowiak, P; Koslowski, O; Ozsancak, C; Blond, S; Destee, A. Effects of subthalamicus nucleus stimulation on parkinsonian dysarthria and speech intelligibility. *Journal of Neurology,* 2004, 251, 327-334.

[229] Samra, K; Riklan, M; Levita, E. Language and speech correlates of anatomically verified lesions in thalamic surgery for parkinsonism. *Journal of Speech and Hearing Research* 1969, 12, 510-514.

[230] Sanabria, J; Ruiz, PG; Gutierrez, R; et al. The effect of levodopa on vocal function in Parkinson´s disease. *Clinical Neuropharmacology,* 2001, 24, 99-102.

[231] Santens, P; De Letter, M; Van Borsel, J; De Reuck, J; Caemaert, J. Lateralized effects of subthalamic nucleus stimulation on different aspects of speech in Parkinson´s disease. *Brain and Language,* 2003, 87, 253-258.

[232] Sapir, S; Pawlas, AA; Ramig, LO; Countryman, S; O´Brien C; Hoehn L; Thompson M. Voice and speech abnormalities in Parkinson disease: Relation to severity of motor impairment, duration of disease, medication, depression, gender, and age. *Journal of Medical Speech-Language Pathology,* 2001, 9, 213-226.

[233] Sapir, S; Spielman, JL; Ramig, LO; Story, BH; Fox, C. Effects of intensive voice treatment (the Lee Silverman Voice Treatment [LSVT]) on vowel articulation in dysarthric individuals with idiopathic Parkinson disease: acoustic and perceptual findings. *Journal of Speech, Language, and Hearing Research,* 2007, 50, 899-912.

[234] Sarno, MT. Speech impairment in Parkinson´s disease. *Archives of Physical Medicine and Rehabilitation,* 1968, 49, 269-275.

[235] Schneider, JS; Diamond, SG; Markham, CH. Deficits in orofacial sensorimotor function in Parkinson´s disease. *Annals of Neurology,* 1986, 19, 275-282.

[236] Schulz, GM; Peterson, T; Sapienza, CM; Greer, M; Friedmann, G. Voice and speech characteristics of persons with Parkinson´s disease pre- and post-pallidotomy surgery: preliminary findings. *Journal of Speech, Language, and Hearing Research,* 1999, 42, 1176-1194.

[237] Schulz, GM; Greer, M; Freidman, W. Changes in vocal intensity in Parkinson´s disease following pallidotomy. *Journal of Voice,* 2000, 14, 589-606.

[238] Schulz, GM. The effects of speech therapy and pharmacological treatments on voice and speech in Parkinson´s disease: a review of the literature. *Current Medicinal Chemistry,* 2002, 9, 1359-1366.

[239] Scott, S; Caird, FI. Speech therapy for Parkinson´s disease. *Journal of Neurology, Neurosurgery, and Psychiatry,* 1983, 46, 140-44.

[240] Scott, R; Gregory, R; Hines, N; Caroll, C; Hyman, N; Papanasstasiou, V; Leather, C; Rowe, J; Silburn, C; Aziz, T. Neuropsychological, neurological and functional outcome

following pallidotomy for Parkinson´s disease: a consecutive series of eight simultaneous bilateral and twelve unilateral procedures. *Brain,* 1998, 121, 659-765.

[241] Shea, BR; Drummond, SS; Metzer, WS; Krueger, KM. Effect on selegiline on speech performance in Parkinson´s disease. *Folia Phoniatrica (Basel),* 1993, 45, 40-46.

[242] Siegert, RJ; Harper, DN; Cameron, FB; Abernethy, D. Self-initiated versus externally cued reaction times in Parkinson´s disease. *Journal of Clinical and Experimental Neuropsychology* 2002, 24, 146-153.

[243] Skodda, S; Schlegel, U. Speech rate and rhythm in Parkinson´s disease. *Movement Disorders,* 2008, 23, 985-992.

[244] Skodda, S; Rinsche, A; Schlegel, U. Progression of dysprosody in Parkinson´s disease: a longitudinal study. *Movement Disorders,* 2009, 24, 716-722.

[245] Skodda, S; Flasskamp, A; Schlegel, U. Vocal rhythm production and acoustical rhythm recognition in Parkinson´s disease. *Movement Disorders submitted*

[246] Skodda, S; Schlegel, U. Formant frequency ratio as a measure of vowel articulation in Parkinson´s disease. *Brain submitted*

[247] Smith, BL; Wasowicz, J; Preston, J. Temporal characteristics of the speech of normal elderly adults. *Journal of Speech and Hearing Research,* 1987, 30, 522-529.

[248] Smith, ME; Ramig, LO; Dromey, C; Perez, KS; Samandari R. Intensive voice treatment in Parkinson´s disease: laryngostroboscopic findings. *Journal of Voice* 1995, 9, 453-459.

[249] Smits-Bandstra, S; de Nil, LF. Sequence skill learning in persons who stutter: Implications for cortico-striato-thalamo-cortical dysfunction. *Journal of Fluency Disorders,* 2007, 32, 251-278.

[250] Solomon, NP; Hixon, TJ.Speech Breathing in Parkinson´s disease. *Journal of Speech and Hearing Research* 1993, 36, 294-310.

[251] Solomon, NP; Lorell, DM; Robin, DA; Rodnitzky, RL; Luschei, ES. Tongue strength and endurance in mild to moderate Parkinson´s disease. *Journal of Medical Speech-Language Pathology,* 1995, 3, 15-26.

[252] Solomon, NP; Robin, DA; Luschei, ES. Strength, endurance and stability of the tongue and hand in Parkinson´s disease. *Journal of Speech, Language, and Hearing Research,* 2000, 43, 256-267.

[253] Solomon, NP. Assessment of tongue weakness and fatigue. *International Journal of Orofacial Myology* 2004, 30, 8-19.

[254] Speech therapy in Parkinson´s disease. *Movement Disorders,* 2002, 17, S163-166.

[255] Spencer, KA; Rogers, MA. Speech motor programming in hypokinetic and ataxic dysarthria. *Brain and Language,* 2005, 94, 347-366.

[256] Stelmach, GE; Worringham, CJ. The control of bimanual aiming movements in Parkinson´s disease. *Journal of Neurology, Neurosurgery, and Psychiatry,* 1988, 51, 223-231.

[257] Steward, C; Winfield, L; Hunt, A; Bressman, SB; Fahn, S; Blitzer, A; Brin, MF. Speech dysfunction in early Parkinson´s disease. *Movement Disorders,* 1995, 10, 562-565.

[258] Stracciari, A; Guarino, M; Cirignotta, F; Pazzaglia, P. Development of palilalia after stereotaxic thalamotomy in Parkinson´s disease. *European Neurology,* 1993, 33, 275-276.

[259] Streifler, M; Hofman, S. Disorders of verbal expression in parkinsonism. In: Hassler RG, Christ JF, eds., *Parkinson-specific motor and mental disorders. Advances in Neurology, Vol. 40.* New York, Raven Press, 1984, 385-393.

[260] Svensson, P; Henningson, C; Karlsson, S. Speech motor control in Parkinson´s disease: a comparison between a clinical assessment protocol and a quantitative analysis of mandibular movements. *Folia Phoniatrica (Basel)* 1993, 45, 157-164.

[261] Taha, JM; Janszen, MA; Favre, J. Thalamic deep brain stimulation for the treatment of head, voice, and bilateral limb tremor. *Journal of Neurosurgery,* 1999, 91, 68-72.

[262] Tasker, RR; Siqueira, J; Hawrylyshyn, P; Organ, LW. What happened to VIM thalamotomy for Parkinson´s disease? *Applied Neurophysiology* 1983, 46, 68-83.

[263] Treisman, M. Temporal discrimination and the indifference interval. Implications for a model of the "internal clock". *Psychological Monographs,* 1963, 77, 1-31.

[264] Troster, AI; Woods, SP; Fields, JA Hanisch, C; Beatty, WW. Declines in switching underlie verbal fluency changes after unilateral pallidal surgery in Parkinson´s disease. *Brain and Cognition* 2002, 50, 207-217.

[265] Tzelepis, GE; McCool, FD; Friedmann, HJ; Hoppin, FG. Jr. Respiratory muscle function in Parkinson´s disease. *American Review of Respiratory Disease,* 1989, 138, 266-271.

[266] Venkatagiri, HS. Slower and incomplete retrieval of speech motor plans is the proximal source of stuttering: Stutters occur when syllable motor plans stored in memory are concatenated to produce the utterance motor plan. *Medical Hypothesis,* 2004, 62, 401-405.

[267] Vercueil, L; Linard, JP; Wuyam, B; Pollak, P; Benchetrit, G. Breathing pattern in patients with Parkinson´s disease. *Respiratory Physiology,* 1999, 118, 163-172.

[268] Volkmann, J; Hefter, H; Lange, H; Freund, HJ. Impairment of temporal organization of speech in basal ganglia diseases. *Brain and Language,* 1992, 43, 386-399.

[269] Wang, E; Verhagen, ML; Bakay, R; Arzbaecher, J; Bernard, B. The effect of unilateral electrostimulation of the subthalamic nucleus on respiratory/phonatory subsystems of speech production in Parkinson´s disease – a preliminary report. *Clinical Linguistics & Phonetics,* 2003, 17, 283-289.

[270] Weiner, P; Inzelberg, R; Davidovich, A; Nisipeanu, P; Magadle, R; Berar-Yanay, N; Carasso, RL. Respiratory muscle performance and the perception of dyspnea in Parkinson´s disease. *Canadian Journal of Neurological Sciences,* 2002, 29, 68-72.

[271] Weismer, G. Articulatory characteristics of Parkinsonian dysarthria: segmental and phrase-level timing, spirantization, and glottal-supraglottal coordination. In: McNeil M, Rosenbeck J, Aronson A, eds., *The Dysarthrias: Physiology, Acoustics, Perception, Management.* San Diego: College-Hill Press, 1984, 101-130.

[272] Weismer, G; Jeng, JY; Laures, JS; Kent, RD; Kent, JF. Acoustic and intelligibility characteristics of sentence production of neurogenic speech disorders. *Folia Phoniatrica et Logopaedica,* 2001, 53, 1-18.

[273] Weiss, P; Stelmach, GE; Hefter, H. Programming of a movement sequence in Parkinson´s disease. *Brain,* 1997, 120, 91-102.

[274] Wise, RJ; Greene, J; Buchel, C; Scott, SK. Brain regions involved in articulation. *Lancet* 1999, 353, 1057-1061.

[275] Wolfe, V; Garvin, J; Bacon, M; Waldrop, W. Speech change in Parkinson´s disease during treatment with l-dopa. *Journal of Communication Disorders* 1975, 8, 271-279.

[276] Wu, JC; Maguire, G; Riley, G; Fallon, J; LaCasse, L; Chin, S; Klein, E; Tang, C; Cadwell, S; Lottenberg, S. A positron emission tomography (18F) deoxyglucose study of developmental stuttering. *Neuroreport,* 1995, 6, 501-505.

[277] Yaryura-Tobias, JA; Diamond, B; Merlis, S. Verbal communication with l-dopa treatment. *Nature,* 1971, 234, 224-225.

[278] Yorkston, KM; Spencer, KA; Duffy, JR. Behavioral management of respiratory / phonatory dysfunction from dysarthria: a systematic review of evidence. *Journal of Medical Speech-Language Pathology,* 2003, 11, 13-38.

[279] Zwirner, P; Barnes, GJ. Vocal tract steadiness: a measure of phonatory and upper airway motor control during phonation in dysarthria. *Journal of Speech and Hearing Research,* 1992, 35, 761-768.

In: Speech Disorders: Causes, Treatment and Social Effects
Editor: Alan E. Harrison, pp. 43-73
ISBN: 978-1-60876-213-2

Chapter 2

SPEECH AND LITERACY: THE CONNECTION AND THE RELEVANCE TO CLINICAL POPULATIONS

Jonathan L. Preston
Haskins Laboratories, New Haven, Connecticut, USA

ABSTRACT

Both speech production and literacy skills are of significant concern to educators and early interventionists. Longitudinal research has shown that children with speech and/or literacy problems remain at significant risk for limited academic, social, and occupational achievement. While these two behavioral domains have often been studied separately (as speech-language disorders and as reading disabilities), the co-occurrence of speech and literacy problems is well-documented, with deficits in one domain often accompanied by (sometimes subtle) deficits in the other. The theoretical link between speech and literacy-related skills in children is reviewed in this chapter, with emphasis on the phonological components of reading. Research is summarized on two main topics: the identification of individuals who are at risk for literacy problems through speech assessment, and the literacy-related skills of children with speech sound disorders. Data are then presented that demonstrate how short-term phonological memory may play an important connecting role between speech and literacy in children with speech sound disorders. Finally, the implications for assessment and intervention for children with speech sound disorders are summarized in an effort to provide a more comprehensive framework for translating research on the speech-literacy link into clinical practice.

Literacy skills, which must be explicitly taught, have their foundations in speech-related skills, which are often learned quite naturally. Alphabetic writing systems take advantage of the fact that there are discernable categories of speech sounds (phonemes) that are produced by speakers of the language. Thus, proficient literacy skills, particularly in an alphabetic orthography, are aided by one's facility with the phonology of the language. That is, successful reading of an alphabetic system involves mapping print to the speech signal, while spelling requires mapping speech to print. The goals of this chapter are to briefly review the well-established connection between speech and literacy, discuss the theoretical and empirical link (based primarily in phonological processing), and extend the discussion of speech and literacy skills to shed light on two clinical populations: children who do not have facility with literacy skills, and children who do not have facility with the productive phonology of their language. It will become apparent that children with literacy problems have been found to have subtle problems with productive phonological skills, and children with speech sound disorders often have problems with literacy-related skills. The implications for clinical research will be addressed throughout the chapter to highlight why the speech-literacy connection is of importance. Phonological short-term memory will be discussed as an important skill in literacy development, and data will be presented to demonstrate how this skill could be assessed in children with poor intelligibility.

The term ***speech sound disorder (SSD)*** will be used to refer to those children who have difficulty producing or using the sounds of their language, but for whom there is no obvious cause (such as hearing impairment, cleft palate, developmental disorder, etc.); other terminology, such as articulation impairment, phonological disorder, or expressive phonological impairment, have been used in the literature. The terms ***dyslexia*** **or** ***reading difficulties*** will be used to refer to children who demonstrate low performance on reading and/or spelling tasks in the absence of an obvious cause (cognitive problems, developmental disabilities, etc.). It should be noted that nearly every study reviewed here uses its own criteria for determining these categories (SSD or dyslexia), and many studies use different terms to refer to the same populations. In addition, both speech production and literacy skills are immensely complex and cannot be thoroughly reviewed here. Both rely on cognitive-behavioral skills that include attention, memory, perception, etc., all of which are the byproduct of genetic and environmental influences; thus, the relationships that will be discussed exist within the context of many other complex neural, psychological, and biological relationships. Accurately measuring the essential parameters of speech and reading is still a challenge even to the most experienced researchers and clinicians

Approximately 50-75% of children with SSD have been found to have long-term academic problems (see Lewis et al., 2006), and approximately 28% of children identified as "at-risk" for literacy problems are referred for speech therapy (Pennington & Lefly, 2001). Thus, the overlap among speech and reading problems is not negligible.

Reading educators often lack sufficient knowledge of phonology (Brady et al., 2009), and some speech-language pathologists judge that they lack sufficient knowledge of reading (e.g., a series of editorials in the *ASHA Leader* 2007-2008). Although this may be a limitation in our professional training programs, research demonstrates a robust relationship between phonological and literacy skills that should be of concern to both professions. Ultimately, we wish to understand speech and reading at the level both of the individual (a particular client or student, etc.) and in populations (persons with SSD, dyslexia, etc.). Thus, beginning with the simple notion that speech skills are a foundation for literacy, it is important to discuss how and why these skills should be considered together.

From a systems-based perspective, both SSD and reading problems have been discussed as arising from weaknesses in the auditory processing or perception of speech, skill automization, and timing mechanisms. For example, individuals with SSD (Jamieson & Rvachew, 1992; Ohde & Sharf, 1988) as well as those with reading problems (Lieberman, Meskill, Chatillon, & Schupack, 1985) have been reported to show below-average identification of synthesized speech, and difficulty encoding the temporal order of perceived speech sounds (Bridgeman & Snowling, 1988; Joanisse, Manis, Keating, & Seidenberg, 2000; Mody, Studdert-Kennedy, & Brady, 1997; Watson & Miller, 1993). Both clinical populations have been shown to struggle with speech- and non-speech rhythmic tasks and motor coordination tasks (Bradford & Dodd, 1996; Fawcett, Nicolson, & Maclagan, 2001; Peter & Stoel-Gammon, 2008). Given that reading skills rely heavily on oral language, it is not surprising that many of the same neural regions needed for speech perception and production are also required for reading and spelling (Constable et al., 2004; Fulbright, et al., 1999; Nicolson, Fawcett, & Dean, 2001; Pugh, et al., 2000).

From an etiological perspective, similar causes have been put forth as contributing to both speech and reading problems. Genetic influences and family histories of the respective disorders likely contribute to the manifestation of both speech and reading problems in children (Campbell, et al., 2003; Lewis, et al., 2006; McGrath, et al., 2007; Shriberg et al., 2005). Additionally, impoverished language environments, often associated with low socioeconomic status or low parental education, likely plays a role in some cases of speech and reading difficulty (Campbell, et al., 2003; McDowell, Lonigan, & Goldstein, 2007).

THE SPEECH-LITERACY CONNECTION: THEORETICAL BASES

There is now ample evidence to support the *phonological deficit hypothesis* of dyslexia, which suggests that poor processing of phonological information is causally related to literacy problems. This is not to say that other processes are never disrupted in individuals with reading problems, but it purports that a specific deficit in the phonological system contributes to reading problems in many individuals (see Scarborough & Brady, 2002 for a review of phonology and reading). It is not surprising, then, that children with a speech production deficit in the phonological domain will be at risk for reading difficulties.

In some approaches, phonological deficits in reading are considered within three general domains of phonological processing: phonological awareness, phonological retrieval/recoding in lexical access (e.g., rapid naming), and phonetic recoding in working memory (e.g., nonword repetition) (Wagner & Torgesen, 1987). In support of the phonological deficit hypothesis is evidence that children with reading problems have more difficulty than children with typical reading skills on (meta)phonological tasks that require attending to the speech signal. Phonological awareness tasks such as rhyming, identifying phonemes in words, manipulating sounds in words (e.g., deleting, substituting, or reversing phonemes), blending sounds to form words, segmenting words into their constituent phonemes, and quickly and accurately recalling/identifying the correct phonological forms of words (particularly words that are longer and more phonologically complex) are good indicators of current reading skills and are also good longitudinal predictors of later literacy (Blachman, 2000; Catts, Fey, Zhang, & Tomblin, 2001; Elbro, Borstrom, & Peterson, 1998; Griffiths & Snowling, 2002; Schatschneider, Fletcher, Francis, Carlson, & Foorman, 2004; Wagner & Torgesen, 1987). Additionally, a multitude of evidence has demonstrated a causal connection, such that explicit instruction in phonological awareness together with training in sound-symbol association (phonics instruction) is beneficial for young children who are struggling to learn to read and spell (Ball & Blachman, 1991; Bradley & Bryant, 1983; Tangel & Blachman, 1992), including those with SSD (Gillon, 2000, 2005).

An obvious question, then, is why some children have poor phonological processing skills. One notion is that children with poor reading skills (as well as those with SSD) may have weak phonological representations (e.g., Goswami, 2000). Phonological representations are stored (internal) representations of the sound features of words (Goswami, 2000; Rvachew & Grawburg, 2006; Stackhouse & Wells, 1997). If such representations are imprecise (inaccurate, weak, fuzzy, or not distinct), children may have difficulty reflecting on those representations to identify the phonological characteristics of words. Thus, mapping print to those representations (or vice versa) would be a challenge. Yet, because phonological representations are internal, it is difficult to empirically measure them and validate the notion that the quality of these representations are at the heart of phonologically-based reading difficulties. Thus, it remains unclear whether the problem is poorly specified representations, impaired access to these representations, or difficulty mapping print to these representations. Figure 1 displays a simple model relating speech production and reading, showing that phonological representations may be the basis for both speech production and phonological processing skills.

The acoustic speech signal is constantly changing, so it is presumed that accurate (precise, clear, distinct) representations are needed in order to recognize and parse the important features of the speech signal (i.e., phonemes) when learning to decode and spell. However, the dynamics of the speech signal makes it difficult to segment into discrete units (i.e., it is helpful for young readers/spellers to segment "pen" into three phonemes, but the acoustic signal is not comprised of three independent units). However, it may be that the ability to focus on articulatory gestures, rather than components of the acoustic signal, is needed for children to develop phonological awareness. Castiglioni-Spalten & Ehri (2003) provide evidence from an intervention study that suggests that awareness of the speech gesture, more than auditory awareness of the speech signal, is helpful in teaching children phonemic awareness. That is, teaching segmenting skills by focusing on articulatory gestures is more beneficial to early reading than teaching children to focus on auditory segmentation. Therefore, meta-knowledge of speech gestures may be more critical than auditory sensitivity for purposes of developing phonemic awareness.

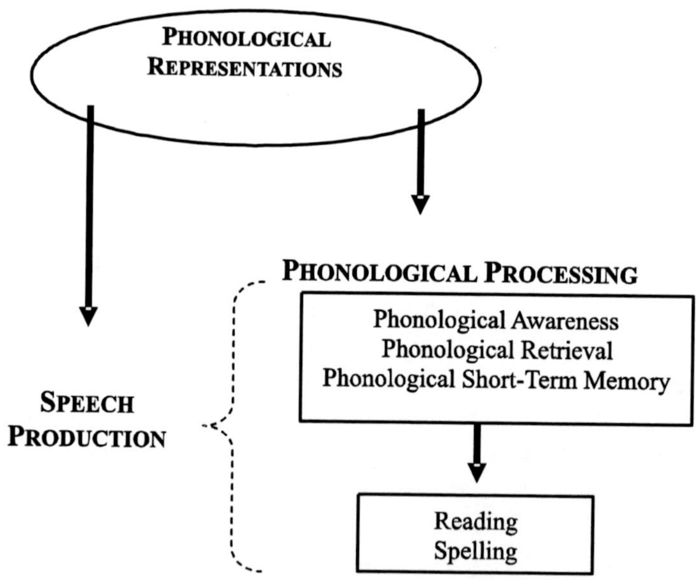

Figure 1. A simple theoretical framework relating speech production and literacy

Elbro (Elbro, 1996; Elbro, et al., 1998; Elbro & Pallesen, 2002) has hypothesized that the distinctness of a child's phonological representations is an important predictor of his/her reading skills. He describes distinctness as the "magnitude of the difference between a representation and its neighbors" (467); that is, the degree to which children know (and can produce) distinct speech sounds in words is presumed to be important in phonological processing. In one study with Danish speaking children, Elbro et al. (1998) measured distinctness of (productive) phonological representations by having kindergarten children teach a puppet the most distinct pronunciation of a word. Distinctness was scored as the percent of selected vowels that were given a maximally distinct pronunciation. The distinctness of a child's (productive) phonological representations in kindergarten was found to be a strong predictor of literacy outcomes in grade two. Similarly, Fowler and Swainson (2004) reported that first and fourth grade poor readers had more trouble than good readers on tasks that required children to imitate pronunciation variations of target words and judge which variant is an acceptable production of the word. Thus, phonological representations, as measured by a child's "best" production of a word, can provide useful diagnostic information.

One topic that has received limited attention is whether a child's facility with phonological awareness tasks is phoneme-specific, and whether phonological awareness problems are associated with the specific phonemes that a child has not yet learned to produce correctly. Sénéchal, Ouellette and Young (2004) speculated that, "the quality of phonemic representations may be reflected in children's expressive phonology or articulation" (243). For example, if a child has difficulty producing /r/, one might assume that the child does not yet have an adult-like representation associated with that sound and might therefore have trouble mentally operating on words with that phoneme. Thomas and Sénéchal (1998) compared groups of three-year-old children on several phonemic awareness tasks; some children consistently produced /r/ correctly, some consistently produced /r/ incorrectly, and some occasionally produced /r/ correctly. They found that three-year-olds who consistently produced /r/ correctly were superior to on several tasks tapping awareness of /r/: phoneme recognition (identifying spoken words beginning with /r/), phoneme judgment (determining whether a puppet's production of a word with /r/ was correct or incorrect), and auditory discrimination (determining whether pairs of nonwords beginning with /r, l, w/ were the same or different). Sénéchal et al. (2004) also reported weak but statistically significant correlations (r ~0.2-0.3) between the accuracy of production of /r/ in the initial position of words and a child's ability to match words that begin with /r/. Thus, phoneme-specific awareness may have a small but significant relationship with phoneme-specific production.

SPEECH-RELATED SKILLS OF CHILDREN WITH LITERACY DIFFICULTIES

Given the influence of phonological skills on reading acquisition, speech-related skills are an important candidate for aiding in the diagnosis of literacy. Other reviews have focused on how meta-phonological skills relate to reading (e.g., Blachman, 2000; Scarborough, 2003); yet, speech production may, to some extent, also reflect reading-related skills. Indeed, children with reading problems, as a group, have been shown to have subtle differences in speech production when compared to children without reading problems. For example, acoustic analysis has shown that adolescents with reading difficulties produce less distinct vowels than adolescents without reading difficulties (Bertucci et al., 2003).

However, the differences in speech production between those with and without dyslexia are revealed primarily when the speech production system is taxed, such as when dyslexics are required to produce speech rapidly or to produce complex articulatory sequences. Figure 2 shows standardized effect size differences (in standard deviations) with the associated 95% confidence intervals from several studies that have used a group-comparison approach in comparing children with and without dyslexia on speech production tasks. It is evident that speech production tasks have been found to relate to reading skills. For example, Fawcett and Nicolson (2002) found that adolescents ages 13 and 16 with dyslexia were slower in their ability to rapidly repeat single syllables (e.g., “puh-puh-puh” or “tuh-tuh-tuh”) and syllable sequences (e.g., “puh-tuh-kuh”) compared to normal readers. Similarly, when asked to repeatedly produce “pa-ta,” “ta-ka,” and “pa-ta-ka” in time to various speeds of a metronome, Wolff, Michel and Ovrut (1990) showed that adolescents and adults with literacy problems were significantly slower than controls, and were also significantly slower than the prescribed metronome speed. In addition, poor readers made more phonemic errors on this repetition task. Catts (1989) reported that dyslexic college students were slower and phonologically less accurate repeating phonologically complex phrases (e.g., *seashells* and *five fruit flies*) than typical readers. Fawcett, Nicolson and Maclagan (2001) found that 8- and 10-year olds with dyslexia were slower than age-matched controls on rapid articulation rate of words. It has also been reported that children with reading problems make more phonological errors when naming pictures (particularly those that are longer or phonologically complex) compared to children without reading problems (Swan & Goswami, 1997). Hence, deficits in speed, timing, and accuracy of speech production and naming have been found in individuals with reading problems. Not surprisingly, similar findings of each of these phenomena have been reported for individuals with SSD (Lewis & Freebairn, 1992; McNutt, 1977; Preston & Edwards, 1999; Williams & Stackhouse, 1998, 2000).

Early Identification

Ideally, speech production measures could prove to be valuable in predicting which children will develop reading problems. Tables 1-3 show correlational evidence of the relationship between speech production and reading-related skills from several studies that do not specifically include children with SSD. It is possible that the relationship between speech sound production accuracy and reading skills is stronger, but that current perceptual (i.e., transcription-based) measures of phonological production are not sensitive enough to consistently detect this relationship.

In general, little information is available on the early speech skills of children who later develop reading problems. One exception is Scarborough (1990), who followed children from 30 months to 60 months of age. The number of consonant errors in a 100-word speaking sample at 30 months was found to correlate with later literacy and phonological awareness skills; however, this measure at 42 and 60 months was not a strong predictor of literacy (Scarborough, 2003). It is possible that observational studies of speech production may be less stable than experimental measures in separating children who will or will not develop literacy problems.

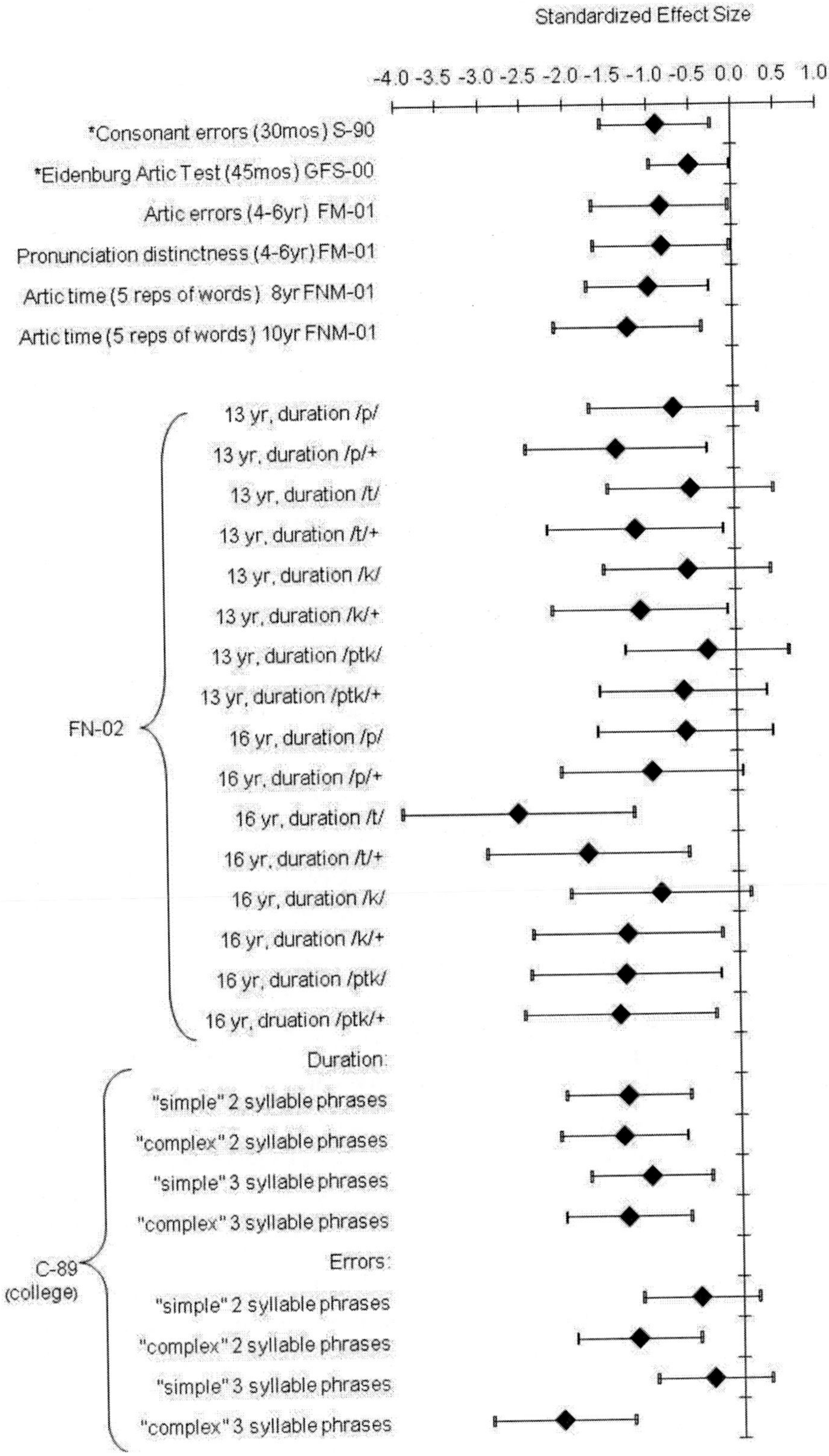

Figure 2. Effect size differences between children with and without literacy problems in speech-related skills

Table 1. Speech production and phonological awareness in children (not specifically SSD)

Study & Participants	n	Speech Measure	Phonological Awareness	Correlation *r*
Scarborough (1990) 30 mo→60 mo	52	Consonant errors in natural production (100 wds)	Phonological awareness (rhyme and initial phoneme matching)	-.34
Foy & Mann (2001) 4-6 yr	40	GFTA consonant errors	Phoneme awareness composite	(.22)
			Rhyme awareness composite	.42
		Pronunciation distinctness	Phoneme awareness composite	(.17)
			Rhyme awareness composite	.42
		Syllable reduction errors	Phoneme awareness composite	(-.21)
			Rhyme awareness composite	-.42
		Phoneme additions	Phoneme awareness composite	(-.10)
			Rhyme awareness composite	(-.13)
		Final consonant deletions	Phoneme awareness composite	(-.12)
			Rhyme awareness composite	(-.22)
		Cluster simplifications	Phoneme awareness composite	(-.10)
			Rhyme awareness composite	(-.18)
Mann & Foy (2003) 4-6 yrs	99	GFTA consonant errors	Phoneme judgment Phoneme manipulation Rhyme awareness	-.23 (.01) -.23
McDowell et al (2007) 2-5 yr	700	Consonants correct on picture naming & nonword repetition	Phonological awareness composite	.65

Notes: → means (predictive) longitudinal correlation; all others are concurrent relationship
( ) means the relationship was not statistically significant

Another example of using early speech production to predict later literacy skills comes from Smith and colleagues (Smith, Lambrecht-Smith, Locke, & Bennett, 2008; Smith, Roberts, Lambrecht-Smith, Locke, & Bennett, 2006). They reported that a child's speaking rate (in syllables/sec) at ages 2-3 was predictive of grade-school literacy achievement. In particular, the time spent pausing during a speaking turn at age 2 was greater for children who were later diagnosed as reading disabled, compared to those who did not develop reading problems. It is possible that this longer pause time reflects slower retrieval of phonological forms and/or planning of articulatory movements. This provides evidence for the notion that speech production skills provide insights into skills that a child may need to support literacy development. That is, rapid access to phonological information during conversation, rather than just the phonological accuracy of output, may be an important consideration in the early years. Future research is needed to delineate the speech variables that are most robust in predicting reading achievement so that children at risk for reading problems can be identified before they begin school.

Table 2. Speech production and literacy in children (not specifically SSD)

Study Participants	n	Speech Measure	Literacy-Related Measure	Correlation *r*
Scarborough (30 mo → 60 mo)	52	Consonant errors in natural production (100 wds)	Letter recognition Letter-sound	-.49 -.37
Griffiths & Snowling (2002) Dyslexics (9-15 yr) & reading-matched controls	11 8	Repetition rate of 1, 2, 3 syllable words	Word reading (word & nonword) Nonword reading Exception word reading	(-.07) .34 (-.07)
Mann & Foy (2003) 4-6 yrs	99	GFTA consonant errors	Word Identification Nonword reading Letter sounds	(-.12) (-.19) (-.06)

Table 3. Speech production and phonological short-term memory in children (not specifically SSD)

Study & Participants	n	Speech Measure	Phonological Short-Term Memory	Correlation r
McDowell et al (2007) 2-5 yr	700	Consonants correct on GFTA	2-4 syllable nonwords	.56
Griffiths & Snowling (2002) Dyslexics (9-15 yr) & reading-matched controls	118	Repetition rate of 1, 2, 3 syllable words	Nonword repetition (2-5 syllables)	.30
Munson et al (2005) 3-6 yr	40	GFTA percentile score	Low frequency nonword sequences High frequency nonword sequences	(.16) (.12)
Mann & Foy (2003) 4-6 yrs	99	GFTA consonant errors	Children's Test of Nonword Repetition (Gathercole et al., 1994)	-.52

Literacy-Related Skills of Children with SSD

Several studies have lead to the conclusion that preschool and school-age children with SSDs, as a group, perform more poorly on phonological processing and literacy tasks when compared to children without SSDs (Bird, Bishop, & Freeman, 1995; Lewis & Freebairn, 1992; Nathan, Stackhouse, Goulandris, & Snowling, 2004; Preston & Edwards, 2007; Raitano, Pennington, Tunick, Boada, & Shriberg, 2004). In an epidemiological investigation, Broomfield and Dodd (2005) found that approximately two thirds of the children with SSD ages 3;6- 16 had delayed phonological awareness. From a longitudinal perspective, the presence of a SSD in childhood is associated with poorer literacy and occupational outcomes as adults (Felsenfeld, Broen, & McGue, 1992, 1994; B.A.; Lewis & Freebairn, 1992). Figure 3 summarizes the magnitude of the difference in literacy-related skills between children with and without SSD across several studies. It is apparent that many of these studies reveal weaknesses in phonological processing and reading skills, including reading of real words (Word Identification) and nonwords (Word Attack).

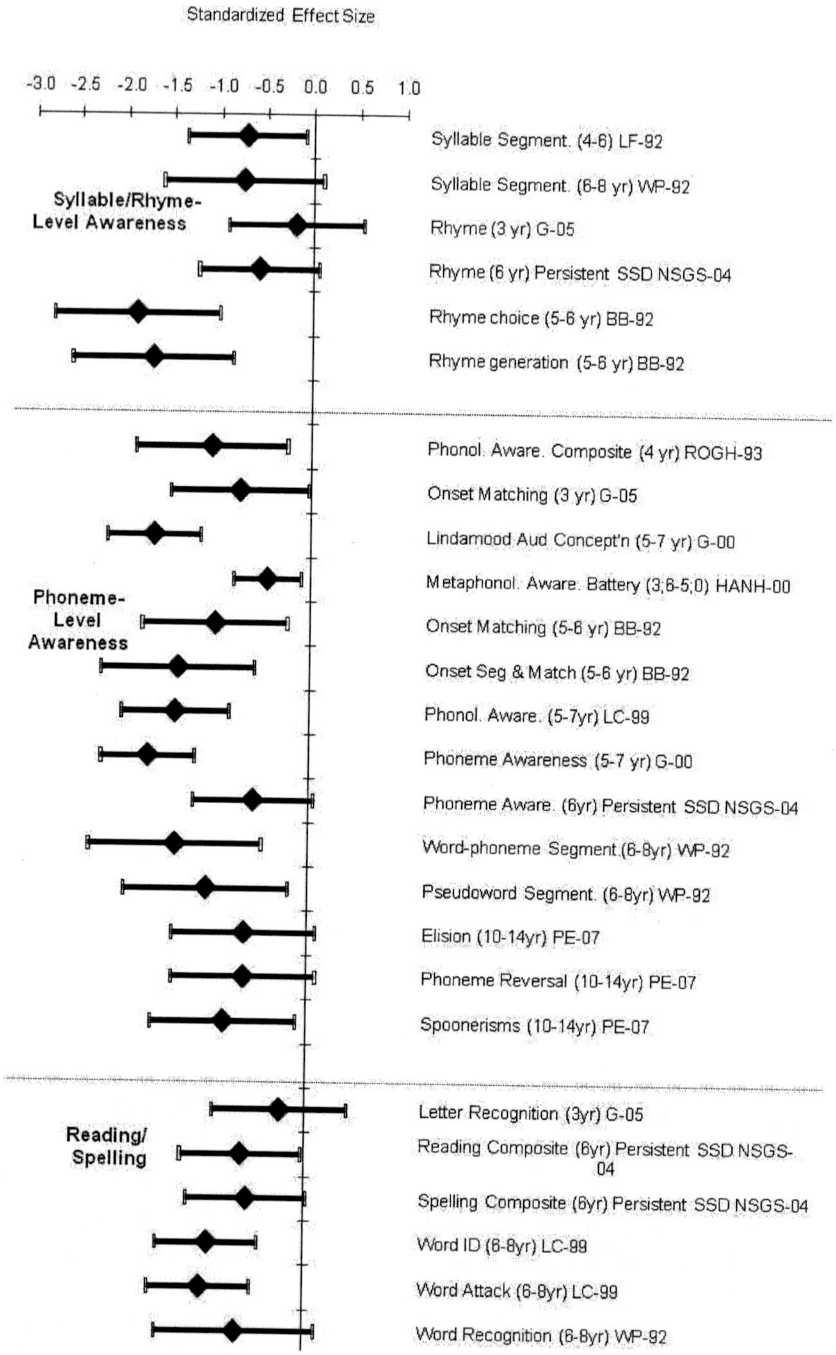

Figure 3. Differences between children with and without SSD in literacy and literacy-related skills (no subgrouping)

Notes: Diamonds show estimated effect size (number of pooled SD between means using Hedge's correction), error bars show 95% CI of the effect size. BB-92: Bird & Bishop, 1992; G-00: Gillon, 2000; G-05: Gillon, 2005; HANH-00: Hesketh et al., 2000; LC-00: Larrivee & Catts, 1999; LF-92: Lewis & Freebairn, 1992; NSGS-04: Nathan et al., 2004; PE-07: Preston & Edwards, 2007; ROGH-04: Rvachew et al., 2004; WP-92: Webster & Plante, 1992;

In particular, residual spelling problems are apparent among individuals with a history of an SSD (Clarke-Klein & Hodson, 1995; Lewis & Freebairn, 1992; Lewis, Freebairn, & Taylor, 2002). Clarke-Klein and Hodson (1995) reported that phonologically-based spelling errors are significantly more common in children with a history of SSD, as compared to children without such a history. However, spelling errors are not necessarily directly related to misarticulation patterns in a child's speech (Snowling & Stackhouse, 1983).

Not all children with SSD have poor reading skills. For example, not all studies find group differences when comparing reading skills of children with and without SSD (Bishop & Clarkson, 2003; Catts, 1993). There has been discussion that other factors, such as delays in other language domains, might mediate the relationship between SSD and literacy problems (see below). What might be most appropriate to state, therefore, is that children with SSD are highly variable in their literacy-related skills, with some children performing within normal limits and others significantly lower. What accounts for this variability? It is clear that factors in addition to a general diagnosis of a SSD are related to literacy skills. That is, there may be subtypes of children with SSD who are at particular risk for literacy problems, or there may be identifiable characteristics within a child that are related to literacy achievement. The next sections describe research that has addressed factors that may be associated with the variability in literacy skills among children with SSD.

Persisting Speech Problems

The critical age hypothesis (Bird, et al., 1995; Bishop & Adams, 1990; Nathan, et al., 2004) postulates that children who fail to achieve normal speech sound production skills by the time they are exposed to formal reading instruction will be at risk for later literacy problems. Thus, children who continue to experience clinically significant speech production problems in kindergarten or first grade and beyond would be at higher risk for literacy problems than would children whose speech production skills normalize by the time they are exposed to literacy instruction. Nathan et al (2004) provided longitudinal evidence that preschoolers whose speech errors persisted until age six had poorer phonological awareness and literacy outcomes than preschoolers whose speech errors had resolved. Similarly, Raitano et al. (2004) reported that children with speech production problems at age 6 had lower phonological awareness skills than did children with a history of SSD whose speech errors had normalized. In a cross-sectional study, Preston and Edwards (Preston & Edwards, 2007, 2009) reported children ages 10-14 with residual SSD performed below typically speaking controls on several measures of phonological processing, including phoneme elision, spoonerisms, nonword repetition, and rapid naming of pictures of multisyllabic words. Thus, persisting speech errors appear to be associated with poor phonological processing skills.

Concomitant Language Skills

Children with SSD often have co-occurring language impairments. In a review, Lewis et al. (2006) reported that the percentage of children with SSD who also have receptive language delay is 6-21%; the percentage of children with SSD who also have expressive language difficulties is estimated to be 38-63%. It appears that, among children with a SSD, a concomitant language disorder (however it might be defined) elevates the risk of literacy problems (Schuele, 2004). This is in line with studies that have shown that general receptive and expressive language skills (i.e., word and sentence-level comprehension and production) are associated with poor literacy skills (Scarborough, 2003; Schuele, 2004).

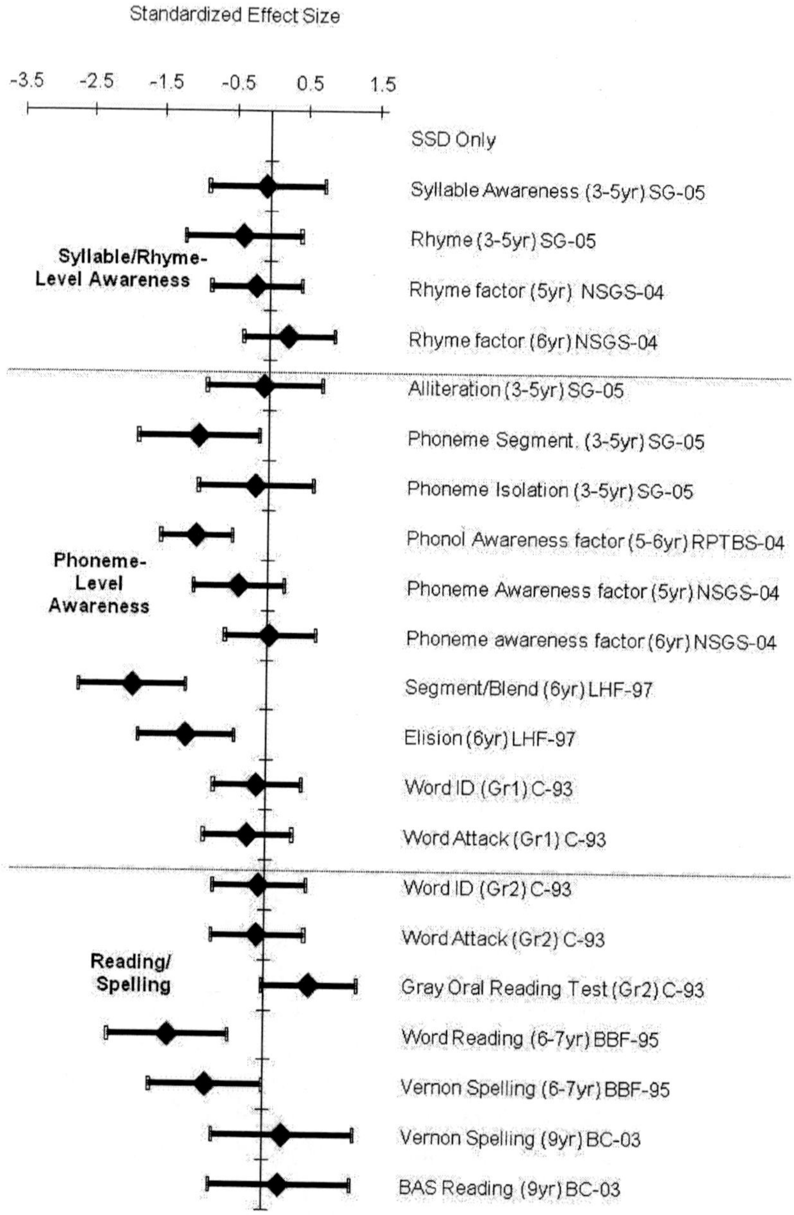

Figure 4. Differences between children with and without isolated SSD in literacy and literacy-related skills (no language impairment)

Notes: Diamonds show estimated effect size (number of pooled SD between means using Hedge's correction), error bars show 95% CI of the effect size. BBF-95: Bird, Bishop & Freeman, 1995; C-93: Catts, 1993; LHF-97: Leitao, Hogben & Fletcher, 1997; NSGS-04: Nathan et al., 2004; RPTBS-04: Raitano et al., 2004; SG-05: Sutherland & Gillon, 2005

Several studies have suggested that children with both a SSD and language impairment are at elevated risk for literacy problems, as compared to children with SSD alone. Various studies have revealed increased risk for literacy problems in subgroups of children with SSD who have concomitant language problems as compared to those who have SSD without associated language impairment (Catts, 1993; Leitao, et al., 1997; Lewis, Freebairn, & Taylor, 2000; Lewis, et al., 2002; Raitano, et al., 2004). For example, Johnson et al (1982) reported that 8-9 year olds with SSD tended to cluster into those with high language/reading skills and those with low language/reading skills.

Figures 4 and 5 show how children with SSD subgrouped based on concomitant language impairment perform on tasks of phonological processing and literacy. It is apparent from these figures that children with SSD and additional language impairments have been more consistently found to struggle with phonological processing and literacy skills; yet, there is also evidence that children with SSD without obvious language problems still have problems with literacy-related tasks. However, because language skills obviously fall on a continuum, the notion of "presence/absence of language impairment" that has been used in many studies is inherently problematic. Thus, statistical comparisons between groups of children with SSD with language impairments and those without will sometimes (but not always) find a group difference. Also, the fact that definitions for SSD and language impairment differ widely from study to study makes it difficult to determine what the critical language skills are that are responsible for elevating the risk for literacy problems. For example, receptive language problems, rather than expressive language problems, might be more strongly associated with literacy development. Thus, one of the most consistent findings is that receptive vocabulary has repeatedly been shown to predict a significant amount of variance (25-30%) in phonological awareness and literacy-related skills in children with and without SSD (Bishop & Adams, 1990; Elbro, et al., 1998; Rvachew, 2006; Rvachew & Grawburg, 2006; Rvachew, Nowak, & Cloutier, 2004). Thus, knowing how a child performed on a vocabulary assessment provides us with *some* indication of how s/he might perform on a test of reading or spelling. Of course, there is much unexplained variance in literacy skills, suggesting that other skills contribute to phonological processing and reading skills as well.

Another interesting notion is described by Bishop and Clarkson (2003), who report that some children with isolated SSD and no concomitant language problems actually perform *above* average on some tests of reading and spelling. Figure 4 shows data from this study, as well as Catts (1993), whose data suggest that there may be children with SSD who are above average in reading/spelling. It may be necessary, therefore, to more specifically define the notion of "isolated" SSD. For example, while some children with rhotic errors have difficult with phonological processing tasks (Preston & Edwards, 2007), it might be the case that children who misarticulate sibilants are less at risk for literacy-related problems. This question has not been fully explored.

Childhood Apraxia of Speech

Childhood apraxia of speech (CAS) is a subtype of SSD is heavily researched, but remains difficult to reliably diagnose. In general, these children are thought to be qualitatively different than other children with SSD. CAS deficits are presumed to be in motor planning/programming of the spatiotemporal parameters of speech, and involve problems with the precision and consistency of movements underlying speech in the absence of neuromuscular deficits (American Speech-Language-Hearing Association, 2007). Their deficits are often described as involving speech sound production errors that are inconsistent, along with phoneme sequencing problems and prosodic disturbances. With regards to literacy development, Stackhouse (1982) reported that 10 children ages 7-11 with CAS performed significantly below age-, gender-, and socioeconomic-matched control children on the Schonell Graded Word Spelling and Reading Tests, as well as a nonword matching task. Additionally, Lewis et al (2004) provided evidence that this subgroup of children is at particular risk for early literacy problems, as compared to other subgroups of children with SSD. In their study, children were diagnosed in preschool with CAS, isolated speech impairment, or speech and language impaired. When followed-up at school-age (8-9 years), the CAS subgroup was significantly lower than the other two subgroups in several measures of reading decoding, reading comprehension, and spelling. Thus, to the extent that CAS can be reliably identified, this diagnosis might usefully predict that these children with SSD will later have literacy problems.

Severity of Speech Disorder

One notion has been that speech sound production accuracy may contribute variance to the prediction of literacy skills. The general assumption is that children who are less accurate (e.g., have a greater percent of sound errors) in their speech production would be more severely impaired, and might therefore be at greater risk for literacy difficulties. Tables 4-5 display correlational evidence between speech sound production accuracy and phonological awareness/literacy. All of the studies rely on perceptual judgment of accuracy, either from picture naming in standardized tests (e.g., the Goldman-Fristoe test of Articulation) or in connected speech (e.g., using Percent Consonants Correct). The wide range of correlation coefficients is likely due, in part, to the fact that speech sound production and phonological awareness/literacy are behaviors that are difficult to reliably measure. The relatively weak relationship may be due to the possibility that speech sound production is not strongly related to literacy, or that our field have yet to identify essential parameters of the speech signal that consistently relate to literacy. Additionally, many studies lack the statistical power to detect a relationship. In general, although some studies report a significant bivariate correlation between global measures of severity of a child's speech disorder and literacy skills, the strength of this relationship appears to be weak.

Given that the simple correlations between speech sound accuracy and literacy measures are inconsistent, it is of interest to determine whether speech production skills contribute variance in predicting literacy skills over time. Several studies have used regression analyses to predict literacy-related skills while including a measure of speech sound accuracy. Bishop & Adams (1990) reported that speech sound accuracy, as measured by percent consonants correct (PCC, Shriberg, Austin, Lewis, McSweeny, & Wilson, 1997; Shriberg & Kwiatkowski, 1982), at both age 4 ½ and age 5 ½ predicted variance in reading accuracy beyond performance IQ and grammatical skills at age 8 ½ (accounting for 5.4 and 9.9% of variance in reading accuracy, respectively). PCC at age 5 ½ predicted 9.9% of the variance in spelling beyond performance IQ and vocabulary at age 8 ½. Additionally, Larrivee and Catts (1999) evaluated speech production, language, and reading skills in first graders with SSD.

They reported that PCC scores from two tasks (picture naming and multisyllable word/nonword repetition) were correlated with Word Identification and Word Attack scores from the Woodcock Reading Mastery Test-Revised. When entered into a regression to predict Word Attack and Word Identification scores, PCC from the mulitsyllable word/nonword repetition task contributed an additional 14% of variance in Word Identification scores beyond the contributions of phonological awareness and general language skills. However, speech production accuracy from the picture naming task did not account for significant variance in either of the reading scores once other language and phonological awareness were controlled.

Speech Sound Error Types

One possibility is that there are specific characteristics of speech production that are more strongly associated with literacy development than others. As just reviewed, global measures of speech sound accuracy, such as number of errors on a standardized test or percent consonants correct, have failed to reveal consistent or robust relationships between speech sound accuracy and literacy achievement. Thus, some studies have explored specific features in a child's speech that relate to phonological processing and literacy development. Some attempts have been made in the literature to classify speech sound error patterns in children with SSD as distortions (e.g., lateralized /s/ or derhoticized /r/), typical phonemic errors (e.g., final consonant deletion, velar fronting) and atypical phonemic errors (e.g., initial consonant deletion, backing of front sounds). It has been discussed that atypical errors may reflect poorly specified phonological representations; thus, those errors might be most strongly related to poor phonological processing skills. For example, McMahon, Stassi and Dodd (1998) reported that the number of unusual phonological errors produced by multiple birth children when they were preschoolers was a significant predictor of their later phonological awareness and literacy skills at approximately 7 years of age. However, they did not report inferential statistics, so the relative contribution of those atypical errors in predicting later literacy-related skills is uncertain.

Preston and Edwards (in press) recorded 43 preschoolers with SSD on a picture-naming task and categorized speech sound errors as distortions (e.g., lateralized /s/ or derhoticized /r/), typical phonemic errors (e.g., final consonant deletion, velar fronting) and atypical phonemic errors (e.g., initial consonant deletion, backing of front sounds). It was found that only atypical errors were correlated with phonological awareness skills. Once receptive vocabulary and age were controlled, atypical errors produced on the picture-naming task were found to contribute an additional 6% of variance in phonological awareness, but the other error types did not. When the same speech sound errors were categorized as correct/incorrect (PCC), speech sound errors did not predict any variance in phonological awareness. Thus, some sound error patterns are more reflective of poor phonological awareness than others, and a global measure of speech sound accuracy was not a useful predictor of phonological awareness.

Additionally, some studies have subtyped children with SSD based on the nature of the speech errors they produce. For example, Leitao and Fletcher (2004) classified children with SSD at age six into two groups: those who produced primarily developmental (typical) speech sound errors and those who produced a significant number of nondevelopmental (atypical) errors. The groups (n=7 per group) were compared at ages 12-13 on several tests of reading, spelling, and phonological processing. Results indicated that the children who originally produced more atypical speech errors performed more poorly on measures of phonological awareness, spelling, and reading comprehension.

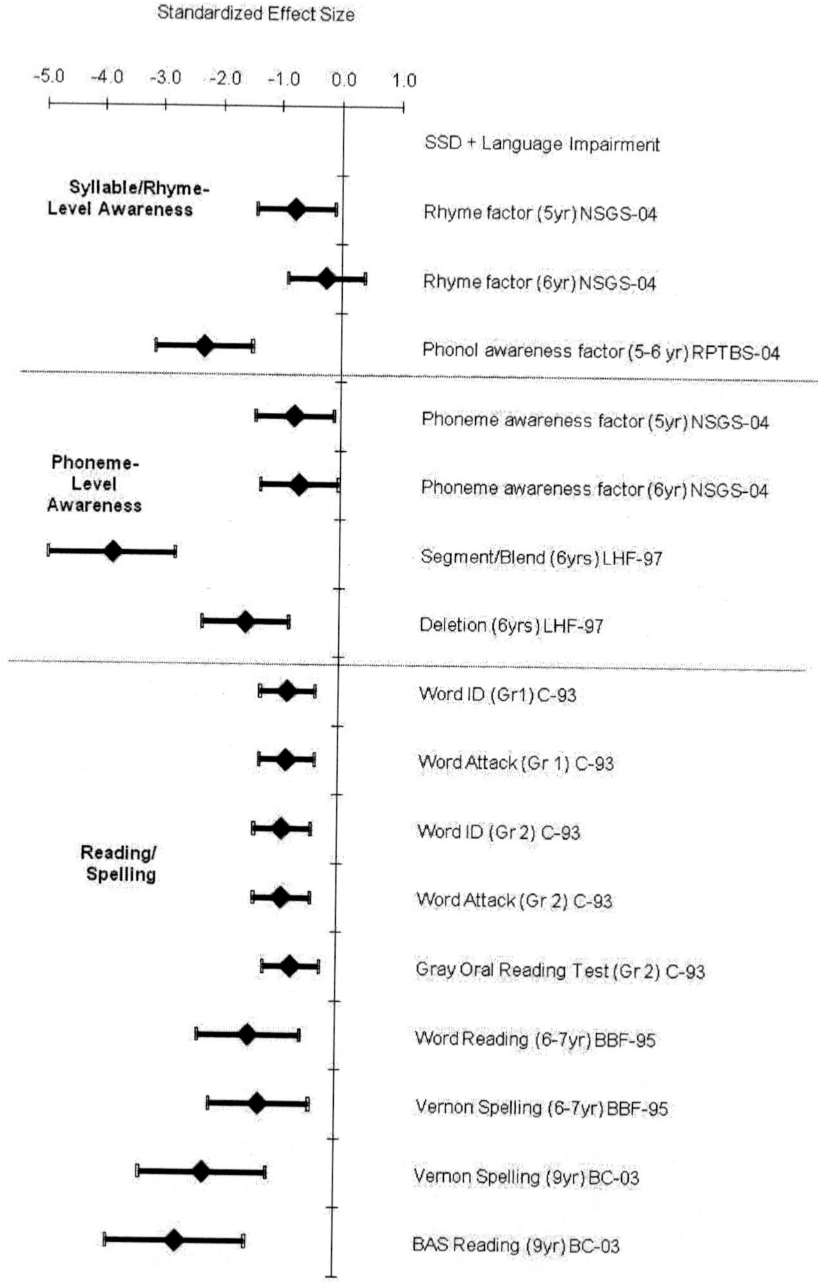

Figure 5. Differences between typically developing children and those with SSD+Language Impairment in literacy and literacy-related skills

Notes: iamonds show estimated effect size (number of pooled SD between means using Hedge's correction), error bars show 95% CI of the effect size. BBF-95: Bird, Bishop & Freeman, 1995; C-93: Catts, 1993; LHF-97: Leitao, Hogben & Fletcher, 1997; NSGS-04: Nathan et al., 2004; RPTBS-04: Raitano et al., 2004

THE ROLE OF PHONOLOGICAL SHORT-TERM MEMORY

Thus far, the focus has been on how speech production is related to phonological awareness or reading/spelling skills. An additional phonological processing skill that has been found to independently contribute to literacy development in young children is phonological short-term memory (Brady, 1991; Wagner & Torgesen, 1987). In general, this refers to the temporary storage of phonological information, which may be needed for many types of phonological processing, reading, and spelling tasks (Scarborough & Brady, 2002). Phonological short-term memory has been found to separate good and poor readers and to correlate with literacy skills such as decoding of nonwords and spelling accuracy (Griffiths & Snowling, 2002; Kamhi, Catts, Mauer, Apel, & Gentry, 1988).

Phonological short-term memory is most commonly assessed via nonword repetition tasks (e.g., repeating sequences such as /naɪ tʃ oɪ taʊ vub/. That is, a child's ability to hold in short-term memory the phonological features of words/nonwords that they just heard, and to then plan and execute those articulatory sequences, has been shown to have a predictive relationship with literacy development. Deficits on nonword repetition tasks are typically assumed to reflect poor articulatory rehearsal; they are often discussed in the context of the "phonological loop" (Baddeley, 2003; Baddeley, Gathercole, & Papagno, 1998), a component of working memory in language in which phonological information is temporarily retained and refreshed via subvocal articulatory rehearsal. That is, there is evidence that people (covertly) repeat linguistic information in order to hold it in memory. With regard to reading, children must hold phonological information in short-term memory when decoding words sound-by-sound; children who are attempting to sound out (decode) a printed word with which they are unfamiliar often rehearse the sounds associated with the letters, either overtly or covertly. Once they reach the end of the word, they must recall all of those sounds.

Phonological Short-Term Memory in Children with SSD

Impairments in phonological short-term memory in children with SSD have been described previously (e.g., Locke & Scott, 1979; Munson et al., 2005; Nijland, 2009; Preston & Edwards, 2007). For example, Locke and Scott (1979) found evidence of an impaired rehearsal mechanism in children with SSD, even when rehearsal is subvocal (i.e., children with SSD had more trouble recalling the names of pictures of rhyming words than typically speaking children). In fact, several recent genetic studies have reported that nonword repetition is important in defining the link between SSD and dyslexia (Smith, Pennington, Boada, & Shriberg, 2005; Stein, et al., 2006; Stein, et al., 2004). Table 6 demonstrates that speech sound production accuracy in (picture naming tasks and in conversation) has consistently been shown to relate to nonword repetition. It is evident that a relatively robust relationship exists between general measures of speech sound accuracy and measures of phonological short-term memory.

Because of this emerging genetic relationship, it is important to have valid measures of phonological short-term memory for children with SSD. Several limitations exist with nonword repetition tasks for children with SSD. Nonword repetition requires the ability to recall phonological input, establish a temporary representation, plan the motor movements of the articulators necessary for the sound sequence, and execute those motor movements. That is, the ability to accurately repeat nonwords not only requires the ability to recall phonemes, but also the ability to perform complex motor movements.

Table 4. Speech production and phonological awareness in children with SSD

Study	n	Speech Measure	Phonological Awareness Measure	Correlation *r*
Preston & Edwards (submitted) 4-5 yr	43	Atypical errors per cons.	PA Principal Component	- .36
		Typical errors per cons.		(- .17)
		Distortions per cons.		(.13)
		GFTA-2 standard score		(.15)
		PCC		(.22)
Bird & Bishop (1992) 5-6 yr	14	Percent distinctive features correct	Onset identification	.60
			Onset segmentation and matching	.47
			Rhyme judgment	(.35)
			Rhyme generation	(.42)
Major & Bernhardt (1998) 3-4 yr	19	PCC-R	Metaphonology composite	ρ=.57
		Consonant Matches (excludes deletions)		ρ= .47
		Percent Vowels Correct		ρ=.64
		Word shape match		ρ=.62
		CVC matches		ρ=.52
		CVCV matches		(<.47)
McDowell et al (2007) 2-5 yr	700	Speech Sound Accuracy (consonants correct on picture naming & nonword repetition	PA composite	.65
Nijland (2009)	21	PCC Percent Vowels Correct	Rhyme judgment	ρ=.48 ρ=.54
Smith et al (2005) 5-6 yr with SSD & siblings 5-8 yr	187	GFTA consonanterrors	Phonological Awareness Principal Component	-.31
		zPCC-R		.10
		Speech1 (log odds of SSD, composite of 7 variables)		-.09
		Speech2 (probability of SSD, composite of 7 variables)		-.11

Table 4. (Continued)

Study	n	Speech Measure	Phonological Awareness Measure	Correlation *r*
Rvachew (2006) Pre-K →Kinder.	47	GFTA-2 consonant errors (Pre-K)	Phonological Awareness Test (cf. Bird et al., 1995) – Pre-K	-.45
		GFTA-2 consonant errors (Kinder.)	Phonological Awareness Test– Kinder.	-.54
		GFTA-2 consonant errors (Pre-K)	Phonological Awareness Test– Kinder.	(-.38)
Rvachew (2007) Pre-K→Gr.1	68	GFTA-2 consonant errors (Pre-K)	Phonological Awareness Test – First Grade	-.47
Rvachew et al (2004) 3-4 yr	34	GFTA-2 consonant errors	Phonological Awareness Test	(-.23)
Webster & Plante (1992) 6-8 yr	22 (11 SSD)	Number of intelligible words	Pseudoword segmentation Word-syllable segmentation Word-phoneme segmentation	.62 (.32) .77

Table 5. Speech production and literacy in children with SSD

Study & Participants	N	Speech Measure	Literacy-Related Measure	Correlation *r*
Catts (1993) Kinder. → Gr.1	56	GFTA consonant errors	Word Attack	(<.29)
			Word Identification	(<.29)
Stein et al (2004) Pre-K SSD & siblings	177	PCC in conversation	Word Attack	.18
			Word Identification	.12
	188	GFTA percentile	Word Attack	.13
			Word Identification	.19
Rvachew (2007) Pre-K → Gr.1	68	GFTA-2 errors (Pre-K) PCC (Pre-K)	First Grade sight word reading	(-.16) (.10)
		GFTA-2 errors (Pre-K) PCC (Pre-K)	First Grade nonword reading	-.39 .30
Lewis et al 2002 ~9 yrs	52	GFTA percentile	Test of Written Spelling-3: Total Predictible Unpredictible	.39 .43 .32
Webster & Plante (1992) 6-8 yrs	22 (11 SSD)	Number of intelligible words	Printed word recognition	(.35)

With regard to preschool assessment of phonological short-term memory, one must consider that children with SSD (as well as typically developing preschoolers) produce many sound errors. A more appropriate task to assess phonological short-term memory would be one that simplifies motor demand and requires children to repeat simple syllables that are likely to be within their repertoire of production. Thus, data are described below demonstrating the assessment of phonological memory in children with SSD without some of the complications associated with previous nonword repetition tasks.

With the use of a more valid task of phonological short-term memory for preschoolers with SSD, we can begin to address the question: *which children with SSD will have poor phonological short-term memory*? In line with previous studies that have suggested that particular speech sound error patterns may be associated with poor phonological processing skills (Preston & Edwards, in press), this brief report investigates how particular speech sound error types (particularly atypical speech sound errors) relate to phonological short-term memory.

The following is a summary of a phonological short-term memory assessment in children with SSD using a nonword repetition task with very limited articulatory demands (i.e., producing only four early developing consonants, /b, m, d, n/). Thus, the phonological complexity of the nonwords is greatly reduced, and performance will not be highly constrained by limitations in a child's production system. This is believed to be a more valid measure of phonological short-term memory for children with SSD because it incorporates syllables that are typically in the productive inventory of such children (Shriberg, Lohmeier, McSweeny, & Kwiatkowski, 2006). We can therefore use such a task to explore skills that are associated with phonological short-term memory without some of the productive complications of prior studies that have relied on stimuli with more complex production demands.

Method

Forty-four preschoolers with SSD were recruited by referrals from local speech-language pathologists. All children were between 4;0 – 5;9 and had no known cause for their speech disorder (such as hearing loss, cleft palate, or developmental disorder). During a screening, all participants were found to have low speech sound production skills, as defined by standard scores below 90 on the Goldman-Fristoe Test of Articulation-2 (Goldman & Fristoe, 2000) (standard score X = 71, SD 12). Additionally, participants did not have severe receptive language delays, as defined by at least two of the following: Standard score above 80 on the Peabody Picture Vocabulary Test-4 (Dunn & Dunn, 2007), scaled score above 6 on the Concepts and Following Directions subtest of the Clinical Evaluation of Language Fundamentals, Preschool-2 (Wiig, Secord, & Semel, 2004), and scaled score above 6 on the Sentence Structure subtest of the CELF:P-2. Nonverbal cognition was also screened, and all participants achieved *T*-scores that were no lower than 1 1/3 SD of the mean on the Pattern Construction subtest of the Differential Ability Scales (Elliott, 1990).

During the experimental session, children participated in phonological processing tasks and a speech production assessment. Speech production was assessed via a picture naming task of 125 words that sampled all phonemes in nearly every position in which they occur, and included many phonologically complex words (multisyllabic words, consonant clusters, etc.). Responses were recorded and were later phonetically transcribed. Speech errors were coded as distortions (sub-phonemic errors, such as dentalized /s/), typical phonemic errors (such as final consonant deletion or velar fronting), or atypical phonemic errors (i.e., those errors that are found rarely, if at all, in typically developing children, such as initial consonant deletion or backing of alveolars, see Preston & Edwards, in press).

Table 6. Speech production and phonological short-term memory in children with SSD

Study & Participants	n	Speech Measure	Phonological Short-Term Memory	Correlation *r*
Current study 4-5 yr	44	Atypical errors per cons.	Syllable Repetition Task (Shriberg et al., 2008)	- .61
		Typical errors per cons.		- .34
		Distortions per cons.		(.03)
		GFTA-2 standard score GFTA-2 percentile		.39 .34
Preston & Edwards (2007) 10-14 yr	13	PCC from pictures	Nonwords (Dollaghan & Campbell, 1998)	(.36)
		PCC-R from pictures		.64
	13	PCC from pictures	English-like nonwords	(.23)
		PCC-R from pictures		.65
Munson et al. (2005) 3-6 yr	40	GFTA percentile	Low frequency nonword sequences High Frequency nonword sequences	.49 .62
McDowell et al (2007) 2-5 yr	700	GFTA consonants correct	2-4 syllable nonwords	.56
Stein et al (2004) Pre-K SSD & siblings	188	GFTA percentile	Nonword repetition (Kamhi & Catts, 1986)	.55
	177	PCC in conversation		.52
Smith et al. (2005) Kinder. SSD & siblings	~187	GFTA consonant errors	Nonwords (Dollaghan & Campbell, 1998)	-.49
		zPCC-R in conversation		.51
		Speech1 (log odds of SSD, composite of 7 variables)		-.52
		Speech2 (probability of SSD, composite of 7 variables)		-.41

Phonological short-term memory was assessed using a repetition task developed by Shriberg and colleagues (Shriberg & Lohmeier, 2008; Shriberg, et al., 2006). The Syllable Repetition Task helps to eliminate problems associated with other nonword repetition tasks because it includes only early developing consonants /b, d, m, n/ and a single vowel /a/. Preschoolers with SSD often have these phonemes in their inventory, and this was confirmed in the present study: all 44 participants produced /b, d, m, n/ in at least two words on the picture naming task. The recorded stimuli range from two to four syllables. Stimuli were presented via laptop and children's responses were digitally recorded and were later transcribed. Responses were later scored based on the percent of consonants produced correctly, using scoring procedures described by Shriberg and Lohmeier (2008).

Results

It was found that phonological short-term memory, as measured by the Syllable Repetition Task, was not predicted by the frequency of occurrence of distortion (subphonemic) errors (r=.03, p=.417). Typical phonemic errors showed a small but significant correlation with phonological short-term memory (r=-.33, p=.015), and atypical phonemic errors were strongly related phonological short-term memory (r=-.60, p<.001).

A multiple regression analysis was then used to predict phonological short-term memory scores from all three speech production variables. The results indicated that atypical errors were the only significant predictor of phonological short-term memory scores (p<.001), and distortions and typical phonemic errors did not predict phonological short-term memory performance (p's >.05). Thus, even though these children were capable of articulating target /b, d, m, n/ in at least some instances, their ability to recall sequences of sounds in nonwords was strongly predicted by the number of atypical errors they produced in the 125 word picture naming task.

To evaluate whether a relationship between atypical errors and phonological short-term memory remained when vocabulary (standard scores on the PPVT-4) and age (in months) were controlled, hierarchical regression analysis was used. Atypical errors remained robust predictors of phonological short-term memory once age and vocabulary were controlled; that is, in step 1, vocabulary and age accounted for 10% of the variance in performance on the nonword repetition task. In step 2, stepwise regression was used to select the speech production variables that were significant predictors of phonological short-term memory. Atypical errors were selected as a significant predictor of phonological short-term memory, and contributed an addition 30% of variance in phonological short-term memory beyond age and vocabulary (ΔR^2 Adj=.30, p <.001).

Discussion

Even when using nonword repetition stimuli that have limited articulatory demands, consonant errors were observed on the nonword repetition task. Thus, sequences of up to four syllables can be challenging for some children with SSD to repeat. The fact that atypical errors on the 125-word picture naming task were so strongly related to phonological short-term memory suggests that there are indeed unique features that can be identified in the productions of preschoolers with SSD that are strongly associated with phonological short-term memory, an important predictor of literacy-related skills.

These data are in line with those of other studies that have investigated short-term phonological memory and speech sound production skills (see Table 6). For example, studies employing factor analysis have indicated that phonological short-term memory and speech sound production skills tend to "hang together" when multiple speech and language variables are considered in children at risk for literacy problems (Foy & Mann, 2001; Gallagher, Frith, & Snowling, 2000). The data presented here indicate that particular types of speech errors may be more strongly linked with poor phonological short-term memory than others.

One interpretation is that the frequency with which children with SSD produce atypical errors may be an appropriate index of the strength of a child's phonological representations (or, perhaps, a child's capability of forming strong phonological representations). Because distortions and typical phonemic errors are common in phonological development, the extent to which we observe *atypical* phonemic errors is noteworthy. Kail (1997) has argued that the *speed* with which children can rehearse phonological information strongly relates to phonological short-term memory skills. Here, the argument is extended to suggest that productive phonological *accuracy* also may be needed for good phonological short-term memory skills. Hence, skills associated with rapid as well as accurate phonological production may be needed for phonological rehearsal. Therefore, speed and accuracy of the phonological system must work together for accurate recall/rehearsal of phonological input (Preston & Edwards, 2009). A causal connection cannot be established here, however. What is known, though, is that these preschoolers with SSD will soon rely on their phonological short-term memory skills for several purposes: (a) to develop sound-symbol associations, (b) to sound out, retain, and blend phonemes when decoding words, and (c) to repeat words phoneme-by-phoneme when learning to spell. Long-term follow-up of these children would help to reveal if atypical errors help to predict later phonological short-term memory and literacy development. Additionally, if indeed atypical errors reflect poorly specified phonological representations and poor phonological short-term memory, then one might expect that improvements in a child's speech production would be linked with improvements in phonological short-term memory. To date, it does not appear that this hypothesis has been tested.

The frequency with which children produce atypical phonemic errors *might* be an appropriate proxy for the strength of phonological representations. However, it might not be the most appropriate metric for children without a SSD. That is, there are some children without a SSD who are also found to develop problems with literacy, and they may not produce atypical phonemic errors. Yet, there may be speech production variables that prove to be strong predictors of literacy-related skills (Smith, et al., 2008). Certainly, further exploration is needed of the predictive nature of speech production factors in determining literacy outcomes.

One limitation that should be acknowledged is that speech sound production assessments in children often involve perceptual judgments of phonemic or phonetic accuracy. While these transcription-based methods are often useful in describing patterns in children's speech, they reduce the continuous speech signal to a series of discrete, ordinal phones and thus fail to capture what is truly happening on an articulatory level. There may be subtleties in gestural movement patterns and coordination that are indicative of poorly specified phonological representations, but that are not easily captured at the level of narrow phonetic transcription.

Conclusion

Speech production skills have the potential to serve as indicators for literacy problems. Greater understandings of the phenotypic and genotypic overlap in SSD and dyslexia will certainly impact our understanding of how assessments and interventions should be tailored. However, it does seem possible to draw some conclusions applicable to clinical practice. For example, it should be evident by now that children with SSD should be evaluated for (pre)literacy skills and should be closely monitored as they progress through school. In addition to weak phonological processing skills, risk factors for (pre)literacy difficulties in children with SSD currently include:

(a) relatively frequent use of atypical speech sound errors (Dodd, 2005; Leitao & Fletcher, 2004; Leitao, et al., 1997; McMahon, et al., 1998; Preston, 2008; Rvachew, Chiang, & Evans, 2007),
(b) features that are consistent with the diagnosis of childhood apraxia of speech (Lewis, et al., 2004; Stackhouse, 1982),
(c) persisting speech production problems (beyond about six years of age) (Bishop & Adams, 1990; Nathan, et al., 2004; Preston & Edwards, 2007; Raitano, et al., 2004),
(d) low vocabulary skills (Preston & Edwards, in press; Rvachew, 2006; Rvachew & Grawburg, 2006) and/or concomitant language delay (Leitao, et al., 1997; Lewis, et al., 2000; Raitano, et al., 2004)

In addition, it appears that weak phonological short-term memory may be important in defining the link between SSD and literacy problems, so assessments of this skill should be careful to avoid complications associated with limited speech sound production capabilities. Direct assessment of phonological awareness skills is critical, as such skills often respond well to treatment.

Interventions that implement phonological awareness training (e.g., rhyming, phoneme identification, segmenting, blending) along with speech sound production therapy have proven to be effective at improving speech production skills and at reducing the risk for literacy problems (Gillon, 2000; Gillon, 2002; Gillon, 2005; Major & Bernhardt, 1998; van Kleeck, Gillam, & McFadden, 1998). Clinicians must be vigilant given that some adolescents with residual speech errors, as well as adolescents and adults with histories of phonological disorders, show signs of literacy-related problems (Lewis & Freebairn, 1992; Preston & Edwards, 2007). Ultimately, these are the outcomes that we wish to prevent. As theory progresses and as measurement techniques improve, more fine-grained analyses of speech production may prove useful in the early identification of children at risk for literacy problems and SSD.

In sum, there is tremendous heterogeneity in literacy skills of children with SSD. Some of the primary factors associated with low phonological processing/literacy have been identified here, but there is much that remains to be determined. For example, it will eventually be necessary to evaluate the relative contribution of each of the characteristics described. That is, variance may be shared among several of these variables (e.g., atypical errors and CAS, or persisting speech problems and low language skills, etc). Ideally, longitudinal studies that evaluate all of these factors would be useful in answering such questions. Additionally, the extent to which any of these factors are associated with response to different types of literacy instruction/intervention remains to be determined.

ACKNOWLEDGEMENTS

Thanks to Carol Fowler, Steve Frost, Laura Raynolds for helpful comments on this manuscript. Preparation of the manuscript was supported by NICHD grant T32HD7548-8, and portions of the data collection were supported by the 2007 American Speech-Language-Hearing Foundation Student grant in Early Childhood Language Development awarded to the author.

REFERENCES

American-Speech-Language-Hearing-Association (2007). Childhood Apraxia of Speech [Technical Report]. available from www.asha.org/policy.

Baddeley, A. (2003). Working memory and language: An overview. *Journal of Communication Disorders, 36*, 189-208.

Baddeley, A., Gathercole, S. & Papagno, C. (1998). The phonological loop as a language learning device. *Psychological Review, 105(1)*, 158-173.

Ball, E. W. & Blachman, B. A. (1991). Does phoneme awareness training in kindergarten make a difference in early word recognition and developmental spelling. *Reading Research Quarterly, 26*(1), 49-66.

Bertucci, C., Hook, P., Haynes, C., Macaruso, P., Bickley, C. (2003). Vowel perception and production in adolescents with reading disabilities. *Annals of Dyslexia, 53*, 174-200.

Bird, J., Bishop, D. V. M. & Freeman, N. H. (1995). Phonological awareness and literacy development in children with expressive phonological impairments. *Journal of Speech and Hearing Research, 38*, 446-462.

Bishop, D. V. M. & Adams, C. (1990). A prospective study of the relationship between specific language impairment, phonological disorders and reading retardation. *Journal of Child Psychology and Psychiatry, 31(7)*, 1027-1050.

Bishop, D. V. M. & Clarkson, B. W. (2003). Written Language As A Window Into Residual Language Deficits: A Study Of Children With Persistent And Residual Speech And Language Impairments. *Cortex, 39(2)*, 215-237.

Blachman, B. A. (2000). Phonological Awareness. In M. L. Kamil, P. B. Mosenthal, P. D. Pearson & R. Barr (Eds.), *Handbook of reading research* (Vol. 3, pp. 483-502). Mahwah, NJ: Lawrence Erlbaum Associates.

Bradford, A. & Dodd, B. (1996). Do all speech-disordered children have motor deficits? *Clinical Linguistics and Phonetics, 10(2)*, 77-101.

Bradley, L. & Bryant, P. E. (1983). Categorizing sounds and learning to read - a causal connection. *Nature, 301*, 419-421.

Brady, S. A. (1991). The role of memory in reading disability. In S. Brady & D. Shankweiler (Eds.), *Phonological processes in literacy: A tribute to Isabelle Y. Liberman* (pp. 129-151). Hillsdale, NJ: Lawrence Erlbaum Ass.

Brady, S., Gillis, M., Smith, T., Lavalette, M., Liss-Bronstein, L., Lowe, E., North, W., Russo, E., Wilder, T. (2009). First grade teachers' knowledge of phonological awareness and code concepts: Examining gains from an intensive form of professional development and corresponding teacher attitudes. *Reading and Writing, 22(4)*, 425-455.

Bridgeman, E. & Snowling, M. (1988). The perception of phoneme sequence: A comparison of dyspraxic and normal children. *British Journal of Disorders of Communication, 23*, 245-252.

Broomfield, J. & Dodd, B. (2005). Epidemiology of speech disorders. In B. Dodd (Ed.), *Differential diagnosis and treatment of children with speech disorders* (2 ed.). London: Whurr Publishers.

Campbell, T. F., Dollaghan, C. A., Rockette, H. E., Paradise, J. L., Feldman, H. M., Shriberg, L. D., et al. (2003). Risk Factors for Speech Delay of Unknown Origin in 3-Year-Old Children. *Child Development, 74(2)*, 346-357.

Castiglioni-Spalten, M. L. & Ehri, L. C. (2003). Phonemic awareness instruction: Contribution of articulatory segmentation to novice beginners' reading and spelling. *Scientific Studies of Reading, 7(1)*, 25-52.

Catts, H. W. (1989). Speech Production Deficits in Developmental Dyslexia. *Journal of Speech and Hearing Disorders, 54(3)*, 422-428.

Catts, H. W. (1993). The relationship between speech-language impairments and reading disabilities. *Journal of Speech and Hearing Research, 36*, 948-958.

Catts, H. W., Fey, M. E., Zhang, X. & Tomblin, J. B. (2001). Estimating the risk of future reading difficulties in kindergarten children: A research-based model and its clinical implementation. *Language, Speech and Hearing Services in Schools, 32(1)*, 38-50.

Clarke-Klein, S. & Hodson, B. W. (1995). A Phonologically Based Analysis of Misspellings by Third Graders With Disordered-Phonology Histories. *Journal of Speech and Hearing Research, 38(4)*, 839-849.

Constable, T., Pugh, K., Berroya, E., Mencl., W.E., Westerveld, M., Ni, W. & Shankweiler, D. (2004). Sentence complexity and input modality effects in sentence comprehension: an fMRI study. *Neuroimage, 22(1)*, 11-21.

Dodd, B. (Ed.). (2005). *Differential diagnosis and treatment of children with speech disorder* (2 ed.). Philadelphia: Whurr Publishers.

Dunn, L. M. & Dunn, D. M. (2007). *Peabody Picture Vocabulary Test* (4 ed.). Minneapolis, MN: Pearson.

Elbro, C. (1996). Early linguistic abilities and reading development: A review and a hypothesis. *Reading and Writing: An Interdisciplinary Journal, 8*, 453-485.

Elbro, C., Borstrom, I. & Peterson, D. K. (1998). Predicting dyslexia from kindergarten: The importance of distinctness of phonological representations of lexical items. *Reading Research Quarterly, 33(1)*, 36-60.

Elbro, C. & Pallesen, B. R. (2002). The quality of phonological representations and phonological awareness: A causal link? In L. Verhoeven, C. Elbro & P. Reitsma (Eds.), *Precursors of Functional Literacy* (Vol. 11). Amsterdam: John Benjamins Publishing

Elliott, C. D. (1990). *Differential Ability Scales*. San Antonio, TX: Psychological Corporation/Harcourt Brace.

Fawcett, A. J. & Nicolson, R. I. (2002). Children with dyslexia are slow to articulate a single speech gesture. *Dyslexia, 8*, 189-203.

Fawcett, A. J., Nicolson, R. I. & Maclagan, F. (2001). Cerebellar Tests Differentiate Between Groups of Poor Readers With and Without IQ Discrepancy. *Journal of Learning Disabilities, 34(2)*, 119-135.

Felsenfeld, S., Broen, P. A. & McGue, M. (1992). A 28-year follow-up of adults with a history of moderate phonological disorder: Linguistic and personality results. *Journal of Speech & Hearing Research, 35(5)*, 1114-1125.

Felsenfeld, S., Broen, P. A. & McGue, M. (1994). A 28-year follow-up of adults with a history of moderate phonological disorder: Educational and occupational results. *Journal of Speech & Hearing Research, 37(6)*, 1341-1353.

Fowler, A. E. & Swainson, B. (2004). Relationships of Naming Skills to Reading, Memory, and Receptive Vocabulary: Evidence for Imprecise Phonological Representations of Words by Poor Readers. *Annals of Dyslexia, 54*, 247-280.

Foy, J. G. & Mann, V. (2001). Does strength of phonological representations predict phonological awareness in preschool children? *Applied Psycholinguistics, 22*(3), 301-325.

Fulbright, R. K., Jenner, A. R., Mencl, W. E., Pugh, K. R., Shaywitz, B. A., Shaywitz, S. E., et al. (1999). The Cerebellum's Role in Reading: A Functional MR Imaging Study. *American Journal of Neuroradiology, 20(10)*, 1925-1930.

Gallagher, A., Frith, U. & Snowling, M. J. (2000). Precursors of literacy delay among children at genetic risk of dyslexia. *Journal of Child Psychology and Psychiatry, 41(2)*, 203-213.

Gillon, G. T. (2000). The efficacy of phonological awareness intervention for children with spoken language impairment. *Language, Speech, & Hearing Services in Schools, 31(2)*, 126-141.

Gillon, G. T. (2002). Follow-up study investigating the benefits of phonological awareness intervention for children with spoken language impairment. *International Journal of Language & Communication Disorders, 37(4)*, 381-400.

Gillon, G. T. (2005). Facilitating phoneme awareness development in 3- and 4-year-old children with speech impairment. *Language, Speech, and Hearing Services in Schools, 36(4)*, 308-324.

Goldman, R. & Fristoe, M. (2000). *Goldman Fristoe Test of Articulation - Second Ed.* Circle Pines, MN: AGS.

Goswami, U. (2000). Phonological representations, reading development and dyslexia: towards a cross-linguistic theoretical framework. *Dyslexia, 6(2)*, 133-151.

Griffiths, Y. M. & Snowling, M. J. (2002). Predictors of exception word and nonword reading in dyslexic children: The severity hypothesis. *Journal of Educational Psychology, 94(1)*, 34-43.

Jamieson, D. G. & Rvachew, S. (1992). Remediating speech production errors with sound identification training. *Journal of Speech Language Pathology and Audiology, 16(3)*, 201-210.

Joanisse, M. F., Manis, F. R., Keating, P. & Seidenberg, M. S. (2000). Language deficits in dyslexic children: Speech perception, phonology, and morphology. *Journal of Experimental Child Psychology, 77(1)*, 30-60.

Johnson, A. F., Shelton, R. L. & Arndt, W. B. (1982). A technique for identifying the subgroup membership of certain misarticulating children. *Journal of Speech and Hearing Research, 25*, 162-166.

Kail, R. (1997). Phonological skill and articulation time independently contribute to the development of memory span. *Journal of Experimental Child Psychology, 67(1)*, 57-68.

Kamhi, A. G., Catts, H. W., Mauer, D., Apel, K. & Gentry, B. F. (1988). Phonological and spatial processing abilities in language- and reading- impaired children. *Journal of Speech and Hearing Disorders, 53*, 316-327.

Larrivee, L. S. & Catts, H. W. (1999). Early reading achievement in children with expressive phonological disorders. *American Journal of Speech-Language Pathology, 8*, 118-128.

Leitao, S. & Fletcher, J. (2004). Literacy outcomes for students with speech impairment: Long-term follow-up. *International Journal of Language & Communication Disorders, 39(2)*, 245-256.

Leitao, S., Hogben, J. & Fletcher, J. (1997). Phonological processing skills in speech and language impaired children. *European Journal of Disorders of Communication, 32*, 91-111.

Lewis, B. A. & Freebairn, L. (1992). Residual effects of preschool phonology disorders in grade school, adolescence, and adulthood. *Journal of Speech and Hearing Research, 35*, 819-831.

Lewis, B. A., Freebairn, L. A., Hansen, A. J., Iyengar, S. K. & Taylor, H. G. (2004). School-age follow-up of children with childhood apraxia of speech. *Language, Speech, and Hearing Services in Schools, 35*, 122-140.

Lewis, B. A., Freebairn, L. A. & Taylor, G. H. (2000). Follow-up of children with early expressive phonology disorders. *Journal of Learning Disabilities, 33(5)*, 433-444.

Lewis, B. A., Freebairn, L. A. & Taylor, H. (2002). Correlates of spelling abilities in children with early speech sound disorders. *Reading and Writing, 15(3-4)*, 389-407.

Lewis, B. A., Shriberg, L. D., Freebairn, L. A., Hansen, A. J., Stein, C. M., Taylor, H. G., et al. (2006). The genetic bases of speech sound disorders: Evidence from spoken and written language. *Journal of Speech, Language, and Hearing Research, 49(6)*, 1294-1312.

Lieberman, P., Meskill, R. H., Chatillon, M. & Schupack, H. (1985). Phonetic Speech Perception Deficits in Dyslexia. *Journal of Speech and Hearing Research, 28(4)*, 480-486.

Locke, J. L. & Scott, K. K. (1979). Phonetically mediated recall in the phonetically disordered child. *Journal of Communication Disorders, 12*, 17-32.

Major, E. M. & Bernhardt, B. H. (1998). Metaphonological skills of children with phonological disorders before and after phonological and metaphonological intervention. *International Journal of Language and Communication Disorders, 33*(4), 413-444.

McDowell, K. D., Lonigan, C. J. & Goldstein, H. (2007). Relations among socioeconomic status, age, and predictors of phonological awareness. *Journal of Speech, Language, and Hearing Research, 50(4)*, 1079-1092.

McGrath, L. M., Pennington, B. F., Willcutt, E. G., Boada, R., Shriberg, L. D. & Smith, S. D. (2007). Gene x Environment interactions in speech sound disorder predict language and preliteracy outcomes. *Developmental Psychopathology, 19(4)*, 1047-1072.

McMahon, S., Stassi, K. & Dodd, B. (1998). The relationship between multiple birth children's early phonological skills and later literacy. *Language, Speech, & Hearing Services in Schools, 29(1)*, 11-23.

McNutt, J. C. (1977). Oral sensory and motor behaviors of children with /s/ or /r/ misarticulations. *Journal of Speech and Hearing Research, 20*, 694-703.

Mody, M., Studdert-Kennedy, M. & Brady, S. (1997). Speech perception deficits in poor readers: Auditory processing or phonological coding. *Journal of Experimental Child Psychology, 64*, 199-231.

Nathan, L., Stackhouse, J., Goulandris, N. & Snowling, M. J. (2004). The development of early literacy skills among children with speech difficulties: A test of the "critical age hypothesis". *Journal of Speech, Language, and Hearing Research, 47*, 377-391.

Nicolson, R. I., Fawcett, A. J. & Dean, P. (2001). Developmental dyslexia: the cerebellar deficit hypothesis. *Trends in Neurosciences, 24(9)*, 508-511.

Nijland, L. (2009). Speech perception in children with speech output disorders. *Clinical Linguistics and Phonetics, 23(3)*, 222-239.

Ohde, R. N. & Sharf, D. J. (1988). Perceptual categorization and consistency of synthesized /r-w/ continua by adults, normal children and /r/-misarticulating children. *Journal of Speech and Hearing Research, 31*, 556-568.

Pennington, B. F. & Lefly, D. L. (2001). Early reading development in children at family risk for dyslexia. *Child Development, 72(3)*, 816-833.

Peter, B. & Stoel-Gammon, C. (2008). Central timing deficits in subtypes of primary speech disorders. *Clinical Linguistics & Phonetics, 22(3)*, 171-198.

Preston, J. L. (2008). *Phonological processing and speech production in preschoolers with speech sound disorders.* Dissertation. Syracuse University, Syracuse, NY.

Preston, J. L. & Edwards, M. L. (2007). Phonological processing skills of adolescents with residual speech sound errors. *Language, Speech and Hearing Services in Schools, 38*, 297-308.

Preston, J. L. & Edwards, M. L. (2009). Speed and accuracy of rapid speech output by adolescents with residual speech sound errors including rhotics. *Clinical Linguistics & Phonetics, 23(4)*, 301-318.

Preston, J.L. & Edwards, M.L. (in press). Phonological awareness and types of sound errors in preschoolers with speech sound disorders. *Journal of Speech, Language & Hearing Research.*

Pugh, K. R., Mencl, W. E., Jenner, A. R., Katz, L., Frost, S. J., Lee, J. R., et al. (2000). Functional neuroimaging studies of reading and reading disability (developmental dyslexia). *Mental Retardation and Developmental Disabilities Research Reviews, 6*, 207-213.

Raitano, N. A., Pennington, B. F., Tunick, R. A., Boada, R. & Shriberg, L. D. (2004). Pre-literacy skills of subgroups of children with speech sound disorders. *Journal of Child Psychology and Psychiatry, 45(4)*, 821-835.

Rvachew, S. (2006). Longitudinal Predictors of Implicit Phonological Awareness Skills. *American Journal of Speech-Language Pathology, 15(2)*, 165-176.

Rvachew, S., Chiang, P.-Y. & Evans, N. (2007). Characteristics of speech errors produced by children with and without delayed phonological awareness skills. *Language, Speech and Hearing Services in Schools, 38(1)*, 60-71.

Rvachew, S. & Grawburg, M. (2006). Correlates of phonological awareness in preschoolers with speech sound disorders. *Journal of Speech, Language, & Hearing Research, 49(1)*, 74-87.

Rvachew, S., Nowak, M. & Cloutier, G. (2004). Effect of phonemic perception training on the speech production and phonological awareness skills of children with expressive phonological delay. *American Journal of Speech-Language Pathology, 13(3)*, 250-263.

Scarborough, H. S. (1990). Very early language deficits in dyslexic children. *Child Development, 61*, 1728-1743.

Scarborough, H. S. (2003). Connecting language and literacy to later reading (dis)abilities: Evidence, theory, and practice. In S. B. Neuman & D. K. Dickinson (Eds.), *Handbook of Early Literacy Research* (Vol. 1, pp. 97-110). New York: The Guilford Press.

Scarboarough, H.S. & Brady, S.A. (2002). Towards a common terminology for talking about speech and reading: A glossary of the "phon" words and some related terms. *Journal of Literacy Research, 34(3)*, 299-336.

Schatschneider, C., Fletcher, J. M., Francis, D. J., Carlson, C. D. & Foorman, B. R. (2004). Kindergarten prediction of reading skills: A longitudinal comparative analysis. *Journal of Educational Psychology, 96(2)*, 265-282.

Schuele, C. M. (2004). The impact of developmental speech and language impairments on the acquisition of literacy skills. *Mental Retardation and Developmental Disabilities Research Reviews, 10(3)*, 176-183.

Sénéchal, M., Ouellette, G. & Young, L. (2004). Testing the concurrent and predictive relations among articulation accuracy, speech perception, and phoneme awareness. *Journal of Experimental Child Psychology, 89(3)*, 242-269.

Shriberg, L. D., Austin, D., Lewis, B. A., McSweeny, J. L. & Wilson, D. L. (1997). The percentage of consonants correct (PCC) metric: Extensions and reliability data. *Journal of Speech, Language, and Hearing Research, 40*, 708-722.

Shriberg, L. D. & Kwiatkowski, J. (1982). Phonological disorders III: A procedure for assessing severity of involvement. *Journal of Speech and Hearing Disorders, 47*, 242-256.

Shriberg, L. D., Lewis, B. A., Tomblin, J. B., McSweeny, J. L., Karlsson, H. B. & Scheer, A. R. (2005). Toward diagnostic and phenotype markers for genetically transmitted speech delay. *Journal of Speech, Language, & Hearing Research, 48(4)*, 834-852.

Shriberg, L. D. & Lohmeier, H. L. (2008). *The syllable repetition task: Technical report* Waisman Center, University of Wisconsin-Madison.

Shriberg, L. D., Lohmeier, H. L., McSweeny, J. L. & Kwiatkowski, J. (2006). *A nonword repetition task for speakers with misarticulations: The Syllable Repetition Task.* Paper presented at the Annual Convention of the American Speech Language Hearing Association, Miami, FL.

Smith, A. B., Lambrecht Smith, S., Locke, J. L. & Bennett, J. (2008). A longitudinal study of speech timing in young children later found to have reading disability. *Journal of Speech, Language, and Hearing Research, 51(5)*, 1300-1314.

Smith, A. B., Roberts, J., Lambrecht Smith, S., Locke, J. L. & Bennett, J. (2006). Reduced speaking rate as an early predictor of reading disability. *American Journal of Speech-Language Pathology, 15(3)*, 289-297.

Smith, S. D., Pennington, B. F., Boada, R. & Shriberg, L. D. (2005). Linkage of speech sound disorder to reading disability loci. *Journal of Child Psychology and Psychiatry, 46(10)*, 1057-1066.

Snowling, M. & Stackhouse, J. (1983). Spelling performance of children with developmental dyspraxia. *Developmental Medicine and Child Neurology, 25*, 430-437.

Stackhouse, J. (1982). An investigation of reading and spelling performance in speech disordered children. *British Journal of Disorders of Communication, 17(2)*, 53-60.

Stackhouse, J. & Wells, B. (1997). *Children's speech and literacy difficulties*. London: Whurr Publishers Ltd.

Stein, C. M., Millard, C., Kluge, A., Miscimarra, L. E., Cartier, K. C., Freebairn, L. A., et al. (2006). Speech sound disorder influenced by a locus in 15q14 region. *Behavioral Genetics, 36(6)*, 858-868.

Stein, C. M., Schick, J. H., Gerry Taylor, H., Shriberg, L. D., Millard, C., Kundtz-Kluge, A., et al. (2004). Pleiotropic effects of a chromosome 3 locus on speech-sound disorder and reading. *American Journal of Human Genetics, 74(2)*, 283-297.

Swan, D. & Goswami, U. (1997). Picture naming deficits in developmental dyslexia: The phonological representations hypothesis. *Brain and Language, 56*, 334-353.

Tangel, D. M. & Blachman, B. A. (1992). Effect of phoneme awareness instruction on kindergarten children's invented spelling. *Journal of Reading Behavior, 24(2)*, 233-261.

Thomas, E. M. & Senechal, M. (1998). Articulation and phoneme awareness of 3-year-old children. *Applied Psycholinguistics, 19(3)*, 363-391.

van Kleeck, A., Gillam, R. B. & McFadden, T. U. (1998). A study of classroom-based phonological awareness training for preschoolers with speech and/or language disorders. *American Journal of Speech-Language Pathology, 7(3)*, 65-76.

Wagner, R. K. & Torgesen, J. K. (1987). The nature of phonological processing and its causal role in the acquisition of reading skills. *Psychological Bulletin, 101(2)*, 192-212.

Watson, B. U. & Miller, T. K. (1993). Auditory perception, phonological processing, and reading ability/disability. *Journal of Speech and Hearing Research, 36(4)*, 850-863.

Wiig, E. H., Secord, W. A. & Semel, E. (2004). *Clinical Evaluation of Language Fundamentals Preschool* (2 ed.). San Antonio, TX: Harcourt/Psych Corp.

Williams, P. & Stackhouse, J. (1998). Diadochokinetic skills: Normal and atypical performance in children aged 3-5 years. *International Journal of Language and Communication Disorders, 33*(Supplement), 481-486.

Williams, P. & Stackhouse, J. (2000). Rate, accuracy and consistency: diadochokinetic performance of young, normally developing children. *Clinical Linguistics & Phonetics, 14(4)*, 267 - 293.

Wolff, P. H., Michel, G. F. & Ovrut, M. (1990). The timing of syllable repetitions in developmental dyslexia. *Journal of Speech and Hearing Research, 33(2)*, 281-289.

In: Speech Disorders: Causes, Treatment and Social Effects
Editor: Alan E. Harrison, pp. 75-96
ISBN: 978-1-60876-213-2

Chapter 3

IMAGING OF BRAIN FUNCTION WITH POSITRON EMISSION TOMOGRAPHY AND ITS ROLE IN APHASIA RESEARCH

Wolf-Dieter Heiss*

Max Planck Institute for Neurological Research, Cologne, Germany

ABSTRACT

Positron Emission Tomography (PET) is at present the only method affording three-dimensional regional quantitation of various physiological, functional and molecular variables in man. Making use of tracers labelled with short lived positron emitting radio-nuclides and coincidence detection of annihilation radiation state of the art technology and advanced computing systems permit quantitative imaging of voluminous organs within one session. By 3-D data acquisition the distribution of small tracer amounts in the brain can be measured with a spatial resolution of down to 2 mm and values of various metabolic, functional and molecular parameters can be calculated applying kinetic and parametric analysis. Over the last 30 years PET has gained importance as a clinical diagnostic procedure yielding information on pathophysiologic mechanisms in various brain diseases. This method has also been used extensively as a tool of functional neuroanatomy when changes of metabolic or perfusional patterns were studied during various stimulations or task performances in healthy subjects or patients with localized brain lesions.

This approach was especially successful in the study of language, which as a complex brain function is based on the interplay of a distributed network in which partial functions are executed in various centres, which are hierarchically organized and lateralized into the dominant hemisphere. Following local brain lesions different language domains are impaired causing the various types of aphasia. Changes in the interactions within the functional network of language are important for the type of aphasia and for the capacity for recovery, e.g. after stroke. In this context, studies of activation patterns during speech tasks in the course after stroke could be used to predict extent of recovery, could demonstrate effects of supportive therapy and may be helpful in

* Corresponding author: Prof. Dr. W.-D. Heiss Max Planck Institute for Neurological Research Gleueler Str. 50 50931 Köln Tel: 49-221-4726-220 Fax: 49-221-4726-349 e-mail: wdh@nf.mpg.de

the development of procedures, e.g. cortical stimulation, for suppression of interfering or for enhancing compensatory effects in rehabilitation.

INTRODUCTION

The utilization of biological probes labelled with short lived radioisotopes makes positron emission tomography (PET) a powerful tool to image function, blood flow, metabolism, transmitter activity, receptor distribution, enzymatic activity, gene expression and other molecular variables in the brain. The high sensitivity allows PET to measure concentrations of molecules in the nano- or picomolar range without affecting the biochemical system being investigated. The wide versatility has made PET an important tool for experimental and clinical neuroscience. PET also played a pioneering role in analyzing the response of brain structures to sensory, motor and cognitive stimulations and thereby providing an insight into the functional organization of the intact brain and the compensatory mechanisms to lesions and diseases. In this context PET identified the various components of the functional network involved in speech perception and production and visualized the effect of damage of eloquent areas on activation patterns, which were also useful for predicting recovery and treatment effects in aphasia.

A SHORT HISTORY OF PET

Positron emission tomography is based on a group of artificial, cyclotron-produced radionuclides (e.g. ^{15}O, ^{11}C, ^{13}N, ^{18}F) with short half-lives and chemical properties permitting labelling of tracers relevant in biology and medicine. Therefore, compounds labelled with these radionuclides have been of interest for a long time, but received special attention when Ter Pogossian et al [1,2] performed the first quantitative measurements of regional cerebral blood flow (rCBF) and regional cerebral oxygen consumption ($rCMRO_2$). Positron-emitting radionuclides are characterized by an unique decay scheme: A positron is emitted from a labelled probe molecule, losing energy by collision with electrons in the tissue until within a very short distance (< 2 mm) it annihilates with one of these electrons. This annihilation converts the mass of the electron and positron into energy which is liberated in the form of two 511-keV gamma rays which are emitted in opposite direction. These gamma rays have sufficient energy to escape the body and can be detected by external detectors connected in and thresholded for "coincidence". By this "coincidence detection" the line along which the annihilation (and therefore the positron emission) took place can be determined. By combining lines of response from many different angles data can be reconstructed into cross-sectional images using mathematical algorithms. For the reconstruction of the distribution of a positron emitting radionuclide in a transverse section filtered back projection [3,4] was developed. This formed the basis for the production of the first PET camera [5], an hexagonal array consisting of 64NaI crystals with photomultipliers and electronics connected in coincidence arrays. The first commercial one-ring camera, the ECAT II became available in 1978 [6] and was distributed to a considerable number of institutions interested in transferring the principle of quantitative tissue autoradiography for blood flow [7] and metabolism [8] to human brain research. Since the first proto-types (review in) [9] the technological advances of PET have been impressive (review) [10]: Multiring cameras permitted simultaneous data acquisition from several brain slices and also allowed limited reconstruction in the axial direction. [11] New detector material (Bismuthgermanate, BGO, Lutetium orthosilicate, LSO) improved light yield and deadtime, new technology (segmented blocks of BGO or LSO detectors coupled to 4 photo multipliers, [12] or recently to avalanche photo diodes (APD) improved spatial resolution and permitted investigations of the whole brain in 3 dimensions with a spatial resolution of 2.5 to 5 mm. [13, 14] However, for a definite anatomic assignment of functional or metabolic values still coregistration to imaging modalities with high resolution of morphology, e.g. MRI, is necessary.

PET Scanners collect data by recording the coincidence combinations between opposing detectors. In order to increase counting efficiency the one-to-one coincidence coupling was soon replaced by a fan beam response from one detector to an array of opposing detectors in the image plane (ECAT II, [6] and with neighbouring rings for acquisition of inter-ring transversal images (e.g. PC-384, 4 rings for 7 slices,[11]). In modern PET scanners multiple rings of detectors allow simultaneous collection of multiple planes of images (e.g. ECAT EXACT HR, 47 slices from 24 rings,[13]). The sensitivity of scanners was further increased by 3 D data acquisition by which all gamma-ray pairs which intersect the PET scanner within a predefined response time are collected and used for reconstruction. Thereby the lines of response are tremendously increased – for the ECAT EXACT HR with nearly 20000 BGO detectors to many millions, for the HRRT with close to 120000 LSO elements to 4.486 x 10^9 possible lines of LORs [14] – and the demands for computing power are accordingly high.

However, also by further increasing the number of detectors spatial resolution attainable with PET is limited. [10] The 180° emission of 511 keV gamma rays is not exact and this deviation impairs the exact localization of an annihilation event by 2 mm for a usual PET system. Before interacting with an electron the positron travels some distance, and the range depends on the energy with which the positron is emitted. The resulting degradation of spatial resolution is between 0.4 (^{18}F) and 1.5 mm (^{15}O). Fortunately, these errors are not additive but convolved together, and the resulting resolution limit is close to 2 mm, as it is already realized in high resolution tomographs for experimental [15] and human applications. [16] However, due to restrictions of injected doses of isotopes, the limited sensitivity (2 – 5 %), the high scatter fraction (40 – 50 %) and the resulting high signal to noise ratio requesting smoothing of data the principally possible spatial resolution can usually not be attained in PET studies

Data Correction and Image Reconstruction

The unmatched capacity of PET is that images can be fully quantitative with a linear relationship between the tissue-concentration of the tracer and the measured counts. In order to utilise this quantifying power a number of corrections must be applied. The most important is attenuation correction caused by the tissue between annihilation event and detector, which can be measured by external positron-emitting sources rotating around the head or calculated from contours of the head and known attenuation coefficients of brain tissue and skull at 511 keV. The coincidence events detected in a PET camera are contaminated by accidental or random coincidences, when two unselected gamma rays activate detectors within the coincidence timing window, and scattered events, when one or both gamma rays are deviated on their way out of the head. Both errors can be measured and are corrected in the recorded data. Further corrections are necessary for different efficiency of the detectors and for count-rate dependent losses due to dead-time of detectors and electronics. [17]

Image reconstruction converts the events detected by the PET scanner into tomographic images of the brain representing the distribution of the tracer. The images are reconstructed from the new data after the correction factors have been applied. Cross-calibration to a source of known concentration allows expressing regional radioactivity in absolute values. In small structures this quantitation is impaired by the partial volume effect due to the limitation in spatial resolution, which can be corrected by coregistration to MRI.

The data set for image reconstruction consists of the projection data for a detector ring as represented in a sinogram, a 2 D matric, where the vertical axis represents the angle of the projection line and the horizontal line represents the displacement of the projection line from the centre of the field of view. From this sinogram cross-sectional images are reconstructed using filtered backprojection [18] applying a spatially invariant filter to the projection data and distributing the counts from a sinogram element along the line in image space it represents. Filtered back projection can be modified for 3 D data sets. [19] In state-of-the-art high resolution scanners iterative methods are applied, which use maximation and minimation criteria to calculate images with the best matches for the measured projection data (Fourier rebinning-FORE-combined with ordered-subsets expectation-maximization – OSEM [20, 19, 21]), but require large computing power [22]).

Parameters for Activation Studies

Functional brain imaging is based on the relationship between changes in neuronal activity and changes in blood flow and metabolism of that region. Compared to other tissue, blood flow and metabolism of the brain, especially the gray matter is very high at rest and metabolic changes during activation are small and for cognitive tasks often less than 5 % of the control condition. [23] Whereas many studies demonstrated a linear relationship between neuronal activity and regional cerebral blood flow (rCBF) (e.g. [24, 25]), these changes in blood flow are not paralleled by appropriate increases in regional cerebral metabolic rate for oxygen ($rCMRO_2$)[26]). This discrepancy results in changes of the local concentration of oxygen in the microcirculation, giving rise to the BOLD (blood oxygen level dependent) signal [27] used in functional magnetic resonance imaging (fMRI). Changes in glucose utilization (CMRGlc) exceed the increase in oxygen consumption. [26] The increase of glycolysis during activation is not only due to the altered spiking activity of neurons, but also affected by synaptic activity as reflected by local field potentials; [28] for excitatory synaptic transmission this increased demand for glucose was attributed to stimulated metabolism of astrocytes necessary for clearance of glutamate from the synapse. [29]

PET measures quantitatively rCBF and rCMRGl at rest and the changes due to functional activation, whereas fMRI observes relative changes in blood oxygenation levels. Regional changes of blood flow due to functional activity were measured with the 2 dimensional inert gas clearance methods using ^{199}Xe (review in [30]). With the introduction of PET it became possible to apply the quantitative autoradiographic deoxyglucose technique [8] to regional measurement of glucose metabolism using ^{18}Fluor-deoxyglucose (FDG). [31] FDG is actively transported into the brain and metabolized by hexokinase to FDG-6-phosphat similarly to glucose. Further steps in the metabolic pathway are blocked by the ^{18}F labelling on position 2, and the rate of the transport and the first metabolic step can be described by a 3-compartment model consisting of plasma pool, FDG in tissue and FDG-6 ph concentration connected by kinetic constants for transport to and into vs out of the brain and phosphorylation / dephosphorylation of the compound. Quantitative determinations of rCMRGl require sequential brain scanning and arterial (or arterialised venous) blood sampling and therefore often relative regional changes of FDG uptake are used in functional activation studies. For reaching the balance between accumulation, trapping and clearing of nonmetabolized FDG 30 min are required, and usually 20 – 30 min are used for image acquisition. Therefore, repeat or rapid studies of functional states are not feasible, and due to the half-life of ^{18}F (110 min) resting and activation studies are usually performed on different days. With the FDG method the first functional studies were performed in the early 80s with visual stimulation. [32]

The strategy to measure blood flow with PET adopted the autoradiographic technique. [33] This required the intravenous injection of a freely diffusible tracer, e.g. $H_2{}^{15}O$, and integration of the activity in the brain by PET over 1 min. [34] The short half-life of ^{15}O (123 sec) allows sufficient tracer to be administered to obtain good counting statistics within this short measuring times with acceptable radiation dose to the subject. Also, repeat measurements of blood flow can be performed every 10 – 15 min permitting follow-up of different activation states in one session. Quantification is straight forward since $H_2{}^{15}O$ accumulates in the brain in a linear fashion with respect to blood flow; usually arterial blood sampling is avoided and regional changes relative to whole brain activity are used for functional studies. [35] $H_2{}^{15}O$-PET assesses the signal from the brain tissue, whereas the BOLD signal for fMRI arises predominantly from blood in draining venules a few millimetres away from the tissue compartment in which neural activity takes place. [36]

Performance and Analysis of Functional Studies

In brain activation studies rCBF or metabolism is measured during the performance of a task and the results are compared with control measurements in order to identify the brain regions involved in the task (Figure 1). The control state should include the same sensorimotor and cognitive activities as the task, except the specific process being investigated. In studies of complex cognitive functions subjects may perform sequential tasks of increasing complexity; each experimental state is compared with the preceding one, so that successive differences reveal brain areas that were recruited serially. For the determination of task related activation subtraction of the "at rest" image from the "task" image has been the preferential method in the beginning, when quantitative metabolic or flow images were used [32, 34]. In order to avoid arterial blood sampling, this approach was replaced by semiquantitative or relative procedures, in which control and task images are normalized to eliminate the effect of global fluctuations. Thus multiple studies can be compared by normalizing each separate study to the same total radioactivity in the brain. [37] A statistical test is then applied to the difference image to determine which changes are statistically significant.

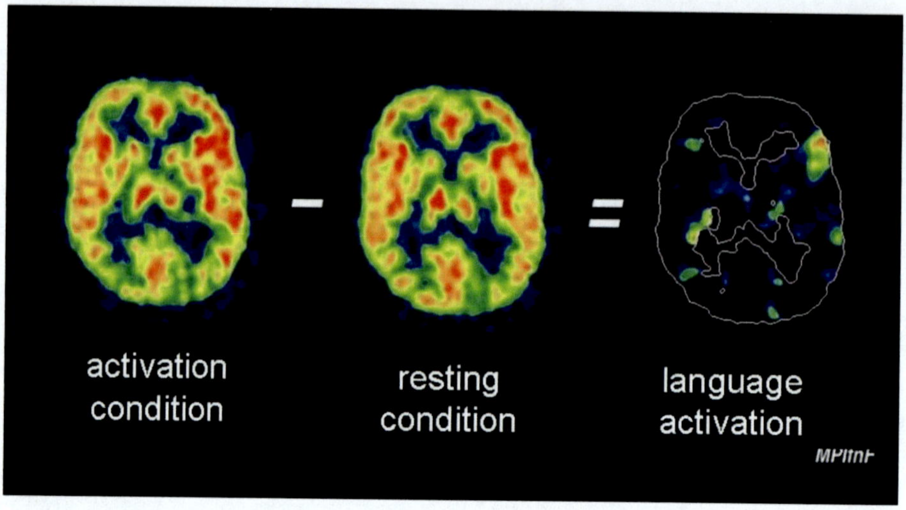

Figure 1. Localization of brain function by activation studies: the resting condition is subtracted from the activation condition.

Anatomical localization of task related changes can be obtained by stereotactic methods: For that purpose the line joining the anterior and posterior commissures of the brain (AP-PC line) is used as a reference for a common coordinate system in both, the PET and the images from a stereotactic brain atlas. [38] Additionally, PET images can be matched to MR images in individual subjects and these can be transformed onto a common anatomical brain representation. [39] For this purpose the images from different persons must be scaled to a common brain size, using linear or, to account for local variations in brain geometry, nonlinear scaling factors. [40] These complex procedures permit the identification of brain structures involved in various tasks, and form the basis for averaging responses in groups of patients, where summed subtraction images show an improved contrast of the local response. With the increased sensitivity of 3 D PET acquisition many runs with different tasks can be done in each individual with relatively low doses [10] which allow the examination of differences in information processing of different subjects, and permits longitudinal studies and investigation of patients with altered brain morphology.

Difference images are noisy and contain signals which might be relevant and irrelevant for the respective task performance. Therefore image analysis strategies are required to select the relevant information. One approach is to place regions of interest within the difference images to test specific hypotheses about areas affected by the specific task. This approach is based on the knowledge how the brain is organized and will miss additional relevant activation sites. It still has great value in the analysis of activation patterns in patients with brain lesions, e.g. strokes or tumors. An alternative approach more open to generating new hypotheses on localization of brain function is the determination of statistically significant responses regardless of their location or magnitude. With a voxel-based assessment PET activation studies were evaluated by change distribution analysis, [41] which provided a mathematical proof for the subtraction paradigm. Most functional imaging studies are now analysed with some form of statistical parametric mapping, a procedure referring to the construction of spatially extended statistical processes to test a hypothesis about involvement of brain regions in particular functions. [42] Statistical parametric maps (SPMs) are images whose voxels are, under a null hypothesis, distributed according to a statistical probability density function. [43] Under the assumption of equivalence of activity (achieved by normalization of data) between resting and task related scans SPMs test defined null hypotheses and yield images of the significance of blood flow change. The simplest tests of significance are t-tests based on repeated measurements, but more sensitive and general approaches use analysis of variance (ANOVA) or analysis of covariance (ANCOVA), which removes the confounding effects of global CBF differences. The ANCOVA generates adjusted mean rCBF values for each experimental and control condition and an associated error variance at each voxel in the data set. These estimates are used to compute statistics for each voxel, and for each comparison of tasks or conditions of interest. This analytical procedure has a high power to identify specialized areas, and to demonstrate interactions among various regions in distributed systems by functional connectivity. Detailed descriptions of methodology, applications and results can be found in the extensive literature.[44]

Limitations for PET Activation Studies

The serious limitation for PET activation studies is radiation exposure, which restricts the number of repeat studies especially in healthy volunteers despite 3D data acquisition and dose fractionation. The complexity of PET requiring a cyclotron for production of short lived isotopes and radio-chemistry for tracer preparation at the site of the scanner further impedes a broad application of this technology for cognitive studies. Therefore, PET activation studies were widely replaced by fMRI which is now the routine for multitask cognitive brain mapping. However, PET's role in this field is not only of historical interest, since it remains the gold standard for the quantification of physiological variables. PET can be used to investigate language production without articulation-related artifacts and – compared to MRI – is a relatively silent technique. It is also equally sensitive to signal throughout the brain, is not affected by inhomogeneities due to air-bone-tissue interfaces and does not – as echo-planar-imaging for fMRI – result in geometric distortion. The wider ring of PET scanners usually does not cause claustrophobia. Additionally, only PET permits to image changes in neurotransmitter and neuromodulator release and their involvement in the performance of complex cognitive tasks and behaviour [45] and the combination of activation studies with other interactions, e.g. transcranial magnetic stimulation. [46]

Functional Activation in Healthy Subjects

Using radiotracer methods a tremendous number of functional studies were performed demonstrating activations in specific brain regions and inter-connected networks (reviews in [47, 48, 49]). In the following only a few examples can be given in which PET was leading for the analysis of functional activation patterns.

Visual System

The first functional mapping studies were performed in the visual system [32] in which increased regional metabolic rates for glucose were demonstrated in relation to intensity and complexity of the stimuli and involvement of visual association cortex was observed with complex interpretation. Topographic representation of different areas of the retina with presentation of central vision near the occipital pole could be shown. [50] In a complex analysis of varying successive visual stimuli Zeki et al (1991) [51] could localize the perception of motion on the convexity of the hemisphere at the junction of the temporal and occipital cortex and the perception of colour to the fusiform gyrus in the inferior part of the occipital gyrus. Matching of faces activated a region of the occipito-temporal cortex while spatial locations were represented in the lateral superior parietal cortex. [52]

Auditory System

Activation of the temporal cortex occurs with a wide variety of auditory stimuli, but distinguishing between two tunes depended on the analysis strategy, where musically naive subjects had greater activation of the right fronto-temporal region and musically sophisticated subjects had greater activations of the left temporal cortex. [53] The characteristics of the auditory stimulus affected the rCBF response in the primary auditory cortex, more complex stimuli including syllables and phonetic discrimination tasks activated additional areas required for further processing, on the superior temporal gyrus bilaterally, the left Broca's area and a superior parietal area. [54]

Motor and Somatosensory Activation

During motor tasks both the pre-central and post-central cortices are activated reflecting the sensory control of movements, [55, 56] but also the premotor cortex is involved in simple and more complex movements of the contralateral arm. Additionally, cerebellar as well as basal ganglia activations are observed. During complex movements of the upper limbs, especially the fingers and the eyes, also activation of the supplementary motor area was detected. [56] More complex tasks – motor planning and learning – involved additional areas in the premotor and prefrontal cortex as well as the superior parietal association cortex. [57] Responses to sensorimotor stimulation of the contralateral hand, face and foot correspond to the somatotopic organization of the primary sensory cortex, [58] but also the supplementary motor area and the cerebellum receive sensory input. The response of the primary cortical area can be modulated by the attentive behaviour of the subject. [59] Brain processes involved in pain activate the thalamus and anterior cingulate, which is attributed to the emotional and attentional components of pain perception. [60]

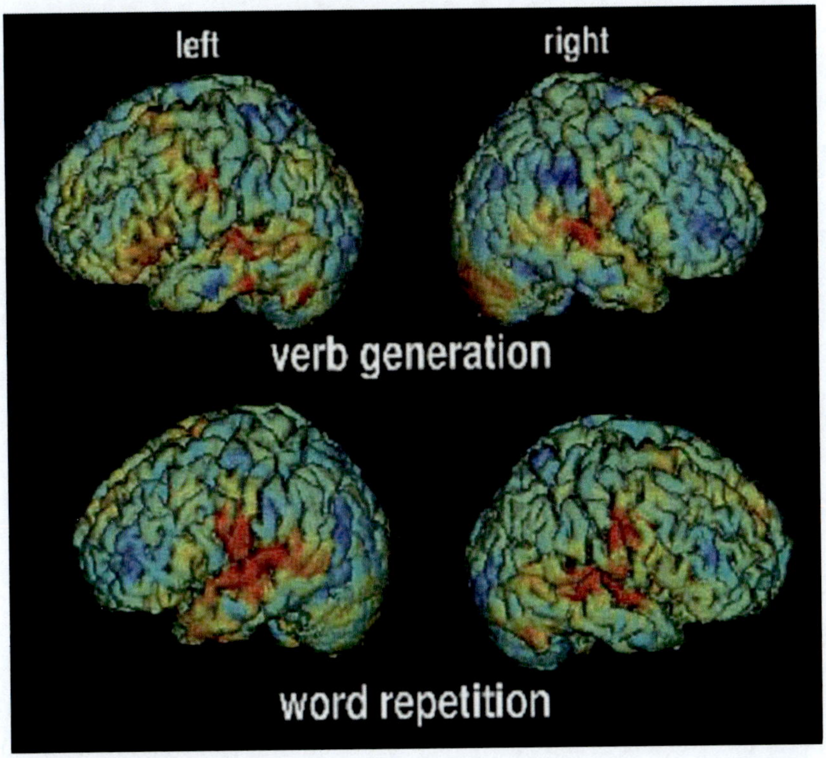

Figure 2. Cortical areas activated by verb generation and word repetition.

Language

PET studies were designed to investigate specific aspects of language processing and speech production. Processing of single words depended on the form of presentation (viewing or listening) and the type of response required (reading or repeating or generating verbs related to a noun). In successive tasks with increasing processing requirements Petersen et al [61] could demonstrate that visual presentation of words activated the primary and extrastriate occipital cortex, listening to words activated the superior temporal cortex bilaterally and the left temporoparietal cortex. Saying nouns activated the primary sensori-motor mouth area, supplementary motor area and left inferior frontal structures (Broca's area) (Figure. 2). The semantic task of generating an appropriate verb activated the left anterior prefrontal and cingulated cortex. Thus, different ways of stimulus presentation involved different primary and association areas, while output and semantic processing activated similar areas regardless of the type of stimulation. Based on additional studies with complex series of stimuli and processing tasks Price [62] has formulated a schematic model of language perception and speech production involving a complex connected network distributed over the whole brain. Further studies including repetitive transcranial magnetic simulation (rTMS) have revealed the influence of transcallosal inhibition for the development of left hemispheric dominance for speech and of the role of the left superior temporal gyrus (Wernicke region) for language interpretation. [46, 63]

Cognition and Memory

PET activation studies have also been performed to study higher cortical functions, as attention, mental imagery and memory (review in [43, 47, 64, 65]) but due to the complex design of these experiments and the necessity of multiple tasks requiring repeated injections of radioactive tracers they are the domain of fMRI. However, PET has also pioneered this field with the first localization of attention to the cingulated cortex [66] and of memory functions to the dorsolateral frontal cortex [67, 68] and the hippocampus. [69] It must be stressed that PET permits to study the effects of various drugs on regional blood flow during memory-tasks, where the effect on serotoninergic nuclei (parahippocampal gyrus) and on dopaminergic areas (dorsolateral prefrontal cortex) could be visualized. [70] In recent experiments even the involvement of synaptic transmission, e.g. in the dopaminergic system, could be directly investigated. [45]

Activation Patterns in Brain Disease

Functional recovery after focal brain lesions is dependent on the adaptive plasticity of the cerebral cortex and of non-affected elements of the functional networks. After cortical injury the adjacent spared cortical tissue as well as more remote areas are altered resulting in changes in both excitatory and inhibitory neurotransmission involved in functional reorganization. One consequence of cortical lesions is reduced collateral and transcallosal inhibition, which is expressed in activation of larger and even contralateral cortical areas during task performance, that are not involved in healthy volunteers. These activation patterns change in the course after a lesion and are related to recovery. Changes in activation patterns and their relationship to recovery were repeatedly studied after ischemic stroke. Due to its outstanding significance for clinical rehabilitation the investigation of motor systems employing active motor tasks has been the focus of several functional imaging studies of post-stroke patients, [71] reviews in [72, 73]. At the site of the injury, cortical responsiveness is reduced, but it increases over time related to the extent of recovery. The reorganisation of central nervous system elements is expressed in increased activity in brain regions distant from the lesion, in an increased activity in the contralateral hemisphere, and in somatotopic shifts within intact cortical regions. How much functional neuroimaging can guide restorative interventions and yield insight into mechanisms of treatment effects is still a matter of debate[74].

Poststroke Aphasia

Aphasia is a severely incapacitating symptom of stroke and is a main cause of functional disturbance. Estimates suggest that more than 20 % of patients suffering a stroke develop aphasia, 10 – 18 % of survivors are left with a persistent speech deficit. [75] Most patients with aphasia due to acute non-progressive brain damage, such as in the case of stroke or head injury, show some degree of recovery of language function during the days, months, or even years following the initial insult. The recuperation is variable, ranging from the hardly noticeable improvement of auditory comprehension of the global aphasia to the apparently complete recovery of the patient with mild fluent aphasia due to small subcortical stroke. It is also well known that improvement can be observed not only in patients submitted to language rehabilitation but also in cases that have not undergone any specific treatment.

Disturbance of Regional Metabolism and Flow versus Severity and Persistence of Language Deficit

Studies of glucose metabolism after stroke [76] have shown metabolic disturbances in the ipsilateral hemisphere caused by the lesion and contralateral hemisphere caused by functional deactivation (diaschisis). [77] Most studies have been performed in right-handed individuals with language dominance in the left hemisphere. The left temporo-parietal region, in particular the angular gyrus, supramarginal gyrus, and lateral and transverse superior temporal gyrus are the most frequently and consistently impaired, and the degree of impairment is related to the severity of aphasia. [78,79] In contrast, metabolic impairment in subcortical structures is related mainly to language fluency and other behavioural aspects, but not to aphasia severity. [80] In patients with aphasia attributable to purely subcortical strokes deactivation of temporo-parietal cortex is regularly found, which is probably responsible for the aphasic symptoms. [81]

Recovery of metabolism in both hemispheres was correlated with recovery of aphasia. One specific region crucial for recovery of language perception has been found in the left temporo-parietal cortex [79, 82] and metabolic disturbance in these areas is related to outcome. [83] Investigations in the subacute state after stroke showed a highly significant correlation with language performance assessed at follow-up after 2 years. [84] The receptive language disorder correlated with rCMRGlc in the left temporal cortex and word fluency correlated with rCMRGlc in the left prefrontal cortex. These results indicate that the functional disturbance as measured by rCMRGlc in speech-relevant brain regions early after stroke is predictive of the eventual outcome of aphasia. However, not only functional deactivation (diaschisis) but also neuronal loss may contribute to metabolic and perfusional changes in the neighbourhood of the infarct, and the condition of the surrounding tissue may affect the recovery of individual patients. In this context it is important to note that early reperfusion to specific areas is able to restore disturbed function, as demonstrated for recovery of naming by reperfusion to the key areas BA37, BA 44/45 (Broca) and BA 22 (Wernicke). [85]

Changes in Activation Patterns versus Recovery of Language Function

On this basis it is not surprising that, in patients with a poor outcome of poststroke aphasia, metabolism in the hemisphere outside the infarct was significantly less than in those with good language recovery, indicating significant cell loss caused by the ischemic episode outside the ischemic core. [86] In addition, the functionality of the network was reduced in patients with an eventual poor outcome; during task performance, patients with an eventual good recovery predominantly activated structures in the ipsilateral hemisphere. It must be kept in mind that aphasia symptoms – and consequently also activation patterns – improve with restoration of regional blood flow. [87]

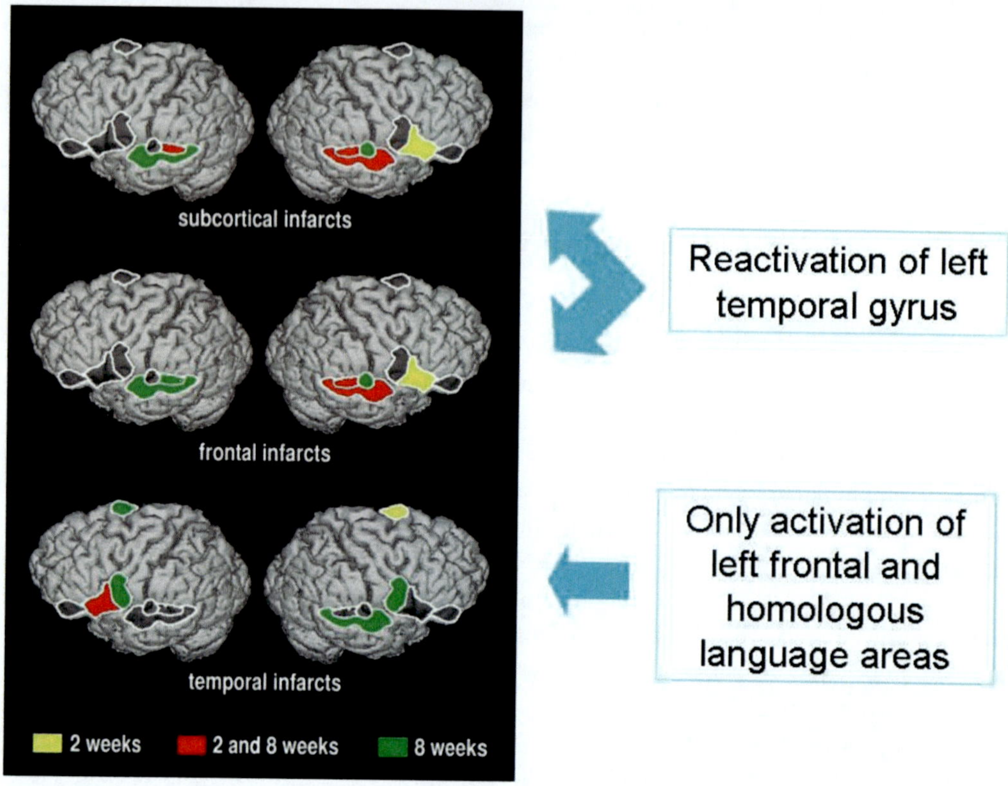

Figure 3. Activation patterns in patients with left hemispheric stroke 2 and 8 weeks after stroke. In the case of subcortical and frontal infarction, the left temporal areas are reactivated correlating to better recovery of language function. From Heiss et al 1999

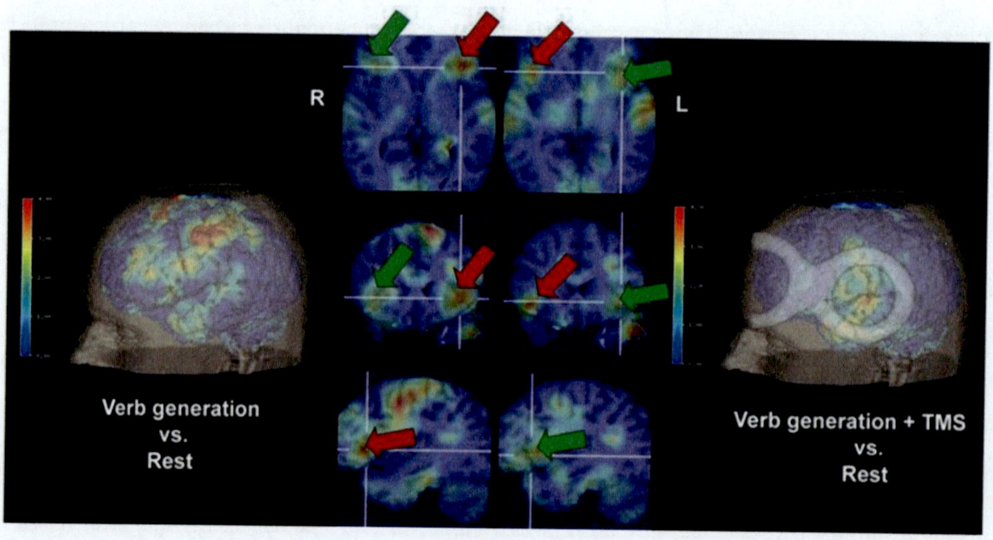

Figure 4. Effect of repetitive transcranial magnetic stimulation on activation pattern by verb generation. Activation pattern (A) and coil position (D) shown in 3 D rendering. Images in 3 dimensions (B) show activation of left inferior frontal gyrus during verb generation (red arrows), images (C) clearly show the decreased activation on the left (green arrow) and increased activity on the right side (red arrows) during rTMS interference. Modified from Thiel et al 2006

One of the central issues of aphasia research is the question why recovery from aphasia is taking place and what the responsible mechanisms for this recovery are. Converging evidence from clinical studies and neural imaging studies of aphasic patients suggest that primary candidates for recovery in right-handed, left-hemisphere language dominant patients include undamaged portions of the language network in the left hemisphere and – to a lesser extent – homologous right-hemisphere areas. [88] Since the language network is not confined to the dominant hemisphere, the role of the right hemisphere after infarcts in the left hemisphere has been addressed in several studies. Generally, more right hemispheric activations were seen in the subacute phase of an infarct with language activation than in normals with the same tasks. [89-92] Despite such responses in the right superior temporal gyrus especially in fluent Wernicke's patients [90, 93] and in the inferior frontal gyrus, [89] efficient restoration of language is usually achieved only if left temporal areas are preserved and can be reintegrated into the functional network. [94] Only the basic function of mere word repetition appears to be sufficiently supported by sole right hemisphere activation. [95] Based on their study in chronic non-fluent aphasia patients Belin et al [96] suggested that the increased activation within the right hemisphere may be a marker of failed or faulty recovery attempts in the sense of maladaptive plasticity or the breakdown of normal interhemispheric control within the distributed neural network. Language recovery in the months immediately after aphasia onset was associated with regression of functional depression (diaschisis) in structurally unaffected regions, in particular in the right hemisphere. [76, 92] Right hemispheric activations after left frontal or temporal parietal damage are not related to the level of recovery [97] but may reflect transcallosal inhibition as a maladaptive neuronal reorganization rather than functional compensation. [91] Despite the brain recruits right hemispheric regions for speech processing when the left-hemispheric centres are impaired, [98] outcome studies reveal that this strategy is significantly less effective than repair of the speech-relevant network in adults. [99]

Changes in the activation pattern induced by repeating words in the course after ischemic stroke were related to recovery from poststroke aphasia. [100] Repeating words activated blood flow in 10 normal controls by more than 10 % relative to resting condition in both upper temporal gyri, by 5 – 10 % in planum temporale and Heschl gyrus of both sides and in the lower part of the central gyrus of the left side, and by less than 5 % in the left Broca area. This test procedure was applied to 23 patients with aphasia of different types. Morphological defects were defined on MRI/CT, and the patients were grouped according to the site of the lesion. Activation PET studies were performed in the subacute stage approximately 2 weeks after the stroke and repeated 6 weeks later. On matched MRIs regions of interest were defined in 14 identified structures of the bilateral language-related network.

The three groups of aphasic patients showed different patterns for activation in the acute and chronic phase, and their improvement was different: Whereas subcortical and frontal infarcts improved considerably in several tests, temporal infarcts showed only little improvement. These differences in improvement of speech deficits were reflected in different patterns of activation in the course after stroke (Figure 3): The subcortical and frontal groups improved substantially and activated the right inferior frontal gyrus and the right superior temporal gyrus (STG) at baseline and regained regional left STG activation at follow-up. The temporal group improved only in word comprehension; it activated the left Broca area and supplementary motor areas at baseline and the precentral gyrus bilaterally as well as the right STG at follow-up, but could not reactivate the left STG. Similar reactivation patterns were observed in smaller groups of patients. [101, 102] A recent study with repeated fMRI and parallel language testing from the acute to the chronic stage after stroke demonstrated a similar pattern. [92] All 14 patients recovered clinically as shown by a set of aphasia tests. In the acute phase (mean: 1.8 days post stroke) group analysis showed little early activation of non-infarcted left-hemispheric language structures, while in the subacute phase (12.1 days post stroke) a large increase of activation in the bilateral language network, with a peak in the right Broca-homologue occured. In the chronic phase (1321 days post stroke) a normalization of activation with re-shift to left-hemispheric areas was observed. This reorganization with recruitment of homologue language zones correlated with improvement, the normalization possibly reflected recovery and consolidation of the language system.

Effect of Treatment in Poststroke Aphasia

Whereas the effect of physiotherapy on improvement of sensorimotor deficits is unchallenged, the efficiency of speech therapy is still controversial, with several randomized controlled trials yielding no difference in outcome between treated and untreated groups. [103, 104] Many trials were undertaken to enhance the recovery from aphasia with adjuvant pharmacotherapy, but again, only a few studies demonstrated efficacy: In a double-blind placebo-controlled study Walker-Batson et al [105] described a significantly increased gain in score in patients treated with dextroamphetamine before speech therapy sessions compared to the placebo group, but the difference was not significant at 6 months follow-up. Similarly, donepezil improved the effect of speech therapy only temporarily. [106] A large Cochrane Review [107] identified piracetam as the only drug with a significant effect on recovery of language, which was also observed in a large multicentre trial. [108] The effect of piracetam is also reflected in altered activation patterns. In a placebo controlled double blind study [109] (2 x 2.4 g piracetam vs placebo) the piracetam group did significantly better especially in subtests reflecting the ability for spontaneous speech. These differences in improvement were also reflected in differences in the achieved activation patterns: In the piracetam group increase in activation was significantly higher in the left transverse temporal gyrus, the left triangular part of the inferior frontal gyrus, and the left posterior temporal gyrus after the treatment period compared with the initial measures. It might be concluded that piracetam as an adjuvant to speech therapy improves recovery of various language functions and that this effect is accompanied by task-related flow activation in eloquent areas of the left hemisphere. Other imaging studies with individualized aphasia treatment in small numbers of patients did not show conclusive changes in fMRI activation patterns (review in [110]).

Combination of Repetitive Transcranial Magnetic Stimulation (rTMS) with Activated Imaging

rTMS is a non-invasive procedure to create electric currents in discrete brain areas [111] which depending on frequency, intensity, and duration can lead to transient increases and decreases in excitability of the affected cortex. Increases in relative cerebral blood volume in contralateral homologous language regions during overt propositional speech fMRI in chronic, non-fluent aphasia patients indicated over-activation of right language homologues. [112] This right hemisphere over-activation may represent a maladaptive strategy, as suggested previously by Belin et al [96] and Rosen et al [88] in their studies with chronic, non-fluent aphasia patients. This over-activation in the right homologous language areas can be interpreted as a result of decreased transcallosal inhibition due to damage of the specialized and lateralized speech areas. [99]

Both types of inhibition – collateral ipsilateral and transcallosal contralateral – can be demonstrated by simultaneous rTMS and PET activation studies. [46] In six normal male volunteers the Broca area, as defined by maximal activation during verb generation in the left inferior frontal gyrus was stimulated by rTMS to interfere with normal language function. During verb generation, rCBF was decreased during rTMS ipsilateral under the coil, but increased ipsilateral outside the coil and in the contralateral homologous area (Figure 4). The effect of rTMS was accompanied by a prolongation of reaction time latencies to verbal stimuli.

The role of activation in the right hemisphere for residual language performance can be investigated by combining rTMS with functional imaging, e.g. PET. [113] Such an approach was used in 11 patients with predominantly non-fluent aphasia 2 weeks after left sided middle cerebral artery infarction. [114] rTMS stimulation sites were selected according to maximum flow activation within left and right inferior frontal gyrus (IFG). Of these patients three activated the left, eight the bilateral inferior frontal gyrus. rTMS (4 Hz for 20 sec.) resulted in increased reaction time latency or error rate in the word generation task in five patients with right IFG activation, indicating essential language function. In a verbal fluency task, these patients had a lower performance than patients with effects of rTMS only over the left IFG, suggesting a less effective compensatory potential of right sided network areas. These results were supported by studies in tumour patients, [115] in which a significant correlation between the laterality index and the performance in a verbal fluency test was observed in the patients without right-positive TMS effect, whereas in patients with a predominant right-positive TMS effect the performance in the verbal fluency test was comparable with that in controls. This result may indicate that in a few patients with left hemispheric brain tumours the slow progression of damage leads to a shift in language function to the right hemisphere which can compensate for the defect on the left side.

Conclusion

The different dynamics of recovery of language function observed in patients after stroke and with tumours in the left hemisphere suggest various mechanisms for compensation of the lesion within the functional network. A hierarchy for effective recovery might be deduced from these data (Figure 4) [116]:

Best, even complete recovery of function can usually only be achieved by the restoration of the original activation pattern within the network of the dominant hemisphere; this is only feasible after small brain damage probably only affecting an area of minor importance permitting functional restitution of the main interconnected components.

If primary functional centres are damaged, reduction of collateral inhibition leads to activation of areas around the lesion; this intrahemispheric compensation involving secondary centres of the ipsilateral network is the basis for incomplete, but often satisfactory improvement of language function.

If ipsilateral network components are severely damaged, reduction of transcallosal inhibition causes activation of contralateral homotopic areas; this interhemispheric compensation involving homotopic contralesional areas contributes to some improvement in function, which is dependent on the extent of the functional shift between the hemispheres, but usually is not as efficient as intrahemispheric compensation. However, in some patients with slowly developing brain damage – and perhaps also an a priori not highly lateralized functional network – the language function can be completely shifted to the right hemisphere, and in these cases speech performance can be preserved or completely recover despite the damage in the left (previously dominant) hemisphere.

It must be shown in larger controlled trials if the blockade of inhibitory interaction by contralateral intact areas with rTMS [117] "increases the ability of the brain to undergo compensatory changes that improve behaviours" [118] and is an effective strategy to improve recovery of language function.

REFERENCES

[1] Ter-Pogossian MM, Eichling JO, Davis DO, Welch MJ, Metzger JM. The determination of regional cerebral blood flow by means of water labeled with radioactive oxygen 15. *Radiology*. 1969;93:31-40

[2] Ter-Pogossian MM, Eichling JO, Davis DO, Welch MJ. The measure in vivo of regional cerebral oxygen utilization by means of oxyhemoglobin labeled with radioactive oxygen - 15. *Journal of Clinical Investigation*. 1970;49:381-391

[3] Cormack AM. Reconstruction of densities from their projections, with applications in radiological physics. *Phys Med Biol*. 1973;18:195-207

[4] Phelps ME, Hoffman EJ, Mullemi NA, Ter-Pogossian MM. Application of annihilation coincidence detection to transaxial reconstruction tomography. *JNuclMed*. 1975;16:210-224

[5] Ter-Pogossian MM, Phelps ME, Hoffman EJ, Mullani NA. A positron emission transaxial tomograph for nuclear imaging (pett). *Radiology*. 1975;114:89-98

[6] Phelps ME, Hoffman EJ, Huang SC, Kuhl DE. Ecat: A new computerized tomographic imaging system for positron-emitting radiopharmaceuticals. *JNuclMed*. 1978;19:635-647

[7] Sakurada O, Kennedy C, Jehle J, Brown JD, Carbin GL, Sokoloff L. Measurement of local cerebral blood flow with iodo(14 c)antipyrine. *AmJPhysiol*. 1978;234:H59-H66

[8] Sokoloff L, Reivich M, Kennedy C, Des Rosiers MH, Patlak CS, Pettigrew KD, Sakurada O, Shinohara M. The (14 c)-deoxyglucose method for the measurement of local cerebral glucose utilization: Theory, procedure, and normal values in the conscious and anesthetized albino rat. *JNeurochem*. 1977;28:897-916

[9] Ter-Pogossian MM. The origins of positron emission tomography. *SeminNuclMed*. 1992;22:140-149

[10] Cherry SR, Phelps ME. Imaging brain function with positron emission tomography. In: Toga AW, Mazziotta JC, eds. *Brain mapping: The methods*. San Diego: Academic Press; 1996.

[11] Eriksson L, Bohm C, Kesselberg M, Blomqvist G, Litton J, Widen L, Bergström M, Ericson K, Greitz T. A four ring positron camera system for emission tomography of the brain. *IEEE Transactions on Nuclear Science*. 1982;29:539-543

[12] Casey ME, Nutt R. A multicrystal two dimensional bgo detector system for positron emission tomography. *IEEE Trans Nucl Sci.* 1986;NS-33:460-463

[13] Wienhard K, Dahlbom M, Eriksson L, Michel C, Bruckbauer T, Pietrzyk U, Heiss WD. The ecat exact hr: Performance of a new high resolution positron scanner. *JComputAssistTomogr.* 1994;18:110-118

[14] Wienhard K, Schmand M, Casey ME, Baker K, Bao J, Eriksson L, Jones WF, Knoess C, Lenox M, Lercher M, Luk P, Michel C, Reed JH, Richerzhagen N, Treffert J, Vollmar S, Young JW, Heiss WD, Nutt R. The ecat hrrt: Performance and first clinical application of the new high resolution research tomograph. *IEEE Transactions on Nuclear Science.* 2002;49:104-110

[15] Cherry SR, Shao Y, Silverman RW, Meadors K, Siegel S, Chatziioannou A, Young JW, Jones WF, Moyers JC, Newport D, Boutefnouchet A, Farquhar TH, Andreaco M, Paulus MJ, Binkley DM, Nutt R, Phelps ME. Micropet: A high-resolution pet scanner for imaging small animals. *IEEE Transactions on Nuclear Science.* 1997;44:1161-1166

[16] de Jong HWAM, van Velden FHP, Kloet RW, Buijs FL, Boellaard R, Lammertsma AA. Performance evaluation of the ecat hrrt: An lso-lyso double layer high resolution, high sensitivity scanner. *PhysMedBiol.* 2007;52:1505-1526

[17] Hoffmann EJ, Guerrero TM, Germano G, al. e. Pet system calibration and corrections for quantitative and spatially accurate images. *IEEE Trans Nucl Sci.* 1989;NS-36:1108-1112

[18] Brooks RA, Di Chiro G. Principles of computer assisted tomography (cat) in radiographic and radioisotopic imaging. *Phys Med Biol.* 1976;21:689-732

[19] Defrise M, Kinahan PE, Townsend DW, Michel C, Sibomana M, Newport D. Exact and approximate rebinning algorithms for 3-d pet data. *IEEE Trans Med Imag.* 1997;16:145-158

[20] Hudson HM, Larkin RS. Accelerated image reconstruction using ordered subsets of projection data. *IEEE Transactions on Medical Imaging.* 1994;13:68-78

[21] Liu X, Comtat C, Michel C, Kinahan P, Defrise M, Townsend D. Comparison of 3-d reconstruction with 3x-osem and with fore + osem for pet. *IEEE Transactions on Medical Imaging.* 2001;20:804-814

[22] Vollmar S, Michel C, Treffert JT, Newport DF, Casey M, Knoess C, Wienhard K, Liu X, Defrise M, Heiss WD. Heinzelcluster: Accelerated reconstruction for fore and osem3d. *Physics in Medicine and Biology.* 2002;47 2651-2658

[23] Clarke DD, Sokoloff L. Circulation and energy metabolism of the brain. In: Siegel G, Agranoff B, Albers RW, Fisher S, eds. *Basic neurochemistry: Molecular, cellular, and medical aspects, 6th ed.* Philadelphia: Lippincott-Raven; 1999:637-669.

[24] Heiss WD, Turnheim M, Vollmer R, Rappelsberger P. Coupling between neuronal activity and focal blood flow in experimental seizures. *ElectroencephclinNeurophysiol.* 1979;47:396-403

[25] Raichle ME. A brief history of human functional brain mapping. In: Toga AW, Mazziotta JC, eds. *Brain mapping: The systems.* San Diego: Academic Press; 2000:33-75.

[26] Fox PT, Raichle ME, Mintun MA, Dence C. Nonoxidative glucose consumption during focal physiologic neural activity. *Science.* 1988;241:462-464

[27] Ogawa S, Lee TM, Kay AR, Tank DW. Brain magnetic resonance imaging with contrast dependent on blood oxygenation. *Proc Natl Acad Sci U S A.* 1990;87:9868-9872

[28] Sharp FR. Relative cerebral glucose uptake of neuronal perikarya and neuropil determined with 2-deoxyglucose in resting and swimming rat. *Brain Res.* 1976;110:127-139

[29] Magistretti PJ, Pellerin L. Cellular bases of brain energy metabolism and their relevance to functional brain imaging: Evidence for a prominent role of astrocytes. *Cereb Cortex*. 1996;6:50-61

[30] Lassen NA, Ingvar DH, Skinhoj E. Brain function and blood flow. *Sci Am*. 1978;239:62-71

[31] Reivich M, Kuhl D, Wolf A, Greenberg J, Phelps M, Ido T, Casella V, Fowler J, Hoffman E, Alavi A, Som P, Sokoloff L. The (18 f)fluorodeoxyglucose method for the measurement of local cerebral glucose utilization in man. *Circulation Research*. 1979;44:127-137

[32] Phelps ME, Kuhl DE, Mazziotta JC. Metabolic mapping of brain's response to visual stimulation: Studies in humans. *Science*. 1981;211:1445-1448

[33] Landau WM, Freygang WH, Jr., Roland LP, Sokoloff L, Kety SS. The local circulation of the living brain; values in the unanesthetized and anesthetized cat. *TransAmNeurolAssoc*. 1955;80:125-129

[34] Herscovitch P, Markham J, Raichle ME. Brain blood flow measured with intravenous h 2 15 o. I. Theory and error analysis. *JNuclMed*. 1983;24:782-789

[35] Fox PT, Mintun MA, Raichle ME, Herscovitch P. A noninvasive approach to quantitative functional brain mapping with h 2 15 o and positron emission tomography. *JCerebBlood Flow Metab*. 1984;4:329-333

[36] Ugurbil K, Toth L, Kim DS. How accurate is magnetic resonance imaging of brain function? *Trends Neurosci*. 2003;26:108-114

[37] Mazziotta JC, Huang SC, Phelps ME, Carson RE, MacDonald NS, Mahoney K. A noninvasive positron computed tomography technique using oxygen-15-labeled-water for the evaluation of neurobehavioral task batteries. *JCerebBlood Flow Metab*. 1985;5:70-78

[38] Talairach J, Tournoux P. *Co-planar stereotaxic atlas of the human brain*. New York: Thieme; 1988.

[39] Seitz RJ, Bohm C, Greitz T, Roland PE, Eriksson L, Blomqvist G, Rosenqvist G, Nordell B. Accuracy and precision of the computerized brain atlas program for localization and quantification in positron emission tomography. *JCerebBlood Flow Metab*. 1990;10:443-457

[40] Friston KJ, Frith CD, Liddle PF, Frackowiak RS. Plastic transformation of pet images. *J Comput Assist Tomogr*. 1991;15:634-639

[41] Fox PT, Mintun MA. Noninvasive functional brain mapping by change-distribution analysis of averaged pet images of h215o tissue activity. *JNuclMed*. 1989;30:141-149

[42] Friston KJ, Frith CD, Liddle PF, Frackowiak RS. Comparing functional (pet) images: The assessment of significant change. *J Cereb Blood Flow Metab*. 1991;11:690-699

[43] Frackowiak RSJ, Friston KJ. Functional neuroanatomy of the human brain: Positron emission tomography - a new neuroanatomical technique. *JAnatomy*. 1994;184:211-225

[44] Friston K, Ashburner J, Kiebel S. *Statistical parametric mapping: The analysis of functional brain images*. Oxford: Elsevier Science & Technology Books; 2007.

[45] Koepp MJ, Gunn RN, Lawrence AD, Cunningham VJ, Dagher A, Jones T, Brooks DJ, Bench CJ, Grasby PM. Evidence for striatal dopamine release during a video game. *Nature*. 1998;393:266-268

[46] Thiel A, Schumacher B, Wienhard K, Gairing S, Kracht LW, Wagner R, Haupt WF, Heiss WD. Direct demonstration of transcallosal disinhibition in language networks. *J CerebBlood Flow Metab*. 2006;26:1122-1127

[47] Herscovitch P. Functional mapping of the human brain. In: Wayner HNJ, Szabo S, Buchanan JW, eds. *Principles of nuclear medicine* Philadelphia: W. B. Saunders 1995:514-531.

[48] Bigler ED, Turkheimer E. *Neuropsychological function and brain imaging*. New York: Plenum; 1989.

[49] Phelps ME. Pet: A biological imaging technique. *NeurochemRes*. 1991;16:929-940

[50] Fox PT, Miezin FM, Allman JM, Van Essen DC, Raichle ME. Retinotopic organization of human visual cortex mapped with positron-emission tomography. *JNeurosci*. 1987;7:913-922

[51] Zeki S, Watson JDG, Lueck CJ, Friston KJ, Kennard C, Frackowiak RSJ. A direct demonstration of functional specialization in human visual cortex. *JNeurosci*. 1991;11:641-649

[52] Haxby JV, Grady CL, Horwitz B, Ungerleider LG, Mishkin M, Carson RE, Herscovitch P, Schapiro MB, Rapoport SI. Dissociation of object and spatial visual processing pathways in human extrastriate cortex. *ProcNatlAcadSciUSA*. 1991;88:1621-1625

[53] Mazziotta JC, Phelps ME, Carson RE, Kuhl DE. Tomographic mapping of human cerebral metabolism: Auditory stimulation. *Neurology*. 1982;32:921-937

[54] Zatorre RJ, Evans AC, Meyer E, Gjedde A. Lateralization of phonetic and pitch discrimination in speech processing. *Science*. 1992;256:846-849

[55] Grafton ST, Woods RP, Mazziotta JC, Phelps ME. Somatotopic mapping of the primary motor cortex in humans: Activation studies with cerebral blood flow and positron emission tomography. *J Neurophysiol*. 1991;66:735-743

[56] Colebatch JG, Deiber MP, Passingham RE, Friston KJ, Frackowiak RSJ. Regional cerebral blood flow during voluntary arm and hand movements in human subjects. *Journal of Neurophysiology*. 1991;65:1392-1401

[57] Seitz RJ, Roland PE. Learning of sequential finger movements in man: A combined kinematic and positron emission tomography (pet) study. *EurJNeurosci*. 1992;4:154-165

[58] Fox PT, Burton H, Raichle ME. Mapping human somatosensory cortex with positron emission tomography. *JNeurosurg*. 1987;67:34-43

[59] Meyer E, Ferguson SSG, Zatorre RJ, Alivisatos B, Marrett S, Evans AC, Hakim AM. Attention modulates somatosensory cerebral blood flow response to vibrotactile stimulation as measured by positron emission tomography. *AnnNeurol*. 1991;29:440-443

[60] Duncan GH, Bushnell MC, Talbot JD, Evans AC, Meyer E, Marrett S. Localization of responses to pain (letter). *Science*. 1992a;255:215 - 216

[61] Petersen SE, Fox PT, Posner MI, Mintun M, Raichle ME. Positron emission tomographic studies of the cortical anatomy of single-word processing. *Nature*. 1988;331:585-589

[62] Price CJ. The anatomy of language: Contributions from functional neuroimaging. *Journal of Anatomy*. 2000;197 Pt 3:335-359

[63] Karbe H, Herholz K, Halber M, Heiss WD. Collateral inhibition of transcallosal activity facilitates functional brain asymmetry. *JCerebBlood Flow Metab*. 1998;18:1157-1161

[64] Cabeza R, Kingstone A. *Handbook of functional neuroimaging of cognition*. London: The MIT Press; 2006.

[65] Law I. Human brain mapping under increasing cognitive complexity using regional cerebral blood flow measurements and positron emission tomography. *Dan Med Bull*. 2007;54:289-305

[66] Pardo JV, Pardo PJ, Janer KW, Raichle ME. The anterior cingulate cortex mediates processing selection in the stroop attentional conflict paradigm. *Proc Natl Acad Sci U S A*. 1990;87:256-259

[67] Petrides M, Alivisatos B, Meyer E, Evans AC. Functional activation of the human frontal cortex during the performance of verbal working memory tasks. *Proc Natl Acad Sci U S A*. 1993;90:878-882

[68] Courtney SM, Ungerleider LG, Keil K, Haxby JV. Object and spatial visual working memory activate separate neural systems in human cortex. *Cereb Cortex*. 1996;6:39-49

[69] Squire LR, Ojemann JG, Miezin FM, Petersen SE, Videen TO, Raichle ME. Activation of the hippocampus in normal humans: A functional anatomical study of memory. *ProcNatlAcadSciUSA*. 1992;89:1837-1841

[70] Grasby PM, Friston KJ, Bench CJ, Frith CD, Paulesu E, Cowen PJ, Liddle PF, Frackowiak RS, Dolan R. The effect of apomorphine and buspirone on regional cerebral blood flow during the performance of a cognitive task-measuring neuromodulatory effects of psychotropic drugs in man. *Eur J Neurosci*. 1992;4:1203-1212

[71] Chollet F, Di Piero V, Wise RJS, Brooks DJ, Dolan RJ, Frackowiak RSJ. The functional anatomy of motor recovery after stroke in humans: A study with positron emission tomography. *AnnNeurol*. 1991;29:63-71

[72] Weiller C. Imaging recovery from stroke. *ExpBrain Res*. 1998;123:13-17

[73] Cramer SC. Repairing the human brain after stroke: I. Mechanisms of spontaneous recovery. *Ann Neurol*. 2008;63:272-287

[74] Cramer SC. Repairing the human brain after stroke. Ii. Restorative therapies. *Ann Neurol*. 2008;63:549-560

[75] Wade DT, Hewer RL, David RM, Enderby PM. Aphasia after stroke: Natural history and associated deficits. *JNeurolNeurosurgPsychiatry*. 1986;49:11-16

[76] Cappa SF, Perani D, Grassi F, Bressi S, Alberoni M, Franceschi M, Bettinardi V, Todde S, Fazio F. A pet follow-up study of recovery after stroke in acute aphasics. *Brain Lang*. 1997;56:55-67

[77] Feeney DM, Baron JC. Diaschisis. *Stroke*. 1986;17:817-830

[78] Metter EJ, Hanson WR, Jackson CA, Kempler D, Van Lancker D, Mazziotta JC, Phelps ME. Temporoparietal cortex in aphasia. Evidence from positron emission tomography. *ArchNeurol*. 1990;47:1235-1238

[79] Karbe H, Herholz K, Szelies B, Pawlik G, Wienhard K, Heiss WD. Regional metabolic correlates of token test results in cortical and subcortical left hemispheric infarction. *Neurology*. 1989;39:1083-1088

[80] Metter EJ, Riege WH, Hanson WR, Jackson CA, Kempler D, Van Lancker D. Subcortical structures in aphasia. An analysis based on (18 f)-fluorodeoxyglucose, positron emission tomography, and computed tomography. *ArchNeurol*. 1988;45:1229-1234

[81] Kumar R, Masih AK, Pardo J. Global aphasia due to thalamic hemorrhage: A case report and review of the literature. *Arch Phys Med Rehabil*. 1996;77:1312-1315

[82] Metter EJ, Kempler D, Jackson CA, Hanson WR, Riege WH, Camras LR, Mazziotta JC, Phelps ME. Cerebellar glucose metabolism in chronic aphasia. *Neurology*. 1987;37:1599-1606

[83] Heiss WD, Emunds HG, Herholz K. Cerebral glucose metabolism as a predictor of rehabilitation after ischemic stroke. *Stroke*. 1993;24:1784-1788

[84] Karbe H, Kessler J, Herholz K, Fink GR, Heiss WD. Long-term prognosis of poststroke aphasia studied with positron emission tomography. *ArchNeurol*. 1995;52:186-190

[85] Hillis AE, Kleinman JT, Newhart M, Heidler-Gary J, Gottesman R, Barker PB, Aldrich E, Llinas R, Wityk R, Chaudhry P. Restoring cerebral blood flow reveals neural regions critical for naming. *J Neurosci.* 2006;26:8069-8073

[86] Heiss WD, Kessler J, Karbe H, Fink GR, Pawlik G. Cerebral glucose metabolism as a predictor of recovery from aphasia in ischemic stroke. *ArchNeurol.* 1993;50:958-964

[87] Jordan LC, Hillis AE. Disorders of speech and language: Aphasia, apraxia and dysarthria. *Curr Opin Neurol.* 2006;19:580-585

[88] Rosen HJ, Petersen SE, Linenweber MR, Snyder AZ, White DA, Chapman L, Dromerick AW, Fiez JA, Corbetta MD. Neural correlates of recovery from aphasia after damage to left inferior frontal cortex. *Neurology.* 2000;55 1883-1894

[89] Ohyama M, Senda M, Kitamura S, Ishii K, Mishina M, Terashi A. Role of the nondominant hemisphere and undamaged area during word repetition in poststroke aphasics - a pet activation study. *Stroke.* 1996;27:897-903

[90] Weiller C, Isensee C, Rijntjes M, Huber W, Müller S, Bier D, Dutschka K, Woods RP, Noth J, Diener HC. Recovery from wernicke's aphasia: A positron emission tomographic study. *AnnNeurol.* 1995;37:723-732

[91] Price CJ, Crinion J. The latest on functional imaging studies of aphasic stroke. *CurrOpinNeurol.* 2005;18:429-434

[92] Saur D, Lange R, Baumgaertner A, Schraknepper V, Willmes K, Rijntjes M, Weiller C. Dynamics of language reorganization after stroke. *Brain.* 2006;129:1371-1384

[93] Musso M, Weiller C, Kiebel S, Müller SP, Bülau P, Rijntjes M. Training-induced brain plasticity in aphasia. *Brain.* 1999;122 1781-1790

[94] Gainotti G. The riddle of the right hemisphere's contribution to the recovery of language. *EurJDisordCommun.* 1993;28:227-246

[95] Berthier ML, Starkstein SE, Leiguarda R, Ruiz A, Mayberg HS, Wagner H, Price TR, Robinson RG. Transcortical aphasia. Importance of the nonspeech dominant hemisphere in language repetition. *Brain.* 1991;114 (Pt 3):1409-1427

[96] Belin P, van Eeckhout P, Zilbovicius M, Remy P, Francois C, Guillaume S, Chain F, Rancurel G, Samson Y. Recovery from nonfluent aphasia after melodic intonation therapy: A pet study. *Neurology.* 1996;47:1504-1511

[97] Fernandez B, Cardebat D, Demonet JF, Joseph PA, Mazaux JM, Barat M, Allard M. Functional mri follow-up study of language processes in healthy subjects and during recovery in a case of aphasia. *Stroke.* 2004;35:2171-2176

[98] Raboyeau G, De Boissezon X, Marie N, Balduyck S, Puel M, Bezy C, Demonet JF, Cardebat D. Right hemisphere activation in recovery from aphasia: Lesion effect or function recruitment? *Neurology.* 2008;70:290-298

[99] Karbe H, Thiel A, Weber-Luxenburger G, Herholz K, Kessler J, Heiss WD. Brain plasticity in poststroke aphasia: What is the contribution of the right hemisphere? *Brain Lang.* 1998;64:215-230

[100] Heiss WD, Kessler J, Thiel A, Ghaemi M, Karbe H. Differential capacity of left and right hemispheric areas for compensation of poststroke aphasia. *AnnNeurol.* 1999;45:430-438

[101] Cao Y, Vikingstad EM, George KP, Johnson AF, Welch KMA. Cortical language activation in stroke patients recovering from aphasia with functional mri. *Stroke.* 1999;30:2331-2340

[102] Warburton E, Price CJ, Swinburn K, Wise RJS. Mechanisms of recovery from aphasia: Evidence from positron emission tomography studies. *JNeurolNeurosurgPsychiatry.* 1999;66:155-161

[103] Greener J, Enderby P, Whurr R. Speech and language therapy for aphasia following stroke (cochrane review). *The Cochrane Library 3.* 2001;Oxford: Update Software

[104] Ferro JM, Mariano G, Madureira S. Recovery from aphasia and neglect. *CerebrovascDis*. 1999;9 (Suppl. 5):6-22

[105] Walker-Batson D, Curtis S, Natarajan R, Ford J, Dronkers N, Salmeron E, Lai J, Unwin DH. A double-blind, placebo-controlled study of the use of amphetamine in the treatment of aphasia. *Stroke*. 2001;32:2093-2098

[106] Berthier ML, Green C, Higueras C, Fernandez I, Hinojosa J, Martin MC. A randomized, placebo-controlled study of donepezil in poststroke aphasia. *Neurology*. 2006;67:1687-1689

[107] Greener J, Enderby P, Whurr R. Pharmacological treatment for aphasia following stroke (protocol for a cochrane review). *The Cochrane Library 3*. 2001;Oxford: Update Software

[108] Orgogozo JM. Piracetam in the treatment of acute stroke. *Cns Drugs*. 1998;9:41-49

[109] Kessler J, Thiel A, Karbe H, Heiss WD. Piracetam improves activated blood flow and facilitates rehabilitation of poststroke aphasic patients. *Stroke*. 2000;31:2112-2116

[110] Crinion JT, Leff AP. Recovery and treatment of aphasia after stroke: Functional imaging studies. *Curr Opin Neurol*. 2007;20:667-673

[111] Pascual-Leone A, Davey N, Wassermann EM, Rothwell J, Puri B. *Handbook of transcranial magnetic stimulation*. London: Arnold Press; 2002.

[112] Naeser MA, Martin PI, Baker EH, Hodge SM, Sczerzenie SE, Nicholas M, Palumbo CL, Goodglass H, Wingfield A, Samaraweera R, Harris G, Baird A, Renshaw P, Yurgelun-Todd D. Overt propositional speech in chronic nonfluent aphasia studied with the dynamic susceptibility contrast fmri method. *Neuroimage*. 2004;22:29-41

[113] Siebner HR, Takano B, Peinemann A, Schwaiger M, Conrad B, Drzezga A. Continuous transcranial magnetic stimulation during positron emission tomography: A suitable tool for imaging regional excitability of the human cortex. *Neuroimage*. 2001;14:883-890

[114] Winhuisen L, Thiel A, Schumacher B, Kessler J, Rudolf J, Haupt WF, Heiss WD. Role of the contralateral inferior frontal gyrus in recovery of language function in poststroke aphasia: A combined repetitive transcranial magnetic stimulation and positron emission tomography study. *Stroke*. 2005;36:1759-1763

[115] Thiel A, Habedank B, Herholz K, Kessler J, Winhuisen L, Haupt WF, Heiss WD. From the left to the right: How the brain compensates progressive loss of language function. *Brain Lang*. 2006;98:57-65

[116] Heiss WD, Thiel A. A proposed regional hierarchy in recovery of post-stroke aphasia. *Brain Lang*. 2006;98:118-123

[117] Naeser MA, Martin PI, Nicholas M, Baker EH, Seekins H, Kobayashi M, Theoret H, Fregni F, Maria-Tormos J, Kurland J, Doron KW, Pascual-Leone A. Improved picture naming in chronic aphasia after tms to part of right broca's area: An open-protocol study. *Brain Lang*. 2005;93:95-105

[118] Ridding MC, Rothwell JC. Therapeutic use of rtms. *Nat Rev Neurosci*. 2007;8:559-567

In: Speech Disorders: Causes, Treatment and Social Effects ISBN: 978-1-60876-213-2
Editor: Alan E. Harrison, pp. 97-118

Chapter 4

USING SPANISH IN THE HOME TO PROMOTE SCHOOL READINESS IN ENGLISH

Virginia Mann, Maricela Sandoval, Lorena Garcia and David Calderon

Department of Cognitive Sciences School of Social SciencesUniversity of California, Irvine, CA

ABSTRACT

This study reports the first five years of a school readiness intervention called 'HABLA' (Home Based Activities Building Language Acquisition), It was designed to increase and enrich speech and literacy activities in the homes of economically and educationally disadvantaged Latino families with children between the age of 2 and 4. A team of trained home visitors provided two years of a 23-week program of visitation in which they met with parent(s) and child twice weekly. Both years presented a Spanish language adaptation of the Parent Child Home Program model; home visitors provide intensive modeling and coaching of non-directive Spanish language use, conversation, and literacy activities. Administration of the PLS-3 in Spanish at the onset and culmination of each year of the program indicates significant increases in receptive and expressive language for each year of visitation (7.8 standard points for the first year, 4.4 for the second) with effect size r ranging from .24 to .41. Participants had significantly improved their levels of oral Spanish skill and scored much higher than a comparison group of untreated peers. A subset of graduates of the two-year program was tested as kindergarteners; they showed a continued advantage over a comparison group of 18 peers who had not received the intervention. For the graduates, both their Spanish PLS-3 scores and English PLS-4 scores were significantly higher, and their parents reported a continued effort to provide literacy experiences at home. The HABLA participants also showed a clear advantage for an English language test of phonological awareness, one of the strongest predictors of school success.

During the early years of their lives, children in affluent and poor families experience a dramatic difference in exposure to speech (Hart & Risely, 1995). On average, those living in poverty hear 300 fewer words per hour and this culminates in a 30 million-word deficit by the time children enter kindergarten. Tied to this deficiency in spoken language exposure is a commensurate deficiency in children's speech that directly relates to the style, quality and diversity of their parent's language (Hart & Risley, 1995). As speech skills are key ingredients in school success (see Duncan et al, 2006; Mann, 1998, Snow, Burns and Griffins 1998), early deficiencies in the speech environment, if left unheeded, may cascade into educational disadvantages and a tragic loss of social capital.

Because the difference in the speech environment between advantaged and disadvantaged children begins so early in their lives, effective intervention must also begin early. An ideal intervention should increase the quality and quantity of parent to child language and should involve shared activities that can become self-sustaining after treatment ceases. The intervention should be home-based, and even if the children are to be English language learners once they begin school, the intervention should target the language of the home since that is the language the parent is most capable of delivering with appropriately rich vocabulary and grammar. Prompted by these considerations, we have developed a home-based intervention program to enrich the Spanish home language and literacy environments of poor Latino children. It is based on the highly successful Parent Child Home Program (PCHP, Levenstein, Levenstein, Shiminski & Stolzberg, 1998).

The Case for Intervention in the Home Language

The participants in this study are native speakers of Spanish whose language and literacy environments in the home are likely to be weak and a limit on the development of children's language. Their academic achievement is likely to suffer from the combined influence of SES, parental education, parental language style and the challenges of ELL; they live in conditions of economic disadvantage (the average family income for the present study is $19,000), low maternal education (average maternal education is 8.7 years of school) and a predominance of directive language use (Laosa, 1982). They live in homes where Spanish is dominant and English is a second language at best (the 2000 census registered our treatment site as having the largest concentration of ELL speakers of Spanish).

Families with low-income, low maternal education, and low proficiency in the English language experience greater hardships, have limited access to resources, and must cope with higher stress levels, all of which diminish the likelihood of their children's school success (Farver, Raver & Knitzer, 2002; Farver Xu, Eppe & Lonigan, 2006), As reviewed by Romero-Contreras, Snow, August, & Calderon (2007), poor, urban, minority, non-English speaking children, particularly those who speak Spanish, have difficulty learning to read and their achievement gap widens as the children progress through elementary school. Both early on and throughout their time in school, Latino children are twice as likely to read below level as European-American children (Kao & Tienda, 1995). The urban school district of concern to this study embodies these observations: it serves a majority of Latino children living below the poverty line , and the students achieve scores in the lowest deciles in the state (API of 3 or lower) where schools in less Latino-dense, more affluent neighboring cities score in the upper deciles (API of 7 or higher).

When intervention and outreach target K-12 students in schools or after school programs, they necessarily operates in English, as that is the language of education. However, when intervention and outreach choose early childhood enrichment it is best done in the homes and in the home language. .Spanish is the home language of the most disadvantaged children in our geographic area (e.g. Southern California) and in the country at large. When Spanish monolingual children enter school they are expected to matriculate into English. Yet their primary language or 'mother tongue' is a scaffold on which to build English matriculation and personal and educational development. Baker (2000), Cummins (2000), Skutnabb-Kangas (2000) and Figuerdo (2006) have each reviewed evidence to the effect that children who come to school with a solid foundation in their mother tongue develop stronger literacy abilities in the school language than those who do not. In Cummins view, in particular, parents and other caregivers (e.g. grandparents) who spend time with their children and tell stories or discuss issues with them in a way that develops their mother tongue vocabulary and concepts have children who come to school well-prepared to learn English and to succeed educationally. This suggests that children's knowledge and skills transfer across languages from the mother tongue they have learned in the home to English in school.

The Intervention

The intervention employed in this study is modeled after the Parent Child Home Program and is delivered by a cadre of students, AmeriCorps members and para-professionals. All receive both pre-service and in-service, all are mentored by university faculty and by specialists in early childhood education. Together they delivered a curriculum whose goal was to enhance primary language development though shared reading, language play and developmentally appropriate activities involving the parent and the child.

The Parent Child Home Program (PCHP) began in the 1960's, when Levenstein and her colleagues began to offer language and literacy remediation in the homes of disadvantaged English speakers. These researchers have since then reported on their program's success as a facilitator of academic achievement in early grades and beyond (Lazar & Darlington, 1982; Kamerman & Kahn, 1995; Levenstein, Levenstein, Shiminski & Stolzberg, 1998). The PCHP's stated goal is to help parents discover their role as a child's first and most important teachers. It helps parents to increase the home literacy environment and to enrich spoken skills. The program consists of two years of intervention beginning when the child is approximately two year of age; each year consists of 23 weeks of home visits with two 30-minute visits per week The stated goal of the PCHP is to prepare parents to actively participate in their children's education by focusing on 6 stated objectives: (i) verbal interaction (ii) in the home (iii) in the primary language of the home (iv) with methods easily learned, (v) using books and toys that stay in the home and (vi) with attention to measurable outcomes that are assessed throughout the program and beyond. Studies of children in English-speaking homes who have received the PCHP show that treated children enter school ready to learn and perform at or above national norms on standardized tests in first grade (Levenstein, Levenstein & Oliver, 2002) and throughout elementary school. They graduate from high school at rates equal to those of middle class students (see Levenstein et al, 1998).

In adapting the PCHP methods to our Spanish-speaking clients, we used the tenents of the PCHP. To make the curriculum as advantageous as possible, we chose our curriculum of books, toys and activities to underscored the eight language and literacy activities recommended by The National Reading Panel. These consist of using language in conversation, listening and responding to stories read aloud, listening to the sounds of spoken language, reading often, learning and using new words, understanding what is read, recognizing and naming the letters of the alphabet and connecting sounds to letters to figure out the "code" of reading. The first six NRP activities were used throughout the two-year program; the final two alphabet-oriented activities were introduced in the second year. As a measure of program outcome, we have tracked expressive and receptive Spanish language skill at baseline and at the completion of each year of treatment. For a sample of children who completed both years of the program we have also measured parents' reports of home literacy activities, and children's Spanish and English language skills and phonological awareness in the kindergarten year.

As the National Reading Council (2001) acknowledged, there is widespread recognition and support of the view that early language intervention can enable children to enter school with the language skills needed to succeed. Such language intervention is especially warranted in the case of children from disadvantaged economic backgrounds, given Hart and Risley's (1995) observations. Children in low SES families are at increased risk for developing both deficient language processing skills (Honig, 1982; Walker, Greenwood, Hart & Carta, 1994) and deficient phonological awareness (Nittrouer, 1996). According to some, their learning of language is constrained by the low values placed upon language in most low-SES sociolinguistic communities (Purcell-Gates, 1998) as well as by parental input that is more directive and immediate (Laosa, 1980; 1982). Lower SES homes are less likely to offer such important home literacy behaviors as shared reading, children's reading materials and age of onset of shared reading (Lonigan, 1994) and the quality of parent to child language can also be influenced of ethnicity, gender and maternal language upon literacy experience (Gauvain, Savage, & McCollum, 2000).

The present study's goal was to provide early intervention and mitigation of the educational disadvantage prevalent in our environment. The program was named 'HABLA', an acronym for "Home-based Activities Building Language Acquisition" which is also the Spanish imperative for "speak!" HABLA's implementation and adaptation of the PCHP targeted the PCHP stated objectives and the NRC recommendations for early reading and school success. Over its first five years of existence, HABLA recruited families with children aged 15 to 30 months to enter a two-year program in order to better prepare their children for school.

At the onset of treatment and at the end of each of the two 23 week programs of home visits, all participants received a measure of outcome, the Spanish PLS-3, which served as a test of expressive and receptive speech. To determine whether the HABLA program sustained its post-treatment gains in Spanish and translated these into an advantage for school success in English, a subset of children who had completed HABLA were evaluated as kindergarteners and compared to a group of untreated peers attending the same school and preschool. The bases of comparison were parental report of home involvement, English and Spanish oral language skills and English and Spanish phonological awareness.

METHOD

Participants

Participants were recruited through family resource centers, flyers distributed in local clinics, schools, faith organizations and by word of mouth. The program was also featured once in the local Spanish language newspaper and three times on public television, and contact information was provided in each case. All participants were required to be economically disadvantaged (maximum income of $30,000 for a family of 5 or more), educationally disadvantaged (maximum education, 11 years) and to be native speakers of Spanish whose parents used Spanish in the home. Children served with the informed consent of their parents who were also required to sign a consent form and a pledge to be present and involved in every home visit. The applicants ranged in age from 12 to 59 months; it was our experience that parents applied to the program even when their children fell out of the age range (children aged 18 – 42 months) we had posted. All children were assessed and their data help to provide a baseline of Spanish skills for the population. Out of an applicant pool of 612 (52.6% male), 537 children met the age criterion and were invited to participate in the two-year HABLA intervention. Five children younger than 18 months were put on a wait list, 70 children 42 months and older were given the option of participating in a foreshortened version of the program which will not be reported here.

Towards the end of the study, we had access to a group of HABLA graduates and a group of untreated peers, all of whom had attended a state preschool program and were currently enrolled in a public school kindergarten. Tracking children into kindergarten proved difficult because there are many schools in the area, kindergarten is optional and the need for affordable housing leads many of our participants to move outside of the area. 38 kindergarteners were tested in the winter of the school year; the average ages of HABLA graduated and the untreated peers were 65.6 mo. and 64.0 mo, respectively, and there were 9 girls and 10 boys in the treated group and 9 and 10 in the untreated group. All served with the written consent of their parents, who also completed a home language and reading questionnaire.

Materials and Procedure

The HABLA curriculum: The curriculum consisted of 46 weeks of home visitation, divided into two programs of 23 weeks each. The first program was given at program entry, and the second program was given approximately one year later. Each program lasted about 7 months. Each week of each programs consisted of two visits: one for presentation of a book or toy that remains permanently in the home and one for assessment and review. Toys and books were chosen for their ability to promote language between parent and child. The same trained home visitor worked with the family for a minimum of one 23-week program and in 70% of the cases where children received both programs. In the first 23 weeks of visitation (e.g. the first year of treatment), the focus was on picture books and materials that emphasized colors, shapes, numbers, animals and common objects as well as basic Spanish grammar and vocabulary. The second set of 23 visits (e.g. the second year) expanded these themes with longer more complex stories, memory activities and the introduction of activities featuring letter names and sounds. The curriculum for each year involved a set order of books and toys chosen to be developmentally appropriate and interrelated. Books and toys alternated and each was provided with a guide sheet that listed the concepts it featured and activities for the parent to do with the child in order to encourage rich language use between parent and child.. All materials remain with the family permanently; the books and all instruction are in the language of the home (Spanish and English are both available)) and were chosen to bridge the gap between preschool and home.

The Home visits: During the initial visit each week the home visitor follows a set of specific guidelines to use the featured book or toy to interact with the child, the instructions for books incorporated the principles of dialogic reading (Arnold, Lonigan and Whitehurst, 1994; Lonigan & Whitehurst, 1998) and shared its focus on building children's knowledge of print as well as on interactive oral language use. The instructions for toys and games focused on expressive language and vocabulary expansion as ell as upon categorization, comparison and memory. Home visitors are taught to coach the parent and child together and to model the verbal interaction and parenting techniques that can occur through reading and educational play. A tip sheet is left for parents to follow, and the parent and child are coached to use the new book or toy for the next several days with the goal of spending at least thirty minutes each day. That same week, two to four days after the initial modeling visit, a second visit occurs. At this time the home visitor assesses parent and child behavior and their ability to sustain verbal play. He or she also provides further coaching and modeling as necessary, and instructs the parent and child to continue to use the toy or book for thirty minutes each day until the next visit. Over time these bi-weekly visits enable the parent to learn how to initiate and sustain the reading and play activities that offer the types of language interaction required for optimal development.

Home Visitors: Home Visitors included UCI students, AmeriCorps members and members of the community who were recruited with flyers, course listings and by word of mouth. The requirements for becoming a home visitor were based on the long history of the PCHP approach (Levenstein et al, 1998); HABLA added the additional requirement that all visitors be bilingual in Spanish and English and culturally compatible with the Latino clientele they were to serve. Home visitors were trained by the director and the site managers who had formal PCHP training as well as extensive experience with the assessment and education of preschool children and parent education. The home visitors were trained for 16 hours before their first visit and required to attend two-hour weekly in-service training sessions thereafter. They were also individually supervised in the home at various points during the delivery of services, and client satisfaction was monitored regularly. Students served between 1 and 3 families per week, AmeriCorps members and paraprofessionals saw between 6 and 10.

Measures of Treatment Effect

The Preschool Language Scale (PLS): The site managers administered the PLS-3 in Spanish to all participants at three points in time: program intake, the end of the first year of treatment, and the end of the second year. At the time that this study began, the PLS-3, Spanish Edition (Zimmerman, Steiner, & Pond, 1993) was the only version available; for consistency, that version was used throughout testing. The PLS is favored in assessment of Head-Start programs (see Kaiser et al, 2000) as well as in longitudinal studies of preschool predictors of reading (see Chaney, 1998) and in clinical and educational settings more generally (see Zimmerman & Castilleja, 2005). It had the virtue of being available in both English and Spanish, though the Spanish version is not standardized owing to the relatively small sample size (N = 181) used in the validation. Zimmerman et al's (1993) validation sample of children for the Spanish version yielded "standardized" scores that averaged 90 instead of 100, and an SEM of 15. In that sample the raw scores of Spanish speaking children had begun to fall behind those of the English speakers by 18 months of age.

Kindergarten testing

Kindergarten testing was administered by two trained research assistants who were familiar with the HABLA program but who had not worked with any of the children involved in the assessment.

The PLS: For the 38 children who participated in the kindergarten study, the PLS-3 in Spanish was used in the winter but the PLS-4 in English was used in the spring. Use of the newer PLS-4 addresses some of the ceiling effects that could arise in the testing of older subject and the problem of inadequately normalized scores for Spanish (Zimmerman, Steiner & Pond, 2002, Zimmerman & Castilleja, 2005), and also provides a measure of the effect of HABLA on children's matriculation into English.

Phonological awareness: Materials for this assessment were adapted from those used in the preschool studies of Foy & Mann, (2001; 2003), and consisted of two parts: a test of rhyme awareness and two tests of phoneme awareness. Rhyme awareness materials included 8 items of an odd-man out rhyme recognition task using pictures of common objects and 5 items of a rhyme production task in which the children were asked to say "what word rhymes with ___" where the prompts consisted of common words (e.g., hop). Words and nonwords were scored as correct as long as they rhymed with the target word.

Phoneme awareness materials were prepared in Spanish and English, and consisted of practice trials and test items for each of four subtests assessing phoneme judgment and phoneme deletion in both initial and final positions. The subtests each consisted of two practice items and five test items. The tests were administered in standard order: phoneme judgment, phoneme deletion, and phoneme substitution.

The scoring followed Foy and Mann (2003): Rhyme awareness was measured as the total of responses on the two rhyme tests, as our primary interest was in the comparison between treated and untreated children, we used Z-transforms so that Spanish testing would not be penalized by the earlier time of testing. For phoneme awareness, phoneme judgment was considered a separate variable from phoneme deletion but we combined z-transforms of the initial and final segment parts within each of these two tasks as the interest was not so much in the effects of age as in the existence of any differences between the two groups in each of the two languages.

Parent survey: A subset of items from Seneschal, Le Fevre, Thomas and Daley (1998) as used in Foy and Mann (2003) were incorporated into a short survey that was made available in Spanish and in English and was given to the parents of the children who participated in the kindergarten assessment. The questions appear in Appendix B; they concern the literacy environment of the family (books available, child's interest in books, frequency child is read to, parental intent to teach).

RESULTS

Rates of Completion and Attrition

A high attrition was anticipated due to the highly mobile nature of the population, which is economically challenged and experiencing an eastward migration towards affordable housing as well as immigration challenges. It was our experience that families were often forced to move at short notice and that some were forced to return to Mexico. In the snapshot of time that this study captures (e.g. January 2001 to January 2006) 537 children between 18 and 42 months were offered the two-year program of treatment. At the time of analysis, data from 393 were available for one year of treatment, of whom 183 had completed the full two-year program. 181 had dropped after one year and 29 were in the process of receiving program two; 89 children were still in program one and 55 had dropped during the first program. We estimate attrition of participants at some point during the full two-year program to be approximately 33.7 %, but that 89.4% of the participants had been able to finish at least the first year of the program.

A series of t-tests revealed very little difference in the demographics of children who completed the full two-year program compared to those who dropped within or after one year. The three groups appear statistically equivalent with respect to gender, PLS-3 baseline, parental education and income. The only significant difference to emerge concerned the type of household: 36% of those who dropped the program came from a household headed by a single mother, compared to 28% of those who continued for the whole program ($t(321)=1.91$, $p<.05$).

The PLS-III in Spanish at Intake and after Each Year of Treatment

Intake: The PLS-3 was given to all 612 children who applied to the program, whether or not they were in the right age range to begin the study (e.g. 18 mo. to three years of age). The mean "standardized" PLS-3 score for the full cohort of children was 91.7 for auditory comprehension and 89.4 for expressive communication, with standard deviation 13.6 in both cases. As a group, the children were equivalent to those seen in Zimmerman et al's (1993) validation sample, which had yielded means of 89.9 and 90.0 for receptive and expressive measures, respectively. In our sample, mean auditory comprehension score was slightly but significantly higher than that of the validation sample, $t(611)= 3.02$, $p<.003$, but the expressive measure was statistically equivalent. Children's average age was 33 months at the time of testing, but age varied between 18 months and 59 months and bivariate correlations showed that age was significantly and negatively correlated with standard receptive skill, ($r(612)=-.277$, $p<.000$, standard expressive skill, $r(612)=-.110$, $p<.005$, and the standard total score, $r(612)=-.213$, $p<.000$. The older children tended to do less well on the PLS-3 relative to what is expected from the English norms and the validation sample. A similar effect of age had been noted in the validation sample (Zimmerle et al, 1993), it may in part be due to the PLS-3 having been created as a Spanish translation of English instead of as a true test of Spanish. Of the 612 children applying to the program, 70 children were 36 months or older. They were too old to be given the treatment program reported in this paper. Their mean age was 46.6 months (*std*=5.74), mean standard Spanish receptive PLS-3 score was 85.87, and mean standard expressive was 86.79. Both of these scores were significantly below the average achieved in the validation sample, $t(69) = -3.37$ and -2.39, respectively, $p<.02$.

For analyses of outcome, we concentrated on 537 children who were offered the HABLA intervention and whose parents gave written consent. These 'treated' children were divided into two cohorts according to the age when they began treatment: those below 30 months (children within six months of being two) and those between 30 and 42 months (children within six months of being three). Each cohort is discussed below. Prior to the start of their HABLA treatment, the treated children had average receptive and expressive scores of 92.47 and 89.88, respectively. Their receptive scores were slightly higher than the validation average (2.5 points, $t(326)= 4.15$, $p<.000$) and the expressive scores were equivalent to the validation average.

Treatment effects of the first year of the program: A total of 393 children completed at least one year of the program at the time of analysis. Their data appear in Tables 1a and b, separated according to the age at which children entered the program (children younger than 30 months compared to those 30 months or older). A 4-way between groups ANOVA revealed a main effect of the first year's treatment, $F(1, 385) = 97.263$, $MSE=22077.76$, $p<.000$; children had gained an average of 7.8 standard points between intake and the end of the first year's treatment. There was also a main effect of the age at entry $F(1,385)=18.28$, $MSE = 9069.41$, $p<.000$); the younger cohort had averaged scores that were 5 points higher than the older cohort. The gains were greater for the older children, who had started with lower scores, $F(1, 385) = 7.868$, $MSE = 1970.55$ $p<.003$. There was a main effect of subtest, $F(1, 385) = 37.50$, $MSE = 2065.45$, $p< .02$); receptive scores averaged 3 points higher, and two-way and three-way interactions revealed this tended to be greater among the younger cohort, $F(1,385)= 7.86$, $MSE = 433.11$, $p<.005$, and greatest at intake, $F(1,385)= 19.29$, $MSE = 865.12$, $p<.000$, especially for younger participants, $F(1,385)=9.78$, $MSE = 439.08$ $p<.002$. There was a marginal effect of gender, $F(1,385)= 3.67$, $MSE = 1820.70$, $p<.056$ reflecting a 2.2 point advantage of the female participants, but this did not interact with any of the other variables. There were no other interactions and no effective difference between children who continued on to the full two-year program and those who did not.

In summary, pre- treatment scores had been close to the validation norm for expressive and 2.5 points higher for receptive, $t(392)=3.88$, $p<.0001$. At the end of the first year's treatment both receptive, $t(392)=12.61$, $p<.000$, and expressive, $t(392)=10.61$, $p<.0001$ language measures gained between 7 and 10 points with the younger children maintaining a persistent advantage on PLS-3 scores.

Table 1a. Mean Standard Scores (and std deviation) on PLS-3 in Spanish: Effect of First Year HABLA treatment children age 15 to 30 months

Time of Evaluation	Expressive	Receptive	Mean age (std)
Program entry N = 153	91.00 (1.07)	97.99 (1.10)	26.38 (2.15) months
End of First Year N = 153	99.98 (1.30)	100.81 (1.21)	33.54 (3.76) months

Table 1b. Mean Standard Scores (and std deviation) on PLS-3 in Spanish: Effect of First Year HABLA treatment on children aged 30 to 42 months

Time of Evaluation	Expressive	Receptive	Mean age (std)
Program entry N = 240	86.70 (0.88)	88.49 (0.86)	34.29 (3.12) Months
End of First Year N = 240	97.31 (1.04)	98.16.(0.97)	40.64 (3.39) Months

Treatment effects for the full two-year program: At the time of analysis, 183 of the participants had completed the full two-year program. Their results appear in Tables 2a and b, as a function of age at entry. A GLM revealed a significant main effect of the second year of treatment, $F(1, 179) = 21.57$, MSE=3502.44, p<.000; between the first and second year, children had gained an average of 4.4 points. There was once again, a significant effect of entry age, $F(1,179)$=12.68, MSE = 6982.45, p<.000; those who started below 30 months averaged 6.2 points higher than those who started between 30 and 42 months, and this pervaded into the second year of the program. There was no difference between the two subtests and all other interactions were not significant, save for a significant effect of gender, F1,179)= 4.85, MSE=2668.54, p<.03, reflecting a 3.8 point advantage among the female participants. All scores were significantly greater than the validation average (p<.000). Paired-t tests indicate that the children had achieved significant gains each year of the program. After the first year, receptive and expressive averaged gains of 6 and 8 standard points, respectively, $t(182)$ =4.55 and 6.83 , p<.000, between the first and second year receptive and expressive averaged gains of 6 and 8 and standard points, respectively, $t(182)$=4.54 and 6.83, p<.0001.

Table 2a. Mean Standard Scores (and std deviation) on PLS-3 in Spanish: Effect of Second Year HABLA treatment on children age 15 to 30 months

Time of Evaluation	Expressive	Receptive	Mean age (std)
End of First Year N = 82	102.02 (1.59)	103.73 (1.46)	33.41 (4.08) Months
End of Second Year N = 82	105.87 (1.60)	106.31 (1.61)	44.99 (4.18) Months

Table 2b. Mean Standard Scores (and std deviation) on PLS-3 in Spanish: Effect of Second Year HABLA treatment on children age 30 to 42 months

Time of Evaluation	Expressive	Receptive	Mean (std)
End of First Year N = 101	95.02 (1.44)	95.91 (1.32)	40.95 (3.37) months
End of Second Year N = 101	101.25 (1.45)	100.91 (1.45)	52.02 (4.14) months

To summarize, the PLS testing reveals a significant effect of the program, for each year of the program. There is also a significant advantage for children who entered before they were 30 months of age. The younger children start with higher scores and maintain an advantage. Girls tend to perform at higher levels but this does not interact with the treatment effect. There is also a tendency for children to have lower expressive scores at the start of treatment and for expressive scores to equal receptive scores as a consequence of treatment. To put these results in terms of treatment effects, we computed *Cohen's d* and *treatment-effect r*. For children completing one year of the program there are medium treatment effects for receptive scores: *Cohen's d*=0.4865, *effect-size r*=.2365, and for expressive: *Cohen's d*=0.6638, *effect-size r*=.3150; for the difference between the first and second year's treatment, there are small treatment effects for receptive scores: *Cohen's d*=0.2670, *effect-size r*=.1393 and expressive *Cohen's d*=0.3592, *effect-size r*=.1768, for the entire two years program, there are medium effects for receptive *Cohen's d*=0.6518, *effect-size r*=.3099 and a large effect for expressive *Cohen's d*=0.9084, *effect-size r*=.4136.

Kindergarten Testing in Spanish and English

PLS: We began our evaluation of kindergarten effects by looking at PLS results for the HALA graduates as compared to untreated classmates. The scaled PLS-3 had been administered in Spanish in the winter and the scaled PLS-4 in English had been administered in the Spring. An ANOVA that considered language (Spanish, English), subtest (expressive, receptive) and treatment group (HABLA, control) revealed a significant effect of group, $F(1,36)=4.806$, $MSE = 1113.57$, $p<.05$: the HABLA-treated children had higher scores, an average advantage of 4.4 points. This advantage is seen in Table 3, where it may also be seen that there was a significant effect of the type of subtest, $F(1,36)=18.02$, $MSE= 1360.934$, $p<.0001$: performance in kindergarten was superior on the tests of expressive language, more so for Spanish than for English $F(1,36)=33.349$, $MSE= 1830.255$, $p<.0001$, and strongest among the HABLA graduates, $F(1,36)=33.349$, $MSE= 423.031$, $p<.0001$. The untreated children had achieved scores at the standard norm on the PLS-3 Spanish expressive but were significantly lower than the standard norm on the Spanish receptive t(18)=- 3.75, $p<.001$, English receptive $t(18)= -2.34$, $p<.03$ and English expressive test $t(18) = -3.82$, $p<.001$. In contrast, the treated children were at the norm on the Spanish receptive test, the English receptive test and the English expressive test and were significantly above the norm on the Spanish expressive test $t(18)= 3.27$, $p<.01$.

Computation of treatment effects indicated medium effects on Spanish receptive scores, *Cohen's d*=0.5743, *effect-size r*=.2760, minimal effects on Spanish expressive, *Cohen's d*=0.0488, *effect-size r*=.0244, medium effects on English receptive scores, *Cohen's d*=0.6393, *effect-size r*=.3045 and minimal effects on English expressive, *Cohen's d*=0.1096, *effect-size r*=.0547.

Rhyme awareness: Using the z-transforms of scores computed separately for Spanish and English for each component of the rhyme awareness tests, we computed an ANOVA for group, language and type of test (judgment, production). The results, as summarized in Figure 1, revealed that HABLA graduates averaged higher scores, $F(1,36)=5.839$, $MSE= 5,839$, $p<.021$, but that no other effects or interactions were significant. Computation of treatment effects indicates medium effects for Spanish *Cohen's d*=0.4622, *effect-size r*=.2252, and English, *Cohen's d*=0.5013, *effect-size r*=.2431.

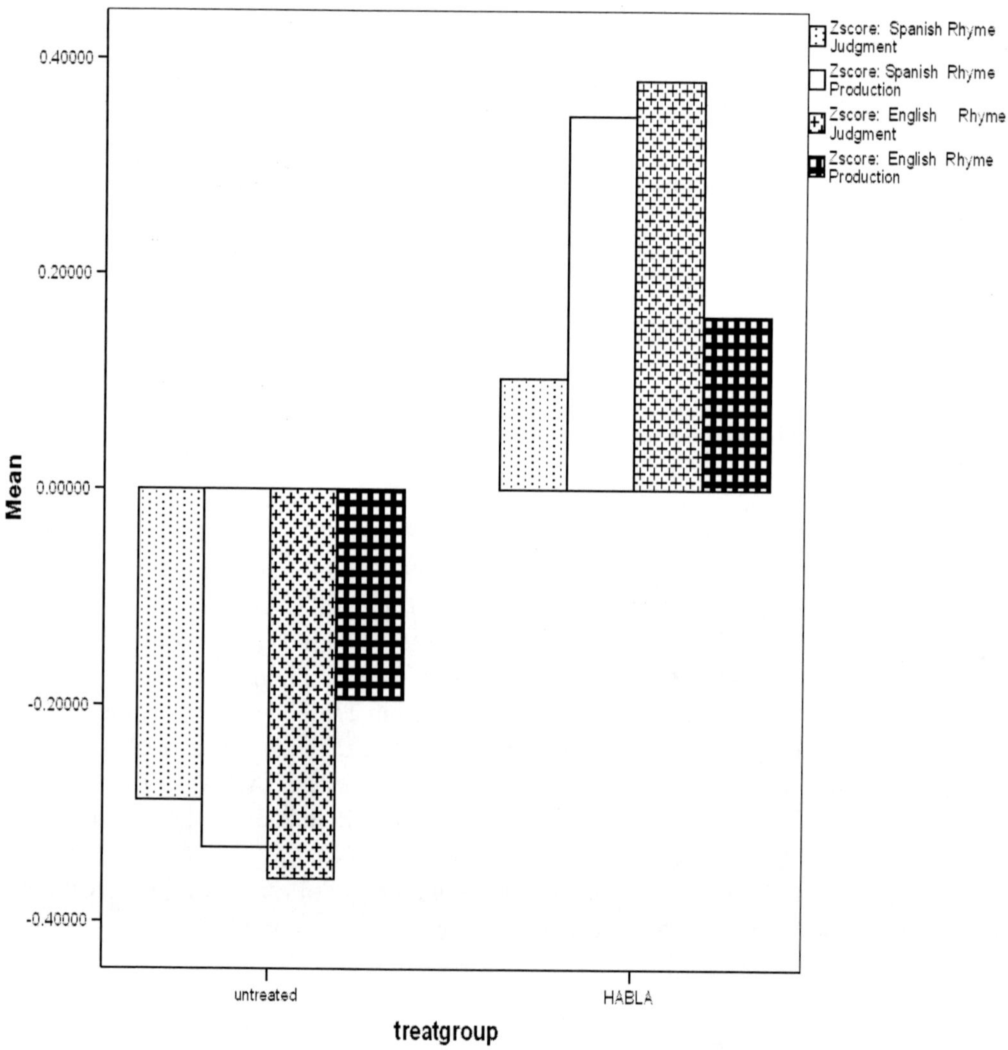

Figure 1. BLA Treatment Effects on Spanish and English: Kindergarten Rhyme Judgment and Production

Table 3. Mean (std dev) Standard Scores on PLS-3 in Spanish and PLS-4 in English: Effect of HABLA 2-year treatment on kindergarten scores

Treatment group	Spanish Expressive	Spanish Receptive	English Expressive	English Receptive
HABLA	108.1 (12.60)	91.9 (10.25)	97.9 (12.91)	96.0 (13.70)
Control	100.15 (14.77)	91.4 (10.26)	90.0 (11.78)	94.6 (11.83)

Table 4. Pearson two-tailed Correlations between Kindergarten Measures

Correlations between Kindergarten measures

	Sp recept.	Sp express.	Eng. recept.	Eng. expr.	Sp rhyme	Sp p. judgm.	Sp. p. manip.	Eng. rhyme	Eng. p. judg.	Eng. p. manip.
Spanish receptive	1	**					*			
Spanish expressive	.530**	1			**	*	*			
English receptive	.206	.151	1	**				**	**	**
English expressive	.019	.183	.620**	1				*		**
Spanish rhyme	.212	.313**	.122	.139	1	**	**			
Spanish p. judgment	.235	.244*	.211	.023	.359**	1	**	*	**	*
Spanish p manip.	.263*	.266*	.026	.064	.501**	.446**	1			**
English rhyme	.002	-.032	.500**	.333*	.105	.355*	.161	1	**	**
English p. judgment	.071	.182	.485**	.069	.192	.532**	.238	.627**	1	**
English p. manip	.197	.237	.525**	.407**	.309	.325*	.417**	.426**	.465**	1

**. o Correlation is siginficant at the 0.001 level (2-tailed)

*. Correlation is significant at the 0.05 level (2-tailed).

Phoneme awareness: Using z-transformations of scores computed separately for each language and each task we examined the effect of treatment group on language (Spanish, English) and task (judgment, deletion). There was a main effect of group, $F(1,36)=4.086$, $MSE=8.68$, $p<.041$, illustrated in Figure 2, reflecting the superior performance of the HABLA treated children. There is no interaction between group and language and no other effects or interactions were significant (owing to the use of Z-transforms). Computation of treatment effects indicate minimal effects for Spanish phoneme judgment *Cohen's* $d=0.0798$, *effect-size* $r=.0393$, and Spanish phoneme manipulation *Cohen's* $d=0.1082$, *effect-size* $r=.0540$, but medium effects for English phoneme judgment, *Cohen's* $d=0.4922$, *effect-size* $r=.2389$, and English phoneme manipulation, *Cohen's* $d=0.6260$, *effect-size* $r=.2987$.

Correlation analyses: As a final analysis of the data, a series of bivariate correlations were conducted to examine the relations between the PLS scores, rhyme and phoneme awareness scores in each language. For this purpose, rhyme judgment and production were combined into a single score but phoneme manipulation and judgment were kept separate. As seen in Table 4, expressive scores in each language were significantly correlated with receptive scores but the correlations between English and Spanish PLS scores failed to reach significance ($p>.1$). Spanish expressive scores were correlated at the $p<.05$ level with Spanish rhyme awareness, phoneme judgment, and phoneme manipulation, Spanish receptive scores were correlated with Spanish phoneme manipulation. English expressive scores were correlated with English rhyme awareness, phoneme judgment, and phoneme manipulation, and English receptive scores were correlated with rhyme awareness and phoneme manipulation. Finally, Spanish measures of rhyme and phoneme awareness were significantly intercorrelated as were measures of English rhyme and phoneme awareness, all at the $p<.003$ level or higher. Of the 9 possible correlations between Spanish and English awareness, only the correlations involve Spanish rhyme awareness failed to reach significance with any of the English scores, but all correlations involving Spanish phoneme awareness were significant at $p<.05$ or higher as was the correlation between English and Spanish phoneme manipulation.

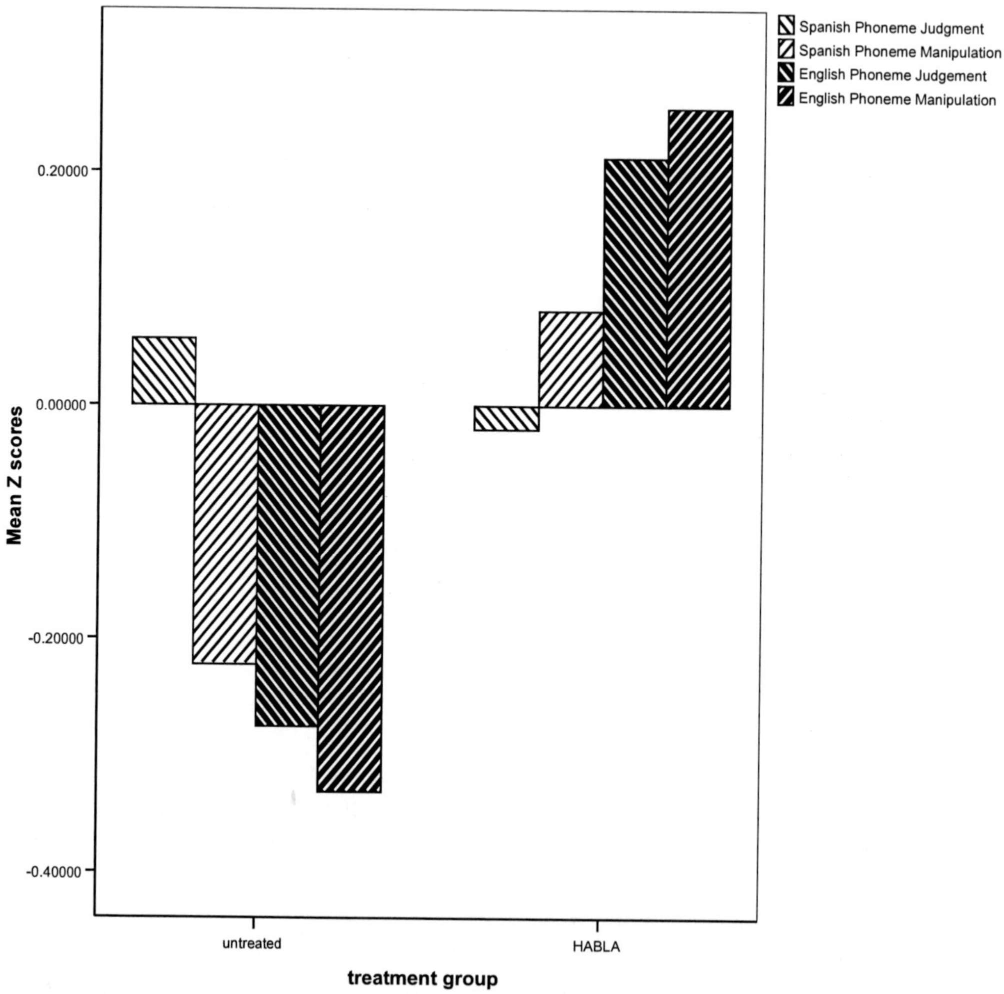

Figure 2. HABLA treatment Effects on Spanish and English Kindergarten Phoneme Judgment and Manipulation

The parent survey: The questions for the Parent Survey appear in Appendix B. Of the 38 children tested as kindergarteners, 34 had parents who completed and returned the questionnaire, 18 treated and 16 untreated. The responses are summarized in Table 5 and indicate that HABLA participants, on average, were living in a richer literacy environment. Their parents had not received significantly more education, but they read to their children more often at bedtime, $t(33)=3.4$, $p<.01$,, and other times, $t(33)=6.1$,

$p<.01$. They provided access to more books, $t(33)=3.1$, $p<.01$, and perceived their children as more frequently asking to be read to, $t(33)=4.9$, $p<.01$. The parents of the treated children were also more likely to report efforts to teach their child to read, $t(33)=4.8$, $p<.01$, and to print, $t(33)=4.3$, $p<.01$. Thus the program's goal of increasing home literacy activities appears to be sustained more than one year after the two-year intervention.

Table 5. Responses to Parent survey in Kindergarten
(lower scores = less activity reported)

Question	HABLA treated	Control
Maternal Education	8.9 (3.8)	7.7 (3.9)
Paternal Education	7.0 (3.6)	7.4 (4.8)
Age when shared reading began	26 months (13.5)	26 months (15.7)
Number of children's books	61-80 (0.96)	21-40 (2.35)
Reading at bedtime	4.0 (2.9)	1.0 (2.23)
Reading at other times	5.6 (1.1)	1.8 (2.2)
Child asks to read	4.8 (0.4)	2.7 (1.6)
Parent teaches printing	4.8 (0.5)	3.2 (1.4)
Parent teaches reading	4.6 (0.7)	2.6 (1.4)

DISCUSSION

Children in low SES families are at increased risk for reading problems due to deficient oral language skills (Honig, 1982; Walker, Greenwood, Hart & Carta, 1994) and deficient phonological awareness (Nittrouer, 1996). Some researchers have speculated that the learning of language is constrained by the low values placed upon language in most low-SES sociolinguistic communities (Purcell-Gates, 1998) as well as by parental input that is more directive and immediate (Laosa, 1980; 1982). Lower SES homes are less likely to offer such important home literacy behaviors as shared reading, provision of children's reading materials, and an early age of onset of shared reading (Lonigan, 1994). The quality of parent to child language can also be influenced of ethnicity, gender and maternal language.

This study aimed to reduce the widening educational gap that faces Latino students. It used home visitation to enrich the home language and literacy activities during children's early preschool years. Home visits provided parents and children with sustainable Spanish language and literacy materials and were spread over two years for a total of 46 weeks of home visitation. The data indicate significant gains in receptive and expressive Spanish language ability. There is also evidence that the parents sustain their enrichment activities at least one year after the program is completed. Like the immigrant parents studied by Farver, Eppe and Ballon (2006), the Latino immigrant parents in this study were able to make the language and literacy environments in their homes begin to approximate middle-class mainstream culture, The data also provide evidence that as kindergarteners, the treated children kept their Spanish advantage yet also developed an advantage for spoken English and literacy skills.

After each 23-week course of treatment, the Spanish PLS-3 scores of children who participated in the program showed significant gains. The average standardized language scores of treated children rose from pre-treatment levels close to the validation sample's average of 90 (Zimmerman et al, 1993) to levels over 100. In contrast, the mean Spanish standard PLS-3 scores for a group of older, untreated children (mean age 47 months) in the community was significantly below the validation sample used to standardize the Spanish PLS-3. The scores of children who participated in HABLA were consistently higher: they did not lose ground and gained as a function of each year's participation. Their average gain of 11 points comes close to the standard deviation of our baseline sample (e.g., 13.5 points) and that of the validation sample (15 points). For the full two-year programs there were medium treatment effects on receptive language and large treatment effects on expressive language.

We do not believe that the gains we observed are a function of test familiarity; the pre-treatment and post-treatment testing were separated by at least 7 months, the second and kindergarten by at least 11 months and there was effectively no overlap in questions. We also do not think they are a test artifact due to specific items being for some reason simpler. Treated children achieved higher scores than the pretreatment scores of untreated children the same age (e.g. the first year of treatment for the younger cohort vs. the baseline for the older cohort, the second year of treatment for both cohorts vs. the scores of untreated children). The PLS-3 data in this study suggest that, all else being equal, younger children in this sample have more age-appropriate language skills than older children but both can benefit from intervention. However, both groups had post-treatment scores that were significantly higher than their pre-treatment scores.

The weakness in language skills that we observed in our pre-treatment data is anticipated by the literature: preschool children living in poverty can be impoverished in oral language skills and the extent of disadvantage widens with age (Hart & Risley, 1995). A similar age-related negative trend was noted in the validation sample (Zimmerman et al, 1993), and is anticipated by research showing that development of a minority language can suffer in the context of bilingual education (Paez, Tabors & Lopez, 2007). Conclusions about the language skills of the older untreated children cannot be drawn from PLS-3 data alone, as the test was constructed as a translation of the English PLS-3 and is not as a true test of Spanish ability. For the future, all evaluations of HABLA participants will be use the PLS-4, a rigorously standardized and normed instrument developed in Spanish. Data in progress suggest that the intake scores on the PLS-4 are higher on average, but that significant gains occur after each year.

The data from the children who had participated in at least one year of treatment suggest that a Spanish language home program can promote Spanish language development during and immediately after treatment, possibly restoring disadvantaged children to an age-appropriate level of Spanish language acquisition. The program appears to create a special advantage for expressive language during and right after treatment. What we have further learned from the data for the children we were able to follow into kindergarten is that a Spanish home program can ultimately promote and facilitate both Spanish and English language acquisition in kindergarten. We also observe that parents who had participated in our treatment program reported a greater number of increased shared reading and greater efforts on the part of parents to teach their child about reading and writing.

Among kindergarten children, the HABLA intervention had associated with higher oral language skills in both Spanish and English. It also associated with superior phonological awareness. Children who had been through HABLA achieved significantly higher standard PLS scores in English, as well as in Spanish. As kindergarteners, the treated children surpassed their untreated peers on two different measures of phonological awareness: rhyme and phoneme awareness. They show higher mean scores on Spanish tests of rhyme awareness and phoneme awareness but also show higher mean scores on English tests of rhyme awareness and phoneme awareness.

Both spoken language skills and phonological awareness have been well recognized as particularly critical for the development of reading (see, for reviews: Adams, 1990; Gottardo, Stanovich, & Siegel, 1996; Foy & Mann, 2001; 2003; Lyon, 1994; Mahony & Mann, 1992; Mann, 1984; 1986; 1993; 1998; Mann & Liberman, 1984; Muter, Hulme, Snowling, & Taylor, 1998; Snow et al, 1998, Stanovich, 1994; Wagner & Torgesen, 1987). For alphabetic readers, phoneme awareness is the strongest correlates of reading success because the alphabet is a transcription of phonemes. Phonological awareness is a language activity that requires something above and beyond the skills of listening and speaking. It is a complex skill that derives from interplays among speech abilities and childhood experiences with word play, books and the ABC's. Phoneme awareness is strongly associated with exposure to literacy activities such as the acquisition of letter-sound knowledge and phonics more generally (Mann & Wimmer, 2002; Morais, Cary, Alegria, & Bertelson, 1979; Read, Zhang, Nie, & Ding, 1986). At the same time it is also associated with the development of primary spoken language skills, as the maturational status of phonological representations and vocabulary is critical for a child to take part in the experiences that instantiate phoneme awareness (Elbro, 1996; Fowler, 1991; Foy & Mann, 2001; 2003; Mann & Wimmer, 2002, Metsala, 1997). Among four- to six-year-olds, for example, factors in the home literacy environment are associated not only with children's awareness of rhyme and of phonemes, but also with their vocabulary, letter knowledge, and performance on such measures of spoken language skill as nonword repetition, rapid naming skill, phonological distinctness, and auditory discrimination. Both a teaching focus in the home and exposure to reading-related activities are directly associated with phoneme awareness and early reading ability, where exposure to a variety of children's literature supports vocabulary learning, more generally (Foy & Mann, 2003).

That an oral language enrichment program for preschoolers can lead to advantages in phonological awareness is consistent with the work of Lonigan (2003) and Foy and Mann (2001) who have shown that children who are advantaged for oral language skills (e.g., the PLS scores) are stronger in emergent literacy skills. The advantage of the HABLA treatment for both English and Spanish phonological awareness as well as the pattern of correlations between English and Spanish skills is consistent with Dickinson, McCabe, Clark-Chiarelli, Wolf (2004) and Quiroga, Lemos-Britton, Mostafapour, Abbott, and Berninger (2002), who observed strong cross-linguistic transfer between Spanish and English phonological awareness skills. That we tend to see fewer correlations involving the rhyme tasks may reflect the fact that materials on this task were real words where those on the phoneme awareness tasks also involved some nonce words.

The bilingual gain in kindergarten that we obtained by treating Latino children in a Spanish home visitation program is reminiscent of the results reported by Campos (1995) who reported that Latino children attending a Spanish-only preschool fared better when it came to reading skills in English than those who were in bilingual programs. It also concurs with Baker (2000), Cummins (2000), and Skutnabb-Kangas (2000) and Figuerdo (2006), all of whom emphasize the role of primary language strength in the acquisition of English as a second language by school children. The present study adds to the accumulating body of work about school readiness by providing evidence that enriching the *oral Spanish language environment in the homes* of very young preschoolers, can effectively raise both their Spanish language skills in the preschool years and their English language and literacy achievements in kindergarten. We agree with Kohnert, Yim, Nett, Kan and Duran (2005) that "systematic instruction in a child's home language during the preschool years supports later academic achievement in English (p.254)." We add that this instruction can occur in the home and appears most effective if it begins around age 2.

ACKNOWLEDGMENTS

This program was made possible through the generous support of the Children and Families Commission of Orange County, and First Five of California. We would like to express our deep gratitude to the over 50 home visitors who made this program possible, and especially to Rocio Santana, Carolina Rodriguez and Jacqueline Arreola, who completed much of the data entry and the additional testing of the kindergarten cohort. We would also like to thank the families who participated; they let us into their homes and gave us access to their children. We thank Judy Foy for her help with the phonological awareness materials and her comments on the manuscript.

REFERENCES

Adams, M. J. (1990). Beginning to read. *Cambridge*, MA: MIT Press.

Arnold, D. H., Lonigan, C. J. & Whitehurst, G. J. (1994). Accelerating language-development through picture book reading – replication and extension to a videotape training format. *Journal of Educational Psychology*, *86*, 235-243.

Baker, C. (2000). A parents' and teachers' guide to bilingualism. 2nd Edition. *Clevedon, England*, Multilingual Matters.

Bradley, L. & Bryant, P. E. (1983). Categorizing sounds and learning to read – a causal connection. *Nature*, *301*, 419-421.

Campos, S. J. (1995). The Carpentería preschool program: A longterm effects study. In E. E. Garcia & B. McLaughlin (Eds.), Meeting the challenge of linguistic and cultural diversity in early childhood education (pp. 34–48). *New York*, : Teachers College.

Chaney, C. (1998). Preschool language and metalinguistic skills are links to reading success. *Applied Psycholinguistics*, *19*, 433-446.

Cummins, J. (2000). Language, power, and pedagogy. Bilingual children in the crossfire. *Clevedon, England*, : Multilingual Matters.

Duursma, E., Romero-Contreras., A., Szuber, P. P., Snow, C., August, D. & Calderon, M. (2007). The role of home literacy and language environment on bilinguals' English and Spanish vocabulary development. *Applied Psycholinguistics*, *28*, 171-190.

Dickinson, D., McCabe, A., Clark-Chiarelli, N. & Wolf, A. (2004). Cross-linguistic transfer of phonological awareness in low-income Spanish and English bilingual children. *Applied Psycholinguistics*, *25*, 323-347.

Elbro, C. (1996). Early linguistic abilities and reading development: A review and a hypothesis. *Reading & Writing*, *8*, 453-485.

Farver, J. M., Eppe, S. & Ballon, D. (2006). Acculturation and family characteristics that facilitate literacy development among Latino children. In M. H. Bornstein & L. R. Cote (Eds.), *Acculturation and parent-child relationships: Measurement and development.* Monographs in Parenting Series. NJ: Erlbaum Press.

Farver, J. A. M., Xu, Y., Eppe, S. & Lonigan, C. L. (2006). Home environments and young Latino children's school readiness Early Childhood Research Quarterly 21 (2006), 196-212.

Figuerdo, L. (2006). Using the known to chart the unknown: A review of first language influence on the development of English-as-a-second-language spelling skill. *Reading and Writing*, *19*, 873-905.

Fowler, A. E. (1991). How early phonological development might set the stage for phoneme awareness. In S. Brady & D. Shankweiler (Eds.), Phonological processes in literacy: A tribute to Isabelle Y. Liberman (pp. 97-117), *Hillsdale*, NJ: Erlbaum.

Foy, J. G. & Mann, V.A. (2001). Does strength of phonological representations predict phonological awareness in preschool children? *Applied Psycholinguistics*, *22*, 301-325.

Foy, J. G. & Mann, V.A. (2003). Home literacy environment and phonological awareness in preschool children: differential effects for rhyme and phoneme awareness. *Applied Psycholinguistics*, *24*, 59-88.

Gauvain, M., Savage, S. & McCollum, D. (2000). Reading at home and at school in the primary grades: Cultural and social influences. Early Education & Development, 11, 447-463.

Gottardo, A., Stanovich, K.E. & Siegel, L.S. (1996). The relationship between phonological sensitivity, syntactic processing and verbal working memory in the reading performance of third grade children. *Child Psychology*, *63(3)*, 563-582.

Hart, B. & Risely, T. R. (1995). Meaningful Differences in the Everyday Lives of Young American Children. Baltimore: Brookes.

Honig, A. S. (1982). Language environments for young children. *Young Children*, *38*, 56-67.

Kamerman, S. B. & Kahn, A. J. (1995). Starting Right. *New York*: Oxford University Press.

Kohnert, K., Yim, D., Nett, K., Kan, P. F. & Duran, K. (2005). Intervention with linguistically diverse preschool children: A focus on developing home language(s). Language, *Speech and Hearing Services in Schools*, *36*, 251-263.

Laosa, L. M. (1980). Material teaching strategies in Chicano and Anglo-American families: the influence of culture and education on maternal behavior. *Child Development*, *51*, 759-765.

Laosa, L. M. (1982). School, occupation, culture and family: The impact of parental schooling on the parent-child relationship. *Journal of Educational Psychology*, *74*, 791-827.

Lazar, I. & Darlington, R. (1982). Lasting effects of early education: A report from the consortium of longitudinal studies. *Monographs of the Society for Research in Child Development*, *47*, (serial 195).

Levenstein, P., Levenstein, S., Shiminski, J. A. & Stolzberg, J. E. (1998). Long-term impact of a verbal interaction program for at-risk toddlers: an exploratory study of high school outcomes in a replication of the Mother-Child- Home Program. *Journal of Applied Developmental Psychology*, *19*, 267-285.

Levenstein, P. & Staff of Verbal Interaction Project. (1976). Child's Behavioiral Traits (CBT). In Johnson, O. G. Ed., Tests and Measurements in Child Development: Handbook II, Vol I. San Francisco: Jossey-Bass.

Levenstein, P., Levenstein, S. & Oliver, D. (2002). First grade school readiness of former child participants in a South Carolina replication of the Parent-Child Home Program. Applied Developmental Psychology, 23,331-353.

Lonigan, C. J. (2003). Development and promotion of emergent literacy skill in preschool children at-risk of reading difficulties. In B. R. Foorman (Ed.), Preventing and remediating reading difficulties: Bringing science to scale (pp. 23-50). Timonium: MD: York Press.

Lonigan, C. J. & Whitehurst, G. J. (1998). Relative efficacy of parent and teacher involvement in a shared-reading intervention for preschool children from low-income backgrounds, *Early Childhood Research Quarterly*, *13*, 263-290.

Lovett, M. W. Steinbach, K. A. & Frijters, J. C. (2000). Remediating the core deficits of developmental reading disability: A double-deficit hypothesis. *Journal of Learning Disabilities*, *33*, 334-358.

Lyon, G. R. (1994). Toward a definition of dyslexia. *Annals of Dyslexia*, *45*, 3-27.

Mach, E. J. & Johnston, C. (1982). A comparison of the mother-child interactions of younger and older hyperactive and normal children. *Child Development*, *53*, 1371-1381.

Mahony, D. L. & Mann, V. A. (1992). Using children's humor to clarify the relationship between linguistic awareness and future reading ability *Cognition*, *45*, 163-186.

Mann, V. A. (1998). Language problems: A key to early reading problems, In B. Y. L. Wong, (Ed.) *Learning About Learning Disabilities*, 2nd Edition (pp. 163-201). *San Diego*, CA: Academic Press.

Mann, V. A. (1993). Phonemic awareness and future reading ability *Journal of Learning Disabilities*, *26*, 259-269.

Mann, V. A. (1986). Phonological Awareness: The Role of Reading Experience. Cognition, 24, 65-92. Also published under the same title in: P. Bertelson (Ed.) *The Onset of Literacy*, 1987. *Cambridge*, Mass.: MIT Press.

Mann, V. A. (1984). Longitudinal prediction and prevention of early reading difficulty. *Annals of Dyslexia*, *34*, 117-136.

Mann, V. A. & Liberman, I. Y. (1984) Phonological awareness and verbal short-term memory: Can they presage early reading problems? *Journal of Learning* Disabilities, *17*, 592-599.

Mann, V. & Wimmer, H. (2002). Phoneme awareness and pathways to literacy: A comparison of German and American children. *Reading & Writing*, *15*, 653-682.

Metsala, J. (1997). Spoken word recognition in reading disabled children. *Journal of Educational Psychology*, *89(1)*, 159-173.

Morais, J., Cary, L., Alegria, J. & Bertelson, P. (1979). Does awareness of speech as a sequence of phones arise spontaneously? *Cognition*, *7*, 323-331.

Muter, V. Hulme, C., Snowling, M. & Taylor, S. (1998). Segmentation, not rhyming, predicts early progress in learning to read. *Journal of Experimental Child Psychology*, *71*, 3-27.

National Reading Council, (2001) Putting Reading First: Helping your Child Learn to Read. Washington, D.C: the Partnership for Reading through the National Institute for Literacy (NIFL) *and the National Institute for Child Health and Human Development (NICHD),* U.S. Department of Education.

Nittrouer, S. (1996). the relation between speech perception and phonemic awareness: Evidence from low SES children and children with chronic OM. *Journal of Speech and Hearing Research*, *39*, 1059-1070.

Páez, M. M., Tabors, P. O. & López, L. M. (2007). Dual language and literacy development *Journal of Applied Developmental Psychology*, *28*, 85-102.

Purcell-Gates, V., McIntyre, E. & Freppon, P. A. (1995). Learning written storybook language in school: A comparison of low SES children in skills-based and whole-language classrooms. *American Educational Research Journal*, *32*, 659-685.

Quiroga, T., Lemos-Britton, Z., Mostafapour, E., Abbott, R. D. & Berninger, V. W. (2002). Phonological Awareness and Beginning Reading in Spanish-Speaking ESL First Graders: Research into Practice. *Journal of School Psychology*, *40*, 1, 85-111.

Raver, C. C, & Knitzer, J. (2002). Ready to enter: What research tells policy makers about strategies to promote social and emotional school readiness among three- and four-year-olds. Washington, DC: National Center for Children in Poverty.

Read, C., Zhang, Y., Nie, H. & Ding, B. (1986). The ability to manipulate speech sounds depends on knowing alphabetic writing. *Cognition*, *24(1-2)*, 31-44.

Seneschal, M., Le Fevre, J., Thomas, E. & Daley, K. (1998). Differential effects of home literacy experiences on the development of oral and written language. *Reading Research Quarterly*, *33*, 96-116.

Skutnabb-Kangas, T. (2000). Linguistic genocide in education-or worldwide diversity and human rights? *Mahwah*, NJ: Lawrence Erlbaum Associates.

Snow, C. E. (1991). The theoretical basis for relationships between language and literacy in development. *Journal of Research in Childhood Education*, *6*, 30-46.

Stanovich, K. E. (1994). Annotation: Does dyslexia exist? Journal of Child Psychology.

Wagner, R. K. & Torgesen, J. K. (1987). The nature of phonological processing and its causative role in the acquisition of reading skills. *Psychological Bulletin*, *101*,192-212.

Walker, D., Greenwood, C., Hart, B. & Carta, J. (1994). Prediction of school outcomes based on early language production and socioeconomic factors. *Child Development*, *65*, 606-621.

Walley, A. C. (1993). The role of vocabulary development in children's spoken word recognition and segmentation ability. *Developmental Review*, *13*, 286-350.

Zimmerman, I. L., Steiner, V. G. & Pond, R. E. (1993). Preschool Language Scale -3, Spanish Edition. San Antonio TX: The Psychological corporation.

Zimmerman, I. L., Steiner, V. G. & Pond, R. E. (2002). Preschool Language Scale, 4th edition. *San Antonio*, TX: The Psychological Corporation.

Zimmerman, I. L. & Castilleja, N. F. (2005). The role of a language scale for infant and preschool assessment. *Mental Retardation and Developmental Disabilities Research Reviews*, *11*, 238-246.

APPENDIX B. MATERIALS FOR PARENT SURVEY:

1. What is the mother's highest level of education: ------ grades
2. What is the father's highest level of education: ------- grades
3. How old was your child when you first started reading picture books to him/her?
4. How many children's books are available in your household?
   None 1-20 21-40 41-60 61-80 more? (estimate----)
5. How often do you, or other members of the family read to your child in a typical week:

a. At bedtime?
   Never once 2 3 4 5 6 7 times -------more? (estimate ----)

b. Other times?
   Neveronce 2 3 4 5 6 7 times -------more? (estimate ---)

6. During a typical week how often does your child ask to be read to?
   Never 1 2 3 4 5 Very often
7. During a typical week, how often do you engage in the following activities?

a. I teach my child to print words:
   1 2 3 4 5
   Never Often

b. I teach my child to read:
   1 2 3 4 5
   Never Often

8. How many children's books are available in your household
   None 1-20 21-40 41-60 61-80 more? (estimate----)

In: Speech Disorders: Causes, Treatment and Social Effects ISBN: 978-1-60876-213-2
Editor: Alan E. Harrison, pp. 119-137

Chapter 5

NEW FRONTIERS IN UNDERSTANDING SPEECH SOUND DISORDER: UNRAVELING THE MYSTERIES OF GENETIC CAUSES

Beate Peter
Department of Speech and Hearing Sciences and Division of Medical Genetics, University of Washington, Seattle

ABSTRACT

The nature of speech sound disorder (SSD) is not yet well understood. Some view it as a single clinical entity, while others propose distinct subtypes, defined variously by criteria such as error types and suspected cause. A universally accepted disorder classification, based on relevant behavioral observations, does not yet exist. An account of genetic substrates would greatly enhance current understanding of SSD, but such an account is not yet available. This chapter reviews the history of genetic research in SSD from the first studies of familial clustering of SSD to the most recent studies in molecular genetics and points to new frontiers in the quest to characterize the biological causes of SSD.

INTRODUCTION

The Quest to Understand the Biological Substrates of Speech Sound Dissorder

In the four short years following an infant's first cry, many remarkable skills emerge and are mastered, among them the ability to convey ideas using spoken language in such a way that even an unfamiliar listener can understand what is being said. Given the complexity of the task, which involves translating a thought into linguistic units, assembling these units into a syntactic frame, and sequencing the requisite sound units and programming the various components of the articulatory musculature to constrain the airstream for purposes of transducing intended speech sounds into actual sound waves, this ability is truly noteworthy. In languages and cultures all over the world, most four-year-olds are capable communicators, having successfully progressed through a set of universally predictable phases of sound production including cry, coo, babble, first words, word combinations, explosive vocabulary growth, and increasingly sophisticated syntactic structures.

Not every child, however, follows this general trajectory. A variety of causes can interfere with speech sound development, including structural abnormalities in the articulatory system, hearing deficits, and psychosocial factors. In the vast majority of cases, no known cause exists. Various terms have been used to describe this type of primary childhood speech disorder, including "articulation disorder," "phonological disorder," "multiple phoneme disorder," "speech delay," "intelligibility impairment" (Shriberg, Tomblin, & McSweeny, 1999), and "speech sound disorder" (e.g., Lewis, Freebairn, & Taylor, 2000). Modifiers such as "functional," "primary," "childhood," and "developmental" are sometimes added to the term to indicate the absence of a known cause and the fact that the disorder manifests during the time when speech is typically acquired. The coexistence of multiple disorder descriptors is one indication that a universally accepted disorder profile and subtype system is not yet available. For the purposes of this text, the term speech sound disorder (SSD) is used to refer to this type of communication disorder.

SSD is fairly common, although published prevalence rates vary. Generally, SSD is more prevalent among boys than among girls, and prevalence decreases with increasing age. Prevalence estimates range from approximately 1% to 15.6% and are not only influenced by age and gender but also by the quantitative criteria selected to identify children with SSD. For example, using a criterion of 75% glossable productions in spontaneous speech, Campbell et al. (2003) estimate that 15.6% of three-year-old children have SSD. Using a z score of -1.14 in a 20-item articulation test as a diagnostic criterion, Shriberg et al. (1999) report a prevalence rate of 3.8% in six-year-old children. Based on a four-stage process of identification, including teacher report and a speech-language pathologist report, McKinnon, McLeod, and Reilly (2007) identified approximately 1.1% of children in an Australian school-age sample in Kindergarten through 6th grade as having SSD. Considerable resources are required to address the needs of children with SSD. According to a survey of school-based speech-language pathologists in the United States (American Speech-Language-Hearing Association, 2004), 94% of the respondents regularly served children with articulation/phonological disorders. Out of a national caseload average of 50 children served each month, 23 were seen for this type of communication disorder.

Despite the size of the affected population and the substantial resources necessary to address speech sound disorders clinically, no universally accepted disorder classification is apparent at this time. One proposed but somewhat controversial subtype of speech disorders of unknown origin is childhood apraxia of speech (CAS), also referred to as developmental apraxia of speech, verbal dyspraxia, and other labels constructed from elements of these terms. As a proposed clinical entity, CAS is generally viewed as interfering with motor planning and/or motor programming processes. A position statement issued by the American Speech-Language-Hearing Association (2007) defines CAS as "a neurological childhood (pediatric) speech sound disorder in which the precision and consistency of movements underlying speech are impaired in the absence of neuromuscular deficits." In addition to a framework that accommodates CAS, a number of classification schemes, based on various theoretical frameworks, coexist in the literature. For instance, Crary's (1993) motolinguistic model of developmental motor speech disorders views SSD from a perspective based on a functional linguistic/motor continuum, where motor execution is modeled at one end of the continuum and linguistic aspects of motor planning are modeled at the other end of the continuum. Dodd's classification of childhood speech disorders (Dodd, 1995) uses error types to distinguish among disorder subtypes such as articulation disorder versus delayed phonological development, or deviant-consistent versus deviant-inconsistent phonological errors. Bauman-Waengler (2000) models speech sound disorders along a phonetic-phonemic continuum, where children allocated close to the phonetic pole of the disorder continuum exhibit mostly distortion errors while those close to the phonemic pole exhibit errors consistent with systematic speech sound substitutions. Shriberg and colleagues (e.g., Shriberg, Lewis, Tomblin, McSweeny, Karlsson & Scheer, 2005) base their disorder classification on suspected etiology, giving rise to subtypes related to genetic factors, otitis media, motor involvement, psychosocial involvement, and speech errors. Each taxonomy is thus defined from a different theory-driven paradigm. It is unknown which of these describes SSD subtypes with the greatest clinical and statistical relevance. A comprehensive account of the biological foundations of SSD, including its genetic liabilities, would greatly enhance our understanding of the nature and subtype structure of this common disorder, but such an account is not yet available.

SSD is frequently seen in the presence of two other types of developmental communication disorders, reading disorder (RD) and language impairment (LI), and more is known about their biological foundations, compared to those of SSD. According to the International Dyslexia Association (Lyon, Shaywitz, & Shaywitz, 2003), RD is a specific learning disability related to written language, characterized by deficits in accurate and/or fluent word recognition, decoding, and spelling. These difficulties are not predicted by other cognitive skills or quality of reading instruction. LI has been defined as a heterogeneous developmental language disorder in the absence of hearing impairment, frank neurological impairment or psycho-emotional disturbance (Leonard, 1998). When comorbidities among certain disorders exceed rates that can be predicted from the joint probabilities of their prevalence rates, an underlying association can be suspected. Given that 3.8% of the children in the Shriberg et al. (1999) study sample were labeled with a speech disorder and 8.1% of the participants were labeled with SLI, the co-occurrence of both, under random conditions, would be 0.31% but the observed co-occurrence was 0.51%, which led the authors to believe that the two disorder types may be mutually associated. According to a review by Peterson, McGrath, Smith, and Pennington (2007), there is general consensus that many children with an early diagnosis of LI struggle with reading later on, and approximately half of them will meet criteria for RD. The overlap between SSD and RD may be slightly less, but there are indications that children with SSD will have difficulty with reading to a greater extent than expected by chance alone, especially in the presence of concomitant LI (Bird, Bishop & Freeman, 1995; reviewed in Pennington & Bishop, 2009; Schuele, 2004). It should be noted that more boys than girls are affected by SSD (Campbell et al., 2003; Fox, Dodd & Howard, 2002; Shriberg et al., 1999), LI (Leonard, 1998; Tomblin, Zhang, Buckwalter, & O'Brien, 2003; Verhoeven & van Balkom, 2004), and RD (Shaywitz, Shaywitz & Fletcher, 1990).

In an attempt to delineate the biological substrates of RD and LI, several studies have evaluated brain structures and functions in these disorders. Magnetic resonance imaging (MRI) studies in children with LI have implicated reduced or absent asymmetry in the planum temporale (e.g., Leonard and seven others, 2002) and in the inferior frontal gyrus (IGF), a region that includes Broca's area (De Fossé and 11 others; 2004). Similar IGF structural abnormalities have also been reported in individuals with RD (Brown, Eliez, Menon, Rumsey, White & Reiss, 2001; Robichon, Levrier, Farnarier & Habib, 2000). More recently, the availability of diffusion tensor imaging has facilitated new discoveries of white matter tract abnormalities in LI and RD. For instance, Jaenoke, Siegenthaler, Preis, and Steinmetz. (2007) showed decreased white matter volumes in the left hemispheres of children with LI, involving the motor cortex, the dorsal premotor cortex, the ventral premotor cortex, and the planum temporale. Motor impairments were seen in most of the applied motor tests. Imaging studies of individuals with RD have found abnormal white matter tracts connecting anterior and posterior perisylvian regions (Deutsch, Dougherty & Bammer, 2005; Klingberg et al., 2000; Richards et al., 2008). Similar structural imaging studies are not yet available in individuals with SSD.

Several functional imaging studies in RD, using positron emission tomography and functional magnetic resonance imaging, have shown abnormal activation in many of the same regions implicated in structural imaging studies. As reviewed by Peterson et al. (2007), findings can be summarized to state that decreased occipitotemporal activation has been observed most often in word recognition deficits, decreased temporoparietal activation has been associated with phonological processing deficits, and increased inferior frontal gyrus activity appears to represent compensation. Fewer functional imaging studies are available in LI. One example is Weismer, Plante, Jones and Tomblin (2005), who showed that adolescents with LI had reduced coactivation of left hemisphere structures, compared to controls, during a verbal working memory task. Virtually no functional imaging studies are available in individuals with SSD.

Characteristic differences in brain structures and functions point to a biological basis underlying LI and RD, which is consistent with a genetic origin in affected individuals. High comorbidity rates with SSD are consistent with a genetic origin in that population as well. Before focusing on the genetics of SSD, a brief review of concepts and procedures relevant for the remainder of this chapter is provided here. Readers familiar with this material should skip over this section.

Terminology and Tools in Genetics

The human genome, consisting of 22 paired autosomal chromosomes and the sex chromosomes X and Y, can be thought of as the biochemical machinery that encodes the formation of all body structures and maintains its functions - in tandem, of course, with environmental factors. An individual's chromosomes can be visualized using microscopy and arranged into a karyotype, showing the paired autosomes and the sex chromosomes.

Each chromosome is a molecule of enormous biochemical complexity, called deoxyribonucleic acid (DNA), a double-stranded, helical-shaped string composed of only four nucleotides: two purines, adenine and guanine, and two pyrimidines, thymine and cytosine, plus a molecular scaffolding structure. Where one strand carries a cytosine, the opposing strand must carry a guanine and vice versa; where one strand carries an adenine, the opposing strand must carry a thymine and vice versa. The two opposing strands thus make up strings of base pairs. Together, the 23 chromosomes make up approximately 3 billion base pairs and, because each chromosome comes in two similar but not quite identical copies, there are approximately 6 million base pairs in a human body cell. It is estimated that humans have approximately 20,000 to 25,000 protein encoding regions called genes. In this respect, the human genome resembles an extremely complex language composed of only four speech sounds. Disruptions in the form of mutations, deletions, insertions, or transpositions of DNA pieces can have substantial effects on the structures or functions of the affected organism. Some disorders result from a variation in just one of the two autosomal gene copies; this pattern is referred to as autosomal dominant. A disorder resulting from changes in both copies of the autosomal gene characterizes an autosomal recessive inheritance pattern. In some cases, a mutation in a single gene can cause a massive disorder. Cystic fibrosis is an example of such a monogenic disease. In other cases, two or more genes are involved and finding them is more complicated. Diabetes and coronary heart disease are examples of polygenic diseases. It is thought that SSD, like LI and RD, are inherited as quantitative traits, where the relevant clinical characteristics vary along a continuum and are influenced by several genes.

The 22 human autosomal chromosome pairs are numbered according to length, with chromosome 1 being the longest and 22, the shortest. Each chromosome has two endpoints called telomeres and a specialized region somewhere along its length called centromere. The shorter arm of the chromosome, i.e., the shorter of the two stretches between the centromere and one telomere, is referred to as the p arm and the longer stretch, as the q arm. The arms can be further described by their banding patterns, visible under a microscope with staining, and a numbering system along each arm, extending from the centromere to each telomere. This nomenclature leads to a rough map of the chromosome that can be used to describe the general location of a gene. According to this convention, the 7p31 address refers to band 31 of the shorter arm of chromosome 7, incidentally, the location of the *FOXP2* gene, which will be mentioned in more detail later.

The human genome contains a large number of DNA regions known to vary among individuals without necessarily causing any particular trait or disease. Because the nature and location of these markers are known, they can be used as signposts to track down the location of an actual disease gene residing close by on the same chromosome. Useful types of markers include single nucleotide polymorphisms (SNPs), where the nature of a single nucleotide can vary among individuals; microsatellites, also referred to as short tandem repeat polymorphisms (STRPs), consisting of variable numbers of base pair sequence repeats; and minisatellites with repeat units that are longer than those in microsatellites. While each SNP occurs in only two variants in the population, microsatellites and minisatellites can have many more variants at each locus. On the other hand, known SNP loci are available in much greater numbers than microsatellites and minisatellites. The proximity of a certain marker of known location to a disease gene of unknown location can be used to map the gene, because the marker tends to be inherited along with the disease gene instead of becoming separated from it through recombination. The likelihood of observing a given configuration of disease in a pedigree, together with a given configuration of a certain marker in a pedigree, is computed under the assumption that the disease and the marker are completely independent from each other, i.e., they are unlinked. This likelihood is then compared to the likelihood of observing the same disease and marker constellation, assuming that they are linked, i.e., the disease and the marker tend to be inherited together. This latter likelihood can be modeled over a range of hypothetical genetic distances. The $\log_{10}$ score of the ratio of the linked over the unlinked likelihood is the log odds score ("lod score"), and the genetic distance with the highest lod score is the best estimate of how closely the marker and the disease gene are linked.

Linkage analysis based on lod scores is only one of many approaches to discovering causative genes. The history of genetics research in populations with SSD illustrates, in part, the evolution of these methodologies.

Reasons to Study SSD Genetics

For RD, a number of genetic regions have been identified, including 1p34-36, 2p15-16, 3p12-q13, 6p21.3-22, 15q15-21, 18p11, and Xq27; regions associated with LI include 13q21, 16q, and 19q; regions associated with traits related to articulation in SSD include 1.p34-36, 3p12-q13, 6p22, and 15q11-13 (reviewed in Lewis and six others, 2006; Pennington & Bishop, 2009; Peterson et al., 2007). Given the substantial amount of comorbidity and the overlap in implicated brain structures and functions, it is surprising that the genetic associations in LI, RD, and SSD do not mirror each other more closely.

The motivation for studying the genetic substrates in SSD, as in many other disorders, is diverse. As mentioned, knowing which genes cause SSD in some or all affected individuals would greatly enhance our understanding of the nature and subtype structure of SSD. This knowledge would translate directly into more accurate diagnostic schemes. Knowing whether a young child carries a genotype that puts him or her at risk for SSD or one of its subtypes is helpful for early intervention, which may prevent the full expression of the disorder. Understanding how genetic factors in SSD interact with genetic factors in other disorders such as LI and RD contributes to our knowledge of the larger picture of disorders in motor, linguistic, and cognitive systems. As in all genetic studies, social and ethical questions arise. For instance, knowledge of a person's disorder genotype could potentially interfere with access to health care. It could also lead to highly controversial practices such as prenatal selection against an affected offspring. The highest ethical standards must be followed in carrying out research in the genetics of communication disorders and in the practice of genetic counseling.

Is gene therapy an option for families with a history of SSD? At the time of this writing, gene therapy is still mostly in its experimental stage. In diseases like cystic fibrosis, where the causative gene is known and has been sequenced, gene therapy has been tried in animal models but not yet in humans. The Food and Drug Administration has not yet approved any gene therapy product for sale in the United States. For SSD, causative genes have not yet been identified and sequenced. Gene therapy continues to be an active area of research,

The following outlines the history of research in the field of SSD genetics. This review highlights the use of various methodologies over the past few decades of research, and the findings to which they have led. As will become evident, the comorbidities and the shared traits among SSD, LI, and RD guided some of the hypotheses regarding suspected gene regions.

Behavioral Genetics Studies in SSD

The earliest indication that difficulties with speech may have a genetic component comes from the observation that they appear to cluster in families. In her 1965 book, *Development and Disorders of Speech in Childhood*, Muriel Morley describes an extensive longitudinal study of speech development in 847 children, of whom 12 were diagnosed with "articulatory apraxia," based on difficulty with imitating the sound sequences of speech. In six of the 12 families, additional family members were affected, not necessarily with the same disorder traits. For instance, one child with speech difficulties had four siblings with typical speech, but the mother had been a late talker and one of her seven brothers also had severe difficulty developing intelligible speech. In another family, a child with disordered speech sound development had a grandfather with a history of stuttering.

Another example of a familial aggregation of communication disorders with varied phenotypic expression is found in Lewis (1992). Her analysis of 87 pedigrees, each with a preschool child with speech difficulties, showed that speech and language disorders aggregate in families, with a higher incidence of males affected than females. Significantly more family members with dyslexia and learning disabilities, but not stuttering or hearing impairment, were found in pedigrees of individuals with phonological disorders than in pedigrees of nondisabled individuals. Determining the mode of inheritance, however, proved to be more difficult. In pedigrees ascertained through 45 probands with a history of speech and language disorders, Lewis, Cox, and Bayard (1993) were unable to determine whether the pattern of affectedness in the pedigrees was more consistent with a major gene model or a multifactorial transmission model.

Felsenfeld, Broen, and McGue (1992) followed up on adults who had participated in a longitudinal speech study, the Templin study, during their childhood 28 years prior. Data had been collected from kindergarten through fourth grade. The participating adults represented two cohorts, one with a childhood history of moderate to severe speech disorder and the other, with average to high speech articulation skills in childhood. The follow-up study showed that the adults with a history of speech difficulties obtained lower scores in articulation, receptive language, and expressive language, compared to the control cohort. To examine whether speech difficulties aggregated in the families of Templin study participants with a history of speech difficulties, Felsenfeld, McGue, and Broen (1995) evaluated articulation abilities, speech error types and history of educational services including speech therapy in the offspring of adults with, and without, a history of speech difficulty. They showed that children of adults who had a history of SSD performed significantly worse on measures of articulation compared to children of adults without a history of SSD. These children were also more likely to have received speech therapy. The speech error types, however, differed from parents to offspring; in other words, the disorder phenotype did not breed true.

One difficulty with genetic SSD studies is that the actual disorder phenotype of an adult cannot easily be measured with standardized articulation test tools because most adults who had speech therapy as children have normalized articulation patterns, and thorough documentation of their speech development in childhood are usually not available. Childhood records of adult study participants such as those evaluated by Felsenfeld et al. (1992; 1995) are rarely available. To study residual effects of SSD in adults whose speech had normalized, Lewis, Freebairn, Hansen, Miscimarra, Iyengar and Taylor (2007) taxed the speech production skills of 147 adults with tasks not normally given during standard articulation and phonology testing, including multisyllabic word imitations, nonword imitations, Pig Latin, and tongue twisters. These adults, of whom 36 reported having received speech therapy in childhood, were the parents of children currently receiving speech therapy. As a group, those parents with a history of speech difficulties obtained lower scores on all measures of speech production, compared to parents who had not received speech therapy. In addition, they also showed lower reading, spelling, and receptive language abilities.

The familial aggregation studies described above are consistent with the interpretation that offspring of individuals with SSD tend to also have SSD, but they could not conclusively isolate the relative contributions of genetic and environmental components. To deliberately distinguish between these two sources of influence, Felsenfeld and Plomin (1997) examined articulation skills in two types of offspring, adopted and biological, and two types of parents, history of SSD and no history of SSD. A biological background of SSD was the best predictor of SSD in the offspring. Twin studies comparing concordance rates for SSD in monozygotic (MZ) and dizygotic (DZ) twins have reported higher concordance rates among the MZ twins, suggesting a substantial genetic contribution (Lewis & Thompson, 1992; Bishop, 2002), but to date, twin studies examining specific traits such as speech sound error types or response to intervention have not been reported.

Molecular Genetics Studies in SSD

Technological advances over the past few decades, for instance the discovery of genetic markers called restriction length polymorphisms (Botstein, White, Skolnick & Davis, 1980) in tandem with sophisticated statistical methods, have enabled geneticists to identify gene regions, individual genes, and even a single nucleotide change as the biological cause of certain diseases. Several studies have addressed the molecular genetics of speech problems. The first set of molecular studies and the only one so far to identify a causative gene for a speech deficit began with a careful analysis of the speech and language deficits in the KE family in the UK. Approximately half of the members in this family in each generation have severe difficulty with speech production and, in addition, with receptive and expressive language, reading, writing, and oral praxis (Hurst, Baraitser, Auger, Graham & Norell, 1990; Vargha-Kadem, Watkins, Alcock, Fletcher & Passingham, 1995; Watkins, Dronkers & Vargha-Khadem, 2002). A series of brain imaging studies (Vargha-Khadem et al., 1998) revealed characteristic structural and functional abnormalities in cortical and subcortical regions, the latter including the basal ganglia.

The co-occurrence of deficits in communication abilities and brain abnormalities in affected individuals suggests a biological disorder substrate, and the pattern of familial aggregation, where half of the offspring of an affected individual is also affected, suggests a dominant mechanism of inheritance, with one mutated copy of a gene sufficient to cause a disorder. This pattern also suggests a monogenic mechanism with full penetrance, such that a single gene causes the disorder and every individual carrying a mutated copy of the gene is affected by the disorder. Following a cytogenetic inspection of the karyotype of some of the affected family members to rule out chromosomal abnormalities, Fisher, Vargha-Khadem, Watkins, Monaco, and Pembrey (1998) performed a genome-wide microsatellite screen in the DNA of 27 members of the family. Statistical analysis of the genotypes, given their position in the pedigree, pointed to a region on the q arm of chromosome 7 as the most likely region to harbor the gene(s) co-segregating with the disorder. The researchers followed up on this result by evaluating a large number of additional markers in this region, leading them to narrow the region to the 7q31 band. Using evidence from an unrelated individual with speech and language deficits similar to those seen in the KE family, the team identified a candidate gene that was found to co-segregate perfectly with the communication disorder seen in the KE family (Lai, Fisher, Hurst, Vargha-Khadem & Monaco, 2001). In accordance with nomenclature conventions, this gene was termed *FOXP2* because it encodes a protein sequence that shows high similarity to the characteristic DNA-binding domain of the forkhead/winged-helix (FOX) family of transcription factors.

The systematic process of arriving at the *FOXP2* gene as causative to the speech and language deficits in the KE family is a textbook example of how a thorough investigation of phenotypes in a multigenerational family can lead to the identification of a single gene. Steps along the way included observing the familial patterns of affectedness, karyotyping, genome-wide microsatellite screening, fine-mapping of candidate regions, identification of candidate genes, and, finally, sequencing the gene in affected individuals. This series of landmark studies doubtlessly benefited from the facts that a large, multigenerational pedigree was available for study, resulting in sufficient statistical power to detect linkage even in a single pedigree; that the disorder was monogenic; and that it was fully penetrant. Subsequent studies in other families with speech and language deficits showed, however, that *FOXP2* mutations are extremely rare. For instance, among 49 individuals with severe SSD, only three had a mutation in this region, a proband, his sibling, and his mother (MacDermot et al., 2005). Furthermore, the mutation seen in the KE family has widely pleiotropic effects not seen in common forms of SSD, where speech is the only affected behavior. The vast majority of SSD cases, hence, are not caused by this mechanism, and it can be concluded that *FOXP2* is necessary but not sufficient for normal speech development.

When substantial chunks of DNA are missing or translocated to a different chromosomal region, serious damage can result, affecting a variety of structures and/or functions. Such pleiotropic mechanisms involving speech production include 22q11.2 deletion syndrome, also referred to as velo-cardio-facial syndrome (reviewed by Widdershoven, Beemer, Kon, Dejockere & Mink van der Molen 2008). This syndrome leads to a number of structural deficits including craniofacial dysmorphisms. Speech production and resonance are affected by velopharyngeal and craniofacial malformations and, additionally, by delayed or disordered speech acquisition. Another example of a chromosomal condition affecting several functions including speech is presented in a case study of three siblings with an unbalanced 4q;16q translocation (Shriberg, Jakielski & El-Shanti, 2008). Findings suggest that duplicated genes on chromosome 16 and/or deletions on chromosome 4 may be associated with the observed traits in these children. Traits included minor dysmorphisms, cognitive delays, and speech abnormalities. Speech was characterized by poor imitative abilities, incomplete sound inventories, multiple vowel errors, inconsistent word productions, increasing number of errors as word length increased, unintelligible conversational speech, slow and dysrhythmic diadochokinetic rates, and fluctuating nasal resonance. The genetic analyses included karyotyping to identify the chromosomal pieces involved in the translocation and microsatellite typing to narrow the regions of the breakpoints. The breakpoints were further investigated with customized microarrays covering the regions of interest with a dense array of SNPs, which allowed the researchers to explore the copy numbers of each probe.

The *FOXP2* mutation, velo-cardio-facial syndrome, and 4q;16q translocation syndrome are examples of rare syndromes where speech is one of several affected functions. The genetic mechanisms causing common forms of speech sound disorder without involvement of other functions are not yet well understood. Several recent studies have sought to identify causative gene regions in individuals with primary SSD by focusing on candidate regions defined through a rationale of pleiotropy, where gene regions implied in another disorder are thought to also influence SSD because the other disorder is frequently comorbid with SSD. Stein et al. (2004) hypothesized that, since many children with SSD present with RD, the same gene region that is associated with RD could also be associated with primary SSD. In sib pairs from 77 families, each ascertained through a proband child with primary SSD, the authors collected data measuring phonological memory, phonological representation, articulation, receptive and expressive vocabulary, reading decoding, reading comprehension. They undertook linkage analysis within a region of interest, 3p12-q13, that had previously been shown to be linked to several traits of RD in one Finnish family (Nopola-Hemmi et al., 2001). Using 15 microsatellite markers spanning a 56 kB (kilobase; equivalent to 56,000 base pairs) stretch within this region, model-free linkage analysis, i.e., without specifying a mode of inheritance such as dominant or recessive, was performed for six reading and language scores and three factor scores that were derived from factor analysis, characterized by phonological short-term memory, articulatory skill, and vocabulary skill, respectively. The statistical analysis was based on the Haseman-Elston method, where squared trait differences in the sibs are regressed on the estimated proportion of marker alleles shared as identical by descent. Significant evidence for linkage within the region of interest was found for the composite factor of phonological short-term memory and for the reading decoding measure. Evidence for the composite factor of articulation skill was suggestive but not statistically significant.

Adding to the rationale of pleiotropy a slightly different rationale, that of genetic proximity, Stein et al. (2006) examined the 15q14-q21 region for linkage to SSD, arguing that this region, in addition to being linked to RD, harbors a gene causing Prader-Willi syndrome and Angelman syndrome, both of which are associated with speech deficits, and that it also has been implicated in autism, which also can affect speech production. A further argument was the finding that, in one family, a duplication in this region has been associated with apraxia of speech, phonological awareness deficits, developmental language disorder, dyslexia, as well as limb apraxia but did not have any dysmorphic clinical features. Participants from 151 families, each ascertained through a proband child with SSD, completed a battery of test measures that included standardized articulation test based on single word production, a measure of consonant accuracy during conversational speech, nonword repetition, multisyllabic word task, oral motor testing, word reading, nonword reading, and reading comprehension. Six microsatellite markers within the region of interest were selected for genotyping. Two model-free types of linkage analysis were performed, a Haseman-Elston regression analysis of sib pairs and an affected sib pair analysis using a conditional logistic model. In the regression analysis, the measure of oral motor ability for single syllable repetitions was tentatively linked at $p = .048$ while the other measures of articulation and reading did not show evidence of linkage. The second linkage analysis confirmed that the region of interest contains a putative locus influencing articulation, phonological memory, and oral motor functioning.

In another example guided by the hypothesis that SSD and RD may share a genetic origin because of frequent comorbidity, Smith et al. (2007) focused on three candidate regions implicated in RD, 1p36, 6p22, and 15q21. Participants were 111 Kindergarten children with a history of SSD and 76 siblings. In each of the candidate regions, standard microsatellite markers were used for genotyping. Measures included speech related measures such as SSD affectation status, standardardized articulation testing, and articulatory accuracy during conversational speech. In addition, nonword repetition ability and phonological awareness were tested. Multiple statistical approaches were used for single point and multipoint linkage, including the revised Haseman-Elston method and the DeFries-Fulker augmented method, which is based on the assumption that, if a trait is linked to a marker, siblings who share more alleles at this marker will have a smaller trait difference than siblings who share no alleles at this marker. Several variants of model-free maximum likelihood linkage analysis were also used. In the candidate region on chromosome 1, only suggestive evidence for linkage to standardized speech scores were seen. Evidence for linkage to speech scores was seen in the candidate region on chromosome 6, using the DeFries-Fulker augmented algorithm, and that on chromosome 15, where linkage peaks were detected with the DeFries-Fulker augmented algorithm and corroborated with maximum likelihood methods.

The candidate locus on chromosome 1, with expanded boundaries to include 1p34-p36, was also evaluated for linkage to SSD by Miscimarra and 11 others (Miscimarra, Stein et al. 2007) . In 151 families, each ascertained through a child with SSD, bivariate predictive modeling showed evidence of comorbidity, familial aggregation, and co-aggregation of SSD and LI were co-morbid. The region of interest was genotyped with ten microsatelliate markers spanning 94 cM (centimorgan, a measure of genetic distance based on recombination probabilities). Measures included standardized articulation testing, nonword repetition, multisyllabic word repetition, errors in difficult- to-articulate phrases, and measures of visual perception and receptive and expressive language. Two statistical analyses were undertaken, affected sib pair (ASP) conditional logistic regression and Haseman-Elston regression of all sib pairs. Two lod score peaks were detected in the candidate region, one with suggestive linkage to verbal short-term memory and articulation and a second one with suggestive linkage to skills more related to language processing than to speech production skills. The authors interpret their findings to suggest that 1p34-p36 could harbor one or more genes with pleiotropic effects on SSD, LI, and RD.

Taken together, the studies summarized here give some indication of gene regions implicated in SSD, but they do not characterize the genetics of SSD fully. The regions on chromosomes 7, 4, and 16 were seen in rare individuals whose speech was disordered but who also showed syndromic involvement in other areas such as language and cognition. These results, hence, suggest that the regions reported as associated with SSD are necessary but not sufficient for the development of normal speech. None of these gene regions can explain primary SSD without syndromic involvement. In studies focusing on individuals with primary SSD and their families, the most frequently reported linkage signals implicated measures of phonological memory, a measure that also has produced linkage signals in families with LI and RD. Deficits in oral articulation, which are pathognomonic for SSD, were linked to candidate regions on chromosomes 1, 6, and 15.

Of all these studies, only the study that led to the discovery of the *FOXP2* mutation used a genome-wide screen, which was done with microsatellite markers and followed up with fine-mapping. The studies reporting linkage to regions on chromosomes 1, 3, 6, and 15 used a candidate region approach, focusing on gene regions defined by linkage to other disorders with SSD comorbitidy. A genome-wide study in common forms of SSD has not yet been reported. To understand the genetic mechanisms in SSD more fully, it will be necessary to expand on previous work, test new hypothesis, and use innovative technologies.

METHODOLOGICAL CHALLENGES AND FUTURE DIRECTIONS

Studying the genetic mechanisms associated with common forms of SSD is extraordinarily challenging for a variety of reasons. First, a universally accepted phenotype profile and diagnostic guidelines for assigning affectation status is not yet available, resulting in variability among participant samples. Similarly, disorder expression may change with age, developmental factors, and therapy effects, introducing additional ascertainment variability in the participant samples. Furthermore, it is unknown whether SSD is caused by common risk alleles acting together (common disease/common variant hypothesis) or by several rare allelic variants giving rise to disorder types of distinct genetic origin but with similar phenotypes (rare disease/rare variant hypothesis). It is therefore difficult to estimate whether SSD in different families is influenced by the same or different genetic mechanisms. One may assume fairly safely that members of a single family who have SSD all share the implicated genetic loci. In a study sample of several families, however, this may not be the case, and this heterogeneity can introduce misleading statistical results. It is therefore imperative to specify phenotypic traits as narrowly as possible (Lander & Schork, 1994). Regarding the two disease/variant hypotheses, quantifying the influence of a multitude of genes, each with a small amount of contribution to the phenotype, is methodologically more challenging than characterizing the action of a single gene contributing a large amount of phenotypic expression. To obtain meaningful results when studying complex traits with multiple contributing genes, it is helpful to study several large pedigrees, where each might only segregate one or two of the relevant genetic variants. Examples of successful analyses of complex traits in large pedigrees include Hasstedt et al. (2004), Riazzudin et al. (2000), and Tomfohrde et al. (1994).

Regarding research techniques, multipoint linkage analysis using microsatellite panels remains a powerful tool for detecting linkage (e.g., Raskind et al., 2008), but it requires pedigrees with informative genotypes, typically multigenerational and large pedigrees. Given that SSD is observable most easily in young children, the practicalities of participant recruitment can create a bias towards linkage algorithms based on sib pair analysis. Another potential reason why sib pairs have been studied more than whole pedigrees is that in linkage analysis based on sib pairs, it is not necessary to specify the mode of inheritance, which is frequently unknown. It is possible to conduct nonparametric linkage analyses in multigenerational pedigrees, especially when affectation status can be assigned unambiguously.

Potential novel approaches to identifying genotype-phenotype associations in SSD include considering functional genetic pathways when forming hypotheses regarding candidate regions or genes; using newly available molecular methodology; and evaluating associated disorder traits that may constitute endophenotypes for SSD and comorbid disorders. An example of an innovative approach to answering questions about the genetic causes of common forms of LI was offered by Vernes and 11 colleagues (2008). Following up on the finding that the *FOXP2* mutation caused a complex and severe communication disorder including components of LI that was rare in the population, this group identified a transcriptional target, *CNTNAP2,* and confirmed its association in a sample of participants with common forms of LI. Members of the same group of researchers (Vernes, MacDermot, Monaco & Fisher, 2009) applied similar reasoning in a sample of individuals with SSD by evaluating the role of the *FOXP1* gene, like *FOXP2* a forkhead-box transcription factor. In this first attempt to evaluate the genetic causes of SSD using a functional rationale, the results were not consistent with mutations in *FOXP1* as a cause of common forms of SSD. Further studies are needed to explore this functional approach in SSD.

Examples of recent advances in molecular technology include genome-wide association studies (GWAS), identification of copy-number variations (CNVs), and next-generation sequencing, none of which have been applied to study SSD genetics to date. GWAS has only recently been used effectively as a tool to identify disease genotypes. With the completion of the Human Genome Project in 2003 and HapMap Project in 2005, a large amount of genome-wide reference data are available to researchers. Using SNP chip technology, it has become possible to obtain a SNP profile for an individual where the readout specifies far more than one million SNPs. The drastic increase in available SNP information has gone alongside with equally drastic decreases in cost. The SNP profiles can be compared to the available reference populations with, and without, the same disease traits, a study design referred to as association study. To detect statistically significant effects of common SNPs on disease risk, large study samples are necessary, especially when studying common disorders. According to a review of GWAS studies in psychiatric disorders (Psychiatric GWAS Consortium Coordinating Committtee, 2009), most initial GWAS studies included 500 to 3,000 cases plus additional control participants, and, in one study, 10,657 participants. Using collaborative approaches, some studies report samples of 8,000 to 20,000 cases, not counting the control participants.

Another new tool, identification of CNVs, also uses SNPs to detect genetic disease variants, but here, identifying longer stretches of deleted or duplicated DNA is the goal of the analysis. In theory, while an unaffected individual has two copies of the chromosomal region, an affected individual may have fewer in the case of deletions, or more in the case of duplications. Velocardiofacial syndrome, mentioned earlier, involving large deletions in 22q11, is an example of such a copy-number variation. Similar to GWAS, to detect meaningful structural abnormalities associated with a given disease, large participant samples are required.

The recent increase of DNA sequence information has been so dramatic that it has been called "meteoric" (Mardis, 2008). Resequencing the entire human genome has become possible and even feasible, but using this wealth of information efficiently to characterize clinically significant differences is a major challenge. Applications in clinical genetics are being developed at the time of this writing. While the technology to sequence the entire genome of an individual is available, applying this information involves handling millions of sequence datapoints while dealing with sequencing errors and naturally occurring variations in the population. Recently, Ng et al. (2009) successfully identified candidate genes for a rare, dominantly inherited disease, Freeman-Sheldon syndrome, using the DNA of only four affected, unrelated individuals, in comparison with the DNA of eight unaffected HapMap individuals. Only protein-coding regions were selected for sequencing. This study demonstrates that candidate genes for rare Mendelian diseases can be identified in a small sample of affected individuals. The authors suggest that the sampe methodology may be extendable to diseases with more complex genetic mechanisms, but larger samples would be necessary in that case.

In terms of disorder traits selected for linkage analyses, the majority of the studies reviewed in this chapter report linkage to traditional core traits for SSD including articulation and phonological awareness, in addition to associated traits such as reading ability and language processing. Pilot work (Peter & Stoel-Gammon, 2008) shows that subgroups of children with SSD have difficulty with various aspects of timing accuracy and that this deficit manifests across motor output systems (oral motor vs. hand claps) and in temporal macrostructures (rhythm) as well as microstructures (vowel durations, clap interval durations). Theoretical and experimental motivation for a potential endophenotype shared by SSD, LI, and RD, slowed motor speeds, is currently being developed by this author. Genetic studies of this type of associated trait, following rigorous validation of the associated trait in the target population, may prove fruitful toward characterizing further the phenotype/genotype association in SSD.

Conclusion

Clearly, there are mutual associations among SSD, LI, and RD. They co-occur at rates greater than expected by chance; all three are seen more frequently in boys than in girls; and some shared anatomical and physiological characteristics have been documented in LI and RD. Even though all three disorders clearly have a genetic component, a genetic cause shared by all three disorders has yet to be identified. The genetic substrates of common forms of SSD have been described in terms of linked regions, but causative genes or sets of genes have not yet been identified. Studying the genetic causes of SSD is extraordinarily challenging, not only because of definitional uncertainties regarding SSD such as the lack of a universally accepted phenotype profile and diagnostic guidelines for assigning affectation status, but also because the underlying disorder framework (common disease/common variant hypothesis or rare disease/rare variant hypothesis) and the associated modes of inheritance are unknown. New ways to approach research by considering functional genetic pathways, using newly available technology efficiently, and considering disorder subclusters defined by associated traits may all aid in unraveling the mysteries of the genetic causes of SSD in the future.

Acknowledgments

Many thanks to Elizabeth E. Marchani for helpful comments on this manuscript. Preparation of this manuscript was supported by NIDCD grant T32DC00033-10 and 11.

References

American Speech-Language-Hearing Association. (2007). *Childhood Apraxia of Speech,* [Position Statement]. Available from www.asha.org/policy.

American Speech-Langue-Hearing Association. (2004). 2004 schools survey. Special report: Caseloads.http://www.asha.org/NR/rdonlyres/35793FB5-99F6-46D9-B2F5-5D5973B05 A95/0/SpecialCaseloads04.pdf

Bauman-Waengler, J. (2000). *Articulatory and Phonological Impairments : A Clinical Focus.* Boston: Allyn and Bacon.

Bird, J., Bishop, D.V. & Freeman, N.H. (1995). Phonological awareness and literacy development in children with expressive phonological impairments. *Journal of Speech and Hearing Research, 38(2)*, 446-462.

Bishop, D. V. M. (2002). Motor immaturity and specific speech and language impairment: Evidence for a common genetic basis. *American Journal of Medical Genetics (Neuropsychiatric Genetics), 114*, 56-63.

Botstein, D., White, R. L. et al. (1980). Construction of a genetic linkage map in man using restriction fragment length polymorphisms. *American Journal of Human Genetics, 32(3)*, 314-31.

Boyar, F. Z., Whitney, M. M., Lossie, A. C., Gray, B. A., Keller, K. L., Stalker, H. J., Zori, R. T., Geffken, G., Mutch, J., Edge, P. J., Voeller, K. S., Williams, C. A. & Driscoll, D. J. (2001). A family with a grandmaternally derived interstitial duplication of proximal 15q. *Clinical Genetics, 60*, 421-430.

Brown, W. E., Eliez, S., Menon, V., Rumsey, J. M., White, C. D. & Reiss, A. L. (2001). Preliminary evidence of widespread morphological variations of the brain in dyslexia. *Neurology, 56*, 781-783.

Campbell, T. F., Dollaghan, C. A., Rockette, H. E., Paradise, J. K., Feldman, H. M., Shriberg, L. D., Sabo, D. L. & Kurs-Lasky, M. (2003). Risk factors for speech delay of unknown origin in 3-year-old children. *Child Development, 74 (2)*, 346-457.

Crary, M. (1993). *Developmental Motor Speech Disorders*. San Diego: Singular Publishing Group.

De Fossé, L., Hodge, S. M., Makris, N., Kennedy, D. N., Caviness, V. S. Jr,, McGrath. L, Steele, S., Ziegler, D. A., Herbert, M. R., Frazier, J. A., Tager-Flusberg, H. & Harris, G. J. (2004). Language-association cortex asymmetry in autism and specific language impairment. *Ann Neurol, 56*, 757-66.

Deutsch, G. K., Dougherty, R. F. & Bammer, R., et al. (2005). Children's reading performance is correlated with white matter structure measured by tensor imaging. *Cortex, 41*, 354-63.

Dodd, B. (1995). Procedures for classification of subgroups of speech disorder. In: B. Dodd (Ed). *The Differential Diagnosis and Treatment of Children with Speech Disorder.* San Diego: Singular Publishing Group.

Felsenfeld, S., Broen, P. A. & McGue, M. (1992). A 28-year follow-up of adults with a history of moderate phonological disorder: linguistic and personality results. *Journal of Speech and Hearing Research, 35(5)*, 1114-1125.

Felsenfeld, S., McGue, M. & Broen, P. A. (1995). Familial aggregation of phonological disorders: Results from a 28-year follow-up. *Journal of Speech and Hearing Research, 38 (5)*, 1091-1107.

Felsenfeld, S. & Plomin, R. (1997). Epidemiological and offspring analyses of developmental speech disorders using data from the Colorado Adoption Project. *Journal of Speech and Hearing Research, 40 (4)*, 778-791.

Fisher, S. E., Vargha-Khadem, F., Watkins, K. E., Monaco, A. P. & Pembrey, M. E. (1998) Localisation of a gene implicated in a severe speech and language disorder. Nat Genet 18, 168-170.

Fox, A.V., Dodd, B. & Howard, D. (2002). Risk factors for speech disorders in children. *International Journal of Language and Communication Disorders, 37(2)*, 117-131.

Hasstedt, S.J., Scott, B.T., Callas, P.W., Vossen, C.Y., Rosendaal, F.R., Long, G.L. & Bovill, E.G. (2004). Genome scan of venous thrombosis in a pedigree with protein C deficiency. *Journal of Thrombosis and Haemostasis, 2*(6), 868-873.

Hurst, J A., Baraitser, M., Auger, E., Graham, F. & Norell, S. (1990). An extended family with a dominantly inherited speech disorder. *Dev Med Child Neurol, 32*, 347-355.

Jaencke, L., Siegenthaler, T., Preis, S. & Steinmetz, H. (2007). Decreased white-matter density in a left-sided fronto-temporal network in children with developmental language disorder: evidence for anatomical anomalies in a motor-language network. *Brain and Language, 102,* 91-98.

Klingberg, T., Hedehus, M., Temple, E., Salz, T., Gabrieli, J. D., Moseley, M. E. & Poldrack, R. A. (2000). Microstructure of temporo-parietal white matter as a basis for reading ability: evidence from diffusion tensor magnetic resonance imaging. *Neuron, 25*, 493-500.

Lai, C. S., Fisher, S. E., Hurst, J. A., Vargha-Khadem, F. & Monaco, A. P. (2001). A forkhead-domain gene is mutated in a severe speech and language disorder. *Nature, 414*(6855), 465-466.

Lander, E.S. & Schork, N.J. (1994). Genetic dissection of complex traits. *Science, 265*(5181):2037-2048.

Leonard, L. (1998). *Children with Specific Language Impairment* (Language, Speech and Communication series). Cambridge, MA: MIT Press.

Leonard, C. M., Lombardino, L. J., Walsh, K., Eckert, M. A., Mockler, J. L., Rowe, L. A., Williams, S. & DeBose, C. B. (2002). Anatomical risk factors that distinguish dyslexia from SLI predict reading skill in normal children. *Journal of Communication Disorders, 35*, 501-531.

Lewis, B. A. (1992). Pedigree analysis of children with phonology disorders. *Journal of Learning Disabilities, 25*, 586-597.

Lewis, B. A., Cox, N. J. & Byard, P. J. (1993). Segregation analysis of speech and language disorders. *Behavior Genetics, 23*, 291-297.

Lewis, B. A., Freebairn, L. A., Hansen, A. J., Miscimarra, L., Iyengar, S. K. & Taylor, H. G. (2007). Speech and language skills of parents of children with speech sound disorders. *American Journal of Speech-Language Pathology, 16(2)*, 108-118.

Lewis, B. A., Freebairn, L. A. & Taylor, H. (2000). Academic outcomes in children with histories of speech sound disorders. *Journal of Communication Disorders, 33*(1), 11-30.

Lewis, B. A., Shriberg, L. D., Freebairn, L. A., Hanson, A. J., Stein, C. M., Taylor, H. G. & Iyengar, S. (2006). The genetic bases of speech sound disorders: Evidence from spoken and written language. *American Journal of Speech-Language Pathology, 49,* 1294-1312.

Lewis, B. A. & Thompson, L. A. (1992). A study of developmental speech and language disorders in twins. *Journal of Speech and Hearing Research, 35*, 1086-1094.

Lyon, G. R., Shaywitz, S. &Shaywitz, B. (2003). A definition of dyslexia. *Annals of Dyslexia, 53,*1-14.

MacDermot, K. D., Bonora, E., Sykes, N., Coupe, A. M., Lai, C. S. L., Vernes, S. C., Vargha-Khadem, F., McKenzie, F., Smith, R. L., Monaco, A. P. & Fisher, S. E. (2005). Identification of *FOXP2* truncation as a novel cause of developmental speech and language deficits. *American Journal of Human Genetics, 76*, 1074-1080.

Mardis, E. R. (2008). The impact of next-generation sequencing technology on genetics. *Trends in Genetics, 24(3)*, 133-141.

McKinnon, D. H., McLeod, S. & Reilly, S. (2007). The prevalence of stuttering, voice, and speech-sound disorders in primary school students in Australia. *Language, Speech, and Hearing Services in Schools, 38,* 5-15.

Miscimarra, L., Stein, Stein, C., Millard, C., Kluge, A., Cartier, K., Freebairn, L., Hansen, A. Shriberg, L., Taylor, H. G., Lewis, B. & Iyengar, S. K. (2007). Further evidence of pleiotropy influencing speech and language: analysis of the DYX8 region. *Human Heredity, 63(1),* 47-58.

Morley, M. E. (1965). The development and disorders of speech in childhood. Baltimore: Williams & Wilkins.

Ng, S.B., Turner, E.H. et al. (2009)/ Targeted capture and massively parallel sequencing of 12 human exomes. *Nature, 461* (7261), 272-276.

Nopola-Hemmi, J., Myllyluoma, B., Haltia, T., Taipale, M., Ollikainen, V., Ahonen, T., Voutilainen, A., Kere, J. & Widen, E. (2001). A dominant gene for developmental dyslexia on chromosome 3. *Journal of Medical Genetics, 38*, 658-664.

Pennington, B. F. & Bishop, D. V. M. (2009). Relations among speech, language, and reading disorders. *Annual Reviews of Psychology, 60*, 283-306.

Peter, B. & Stoel-Gammon, C. (2008). Central timing deficits in children with primary speech disorders. *Clinical Linguistics & Phonetics, 22(3)*, 171-198.

Peterson, R. L., McGrath, L. M. Smith, S. D. & Pennington, B. F. (2007). Neuropsychology and genetics of speech, language, and literacy disorders. *Pediatric Clinic of North America, 54,* 543-561.

Psychiatric GWAS Consortium Coordinating Committtee. (2009). Genomewide association studies: History, rationale, and prospects for psychiatric disorders. *American Journal of Psychiatry,* 2009 April, Epub ahead of print.

Raskind, W.H., Matsushita, M., Peter, B., Biberston, J., Burbank, R., Wolff, J., Lipe, H., & Bird, T. (2008). Familial Dyskinesia and Facial Myokymia (FDFM): Follow-up of a large family and linkage to chromosome 3p21-3q21.

Riazuddin, S., Castelein, C.M., Ahmed, Z.M., Lalwani, A.K., Mastroianni, M.A., Naz, S., Smith, T.N., Liburd, N.A., Friedman, T.B., Griffith, A.J., Riazuddin, S. & Wilcox, E.R. (2000). Dominant modifier DFNM1 suppresses recessive deafness DFNB26. *Nature Genetics, 26*(4), 431-434.

Richards, T., Stevenson, J., Crouch, J., Johnson, L. C., Maravilla, K., Stock, P., Abbott, R. & Berninger, V. (2008). Tract-based spatial statistics of diffusion tensor imaging in adults with dyslexia. *American Journal of Neuroradiology, 29,* 1134-1139.

Robichon, F., Levrier, O., Farnarier, P. & Habib, M. (2000). Developmental dyslexia: atypical cortical asymmetries and functional significance. *European Joural of Neurology*, *7*, 35-46.

Schuele, C. M. (2004). The impact of developmental speech and language impairments on the acquisition of literacy skills. *Mental Retardation and Developmental Disabilities Research Reviews, 10,* 176-183.

Shaywitz, S., Shaywitz, B., Fletcher, J. & Escobar, M. (1990). Prevalence of reading disability in boys and girls. Results of the Connecticut longitudinal study. *Journal of the American Medical Association, 264,* 998-1002.

Shriberg, L. D., Jakielski, K. J. & El-Shanti, H. (2008). Breakpoint localization using array-CGH in three siblings with an unbalanced 4q;16q translocation and childhood apraxia of speech (CAS). *American Journal of Medical Genetics Part A, 1;146A(17)*, 2227-2233.

Shriberg, L. D., Lewis, B. L., Tomblin, J. B., McSweeny, J. L., Karlsson, H. B. & Scheer, A. R. (2005). Toward diagnostic and phenotype markers for genetically transmitted speech delay. *Journal of Speech, Language, and Hearing Research, 48(4)*, 834-852.

Shriberg, L. D., Tomblin, J. B. & McSweeny, J. L. (1999). Prevalence of speech delay in 6-year-old children and comorbidity with language impairment. *Journal of Speech, Language, and Hearing Research, 42(6)*, 1461-1481.

Stein, C. M., Millard, C., Kluge, A., Miscimarra, L. E., Cartier, K. C., Freebairn, L. A., Hanson, A. J., Shriberg, L. D., Taylor, H. G., Lewis, B. A. & Iyengar, S. K. (2006). Speech sound disorder influenced by a locus in 15q14 region. *Behavioral Genetics, 36*(6), 858-868.

Stein, C. M., Schick, J. H., Taylor, H., Shriberg, L. D., Millard, C., Kundtz-Kluge, A., Russo, K., Minich, N., Hansen, A., Freebairn, L. A., Elston, R. C., Lewis, B. A. & Iyengar, S. K. (2006). Pleiotropic effects of a chromosome 3 locus on speech-sound disorder and reading. *American Journal of Human Genetics, 74(2)*, 283-297.

Tomblin, J. B., Zhang, X., Buckwalter, P. & O'Brien, M. (2003). The stability of primary language disorder: four years after kindergarten diagnosis. *Journal of Speech, Language, and Hearing Research, 46(6)*, 1283-1296.

Tomfohrde, J., Silverman, A., Barnes, R., Fernandez-Vina, M.A., Young, M., Lory, D., Morris, L., Wuepper, K.D., Stastny, P. & Menter, A., et al. (1994). Gene for familial psoriasis susceptibility mapped to the distal end of human chromosome 17q. *Science, 264,* 1141-1145.

Vargha-Khadem, F., Watkins, K., Alcock, K., Fletcher, P. & Passingham, R. (1995). Praxic and nonverbal cognitive deficits in a large family with a genetically transmitted speech and language disorder. *Proceedings of the National Academy of Sciences United States of America, 92,* 930-933.

Vargha-Khadem, F., Watkins, K. E., Price, C. J., Ashburner, J., Alcock, K. J., Connelly, A., Frackowiak, R. S. J., Friston, K. J., Pembrey, M. E., Mishkin, M, Gadian, D. G. & Passingham, R. E. (1998). Neural basis of an inherited speech and language disorder. *Proceedings of the National Academy of Science United States of America, 95(21)*, 1269512700.

Verhoeven, L. & van Balkom, H. (2004). Developmental language disorders: Classification, assessment, and intervention. In: L. Verhoeven and H. van Balkom (eds), *Classification of Developmental Language Disorders: Theoretical Issues and Clinical Implications.* Mahwah, NJ: 45Lawrence Erlbaum Associates.

Vernes, S. C., MacDermot, K. D., Monaco, A. P. & Fisher, S. E. (2009). Assessing the impact of FOXP1 mutations on developmental verbal dyspraxia. Vernes, S. C., Macdermot, K. D, Monaco, A. P, Fisher, S. E. *European Journal of Human Genetics*, 2009 Apr 8. [Epub ahead of print].

Vernes, S. C., Newbury, D. F., Abrahams, B. S., Winchester, L., Nicod, J., Groszer, M., Alarcón, M., Oliver, P. L., Davies, K. E., Geschwind, D. H., Monaco, A. P. & Fisher, S. E. (2008). A functional genetic link between distinct developmental language disorders. *New England Journal of Medicine, 359(22)*, 2337-2345.

Watkins, K. E., Dronkers, N. F. & Vargha-Khadem, F. (2002). Behavioural analysis of an inherited speech and language disorder: comparison with acquired aphasia. *Brain, 125*, 452-464.

Weismer, S. E., Plante, E., Jones, M. & Tomblin, J. B. (2005). A functional magnetic resnance imaging investigation of verbal working memory in adolescents with specific language impairment. *Journal of Speech, Language, and Hearing Research, 48(2)*, 405-425.

Widdershoven, J. C., Beemer, F. A., Kon, M., Dejockere, P. H. & Mink van der Molen, A. B. (2008). Possible mechanisms and gene involvement in speech problems in the 22q11.2 deletion syndrome. *Journal of Plastic, Reconstructive, and Aesthetic Surgery, 61(9)*, 1016-1023. Epub 2008 Jun 12.

In: Speech Disorders: Causes, Treatment and Social Effects
Editor: Alan E. Harrison, pp. 139-159
ISBN: 978-1-60876-213-2

Chapter 6

Treatment Outcomes of the Intensive Stuttering Therapy for Adolescents and Adults

Rodney Gabel, Farzan Irani, Scott Palasik, Eric Swartz and Charlie Hughes
Bowling Green State University Bowling Green, OH, USA

Abstract

Stuttering is a multifaceted communication disorder that not only affects the individual's speech fluency, but also impacts how he or she feels and thinks about themselves and communication. Thus, coping effectively with stuttering during adulthood often requires a multifaceted approach. The purpose of this chapter is to describe an intensive therapy program, the Intensive Stuttering Therapy for Adolescents and Adults, which utilizes such an approach. This proposed chapter is broken into three parts. First, the complex nature of stuttering and the rationale for a multifaceted approach will be discussed. Next, the author will describe the approach and the initial outcome data from this clinic. Finally, future directions for this clinical program will be explained, including the rationale and need for using telepractice as an adjunct to the intensive clinic.

Introduction

The Problem of Stuttering

Stuttering, if it persists into adolescence and adulthood, is often a chronic disorder that requires the help of a skilled clinician to assist individuals in developing the skills necessary to cope with the problem. Unfortunately, there is perhaps no other disorder in our field that continues to baffle most speech-language pathologists (SLPs). In fact, studies have found that many SLPs do not feel comfortable working with people who stutter (PWS) (Brisk, Healey, & Hux, 1997; St. Louis & Durrenberger, 1993). This discomfort may be due to a reduction in coursework and clinical training in stuttering offered in graduate programs (Yaruss & Quesal, 2002). To compound these issues, there are relatively few SLPs who identify themselves as specialists in stuttering (Manning, 2001; Tellis, Bressler, & Emerick, 2008). Thus, there are many obstacles for adults and adolescents who stutter that are attempting to access appropriate services.

For decades, there has been agreement that stuttering is a multidimensional communication disorder (Bloodstein & Bernstein-Ratner, 2008). Certainly, the most obvious dimension of stuttering is the disruption in speech fluency. Also, there is a potential for a variety of negative reactions by both the person who stutters and their listeners (Cooper, 1993). There are several different ways to define stuttering and the accompanying behaviors. One of the most detailed definitions of stuttering was forwarded by Wingate (1964). In this definition, stuttering has seven components:

1. Disruption of fluency of verbal expression.
2. Characterized by involuntary, audible, or silent repetitions or prolongations in the utterance of short speech elements.
3. Disruptions usually occur frequently.
4. Disruptions are not readily controllable.
5. Disruptions are sometimes accompanied by accessory activities involving the speech apparatus, and related or unrelated body structures.
6. Indications of the presence of an emotional state, fear, embarrassment, and irritation.
7. Discoordination in the peripheral speech mechanism.

A simple definition of chronic stuttering was suggested by Cooper (1993). In this definition, Cooper suggests that as someone continues to stutter throughout childhood, adolescence, and adulthood they develop a complex array of reactive behaviors to the problem. These reactions take the form of affective (emotional), behavioral (physical), and cognitive (beliefs and attitudes) behaviors. For these individuals, coping positively with stuttering will take a considerable amount of effort, which will most likely require the services of a speech-language pathologist (SLP).

From these definitions, and those of other authors (Guitar, 2006; Manning, 2001), it appears to be widely accepted that adolescents and adults who stutter experience much more when they stutter than just the disfluencies in their speech. Another definition that provides further explanation of these experiences was proposed by Yaruss (2007). This definition utilizes the International Classification of Impairments, Disabilities, and Handicaps (ICIDH) framework. The ICIDH includes not only the surface behaviors of stuttering or the impairment, but also includes a description of difficulties a speaker might experience in daily communication (disability) and the overall consequences this disability could have on the speaker's life experiences (handicap) (Yaruss, 2007).

This more broad-based framework of stuttering as described by the ICIDH is further supported by reports of the lack of long-term maintenance of gains made in therapy (St. Louis & Westbrook, 1987; Cordes., 1998; Bloodstein & Ratner, 2008). Crichton-Smith (2002) report that speech management strategies taught in therapy are employed variably across different situations with a distinct possibility that the client's original strategies of avoidance and escape might reoccur leading to the possibility of relapse. The study by Critchton-Smith explored the communicative experiences and coping strategies used by 14 adults who stutter via in-depth qualitative interviews. Although the results might not generalize to a population of PWS, it is important to realize that certain mechanisms, beyond the surface behaviors of stuttering can influence treatment outcomes and could possibly lead to relapse or a loss of treatment gains made over a period of time. Similarly, Klompas and Ross (2004) investigated life experiences of 16 PWS from South Africa using a qualitative framework to explore the impact stuttering had on their quality of life. The results of this study indicate that most participants reported negative effects of stuttering on their self-esteem and self-image that had evoked strong emotions in them.

Another study by Stewart and Richardson (2004) investigated the effects of therapy from a patient perspective by interviewing 13 PWS who had received group therapy between 1995 and 1999 that comprised a combination of "speak more fluently" and "stutter more fluently" approaches grounded in a client-centered and personal construct therapy. The results of this study indicated that most clients did benefit from the therapy program; however, they also felt the need for continued support following discharge from therapy. In addition, Yaruss, et al. (2002) surveyed members of the National Stuttering Association (NSA) to learn about their experiences in support groups as well as their experiences in speech therapy. The results of this study indicated that most individuals surveyed had received speech therapy several times in their lives. Responses suggested that individuals who had received fluency-shaping treatments were more likely to experience relapse as opposed to individuals who received stuttering modification or a combination of approaches.

Intensive Therapy for Adults and Adolescents Who Stutter

Due to the multifaceted nature of stuttering, it is very important to develop appropriate therapy programs for adolescents and adults who stutter. It is equally important that these programs be easily accessible and allow PWS opportunities to interact with a specialist in stuttering. As stated earlier in this chapter, it is unfortunate that many PWS will have difficulties accessing therapy because many speech-language pathologists (SLPs) report being uncomfortable or ill-prepared to work with PWS (Brisk, et. al, 1997; St. Louis & Durrenberger, 1993; Tellis, et. al, 2008), there is a continuing reduction in educational and clinical experiences related to stuttering (Yaruss & Quesal, 2002) and few SLPs specialize in treating individuals who stutter (Manning, 2001, Tellis, et. al, 2008). These issues, along with the difficult nature of stuttering and the length of therapy, make identifying appropriate treatment very difficult.

One way to provide treatment to adults and adolescents who stutter is through intensive therapy programs (Boberg & Kully, 1994; Langevin, & Kully, 2003; Kully, Langevin, & Lomheim, 2007; O'Brian, Packman, & Onslowe, 2008). Intensive programs require individuals to live in close proximity to a clinic, which usually employs specialists in stuttering, for a short period of time (i.e. generally three weeks or fewer). Many intensive programs report positive outcomes (Boberg & Kully, 1994; Langevin & Kully, 2003; Kully, et. al, 2007; O'Brian, et. al, 2008), especially when traditional, follow-up therapy is included in the treatment program (St. Louis & Westbrook, 1987).

Structure of the Multifaceted Program for People Who Stutter

At Bowling Green State University, an intensive clinic for adolescents and adults has been developed. Over the past seven years, the intensive portion of the clinic has been offered on five occasions. In all, 24 individuals between the ages of 12 and 39 have participated. Though there have been subtle differences in the schedule and approaches utilized, each offering has included between 75 and 80 hours of direct treatment over a 15-day period.

The clinic employs a multifaceted therapy program, which includes speech restructuring (i.e., fluency shaping), stuttering modification, and counseling (i.e., self-help) approaches. The program was initially developed based on therapy models described by several authors (Gregory, 2003; Guitar, 2006). Prior to initiating therapy, each client is engaged in a diagnostic. During this assessment, several speech samples are gathered in both clinical (reading, monologues, and conversations) and extra-clinical contexts (conversations and phone calls). The clinicians complete standard measurements of speech fluency (i.e., syllables stuttered), speech naturalness, and stuttering severity. Additionally, pencil-and-paper questionnaires such as the *Erickson S-24* (Andrews & Cutler, 1974), the *Locus of Control of Behavior (LCB)* (Craig, Franklin, & Andrews, 1984), *The Speech Locus of Control (SP-LOC)* (McDonough & Quesal, 1988), and the *Overall Assessment of the Speaker's Experience with Stuttering* (Yaruss & Quesal, 2008) are used to assess the clients' affective and cognitive reactions to stuttering and readiness for change. Each clinical measure is completed during the start of the intensive program, again at the end of the program, and during any follow-up therapy.

As a part of the clinic, the client's values and perspectives related to stuttering and therapy are assessed. The importance of understanding the needs of our clients' has been underscored as an important piece of evidence in understanding the effectiveness of our therapy (ASHA, 2004; 2005). To complete this assessment, each client is engaged in a semi-structured interview. During the interview, the clients discuss how stuttering has affected their lives, the experiences they have had with stuttering, and their expectations for therapy. Each interview is analyzed using qualitative procedures (Patton, 2002) and this data is used as a benchmark for tailoring the therapy program to meet the needs of the clients. At the end of the program, the interview is repeated and the clients are asked to reflect on their experiences in therapy and their expectations for the future. This narrative is analyzed similarly to the initial interview.

The therapy program is delivered in three phases. Phase I of the program is generally initiated on the first day of therapy. During this phase, the clients are engaged in a process of increasing their awareness and understanding of stuttering. During both individual and group sessions, the clinicians guide the clients in identifying the behaviors that make up their stuttering problem: types of disfluencies, secondary physical reactions and tension, negative emotional reactions, and negative communication attitudes (Van Riper, 1982). During Phase 2 of the program, initiated during the first three to four days of therapy, the clients learn ways in which they might reduce the tension in their speech and stuttering. Approaches such as open and honest stuttering, as well as voluntary stuttering are utilized to assist clients in learning new ways to stutter without tension (Van Riper, 1982). In the later stages of Phase II, which generally spans the entire program, the clients practice modification skills such as pull-outs and cancellations (Van Riper, 1982). During the third phase of therapy, clients learn speech restructuring techniques. Specifically, clients learn behaviors such as easy onsets, deliberate phonation, airflow management, and reduced rate. The clients learn to use each technique at a very slow speech rate, and then these new behaviors are generalized in the clinic at increasing speech rates, and finally at more normal speech rates in extra-clinical settings. This phase of treatment begins early in the second week of therapy and is a focus until the end of therapy.

Throughout the clinic, the clients are engaged in discussions that direct them to develop an individual maintenance program, which often includes a suggestion for follow-up therapy. In fact, clients are offered a variety of options for follow-up therapy. First, they can attend weekly or bi-weekly sessions at the Bowling Green Speech and Hearing Clinic or off-site at their school or another setting. In addition, clients have attended 10-hour intensive follow-up sessions offered 3 times a year. Also, clients have used telepractice sessions, either through phone calls or teleconferencing, to guide their follow-up therapy.

There has been one initial outcome study published about this program. Gabel, Daniels, and Hughes (2008) explored outcomes of four clients who attended the clinic. Therapy measurements, aside from the *OASES* (Yaruss & Quesal, 2008), were completed at the beginning of therapy and at the end of therapy. At six-months following the end of the intensive clinic, the clients provided speech samples for analysis and completed a follow-up questionnaire regarding their experiences since therapy and perceptions of the benefits of treatment. Results of the study suggested that all of the clients made reductions in percentage of syllables stuttered and stuttering severity following therapy and these changes were maintained at 6-months. In addition, each client was perceived to have speech that sounded more natural. There were mixed findings related to the three pencil and paper questionnaires, but qualitative analysis of the pre and post interviews suggested that the participants had made positive changes in their feelings about stuttering, experienced an increased sense of control, increased understanding of stuttering, and a realization that therapy was a process still to be worked on. These changes were maintained at six-months, as evidenced by the responses on the follow-up questionnaire.

The primary weakness of this initial study is that the participants did not complete follow-up analysis of their speech at 12-months post therapy, which has been done in other outcome studies (Boberg & Kully, 1994; Kully, et. al, 2007; O'Brian, et. al, 2008; St. Louis & Westbrook, 1987). This paper will report on an additional phase I study with a different group of participants who attended clinic. This study will be similar to Gabel, et al. (2008), but will include follow-up measures at six and 12 months post therapy. The following questions guided this research:

1. What are the benefits of the Intensive Stuttering Therapy for Adolescents and Adults?
2. What types of changes did clients maintain following this clinic?
3. What do clients report as the benefits of the therapy program?

METHODS

This study utilized a treatment effectiveness approach, also known as a treatment outcome approach (Yaruss, 1998). Some suggest that treatment efficacy designs should be the only approach used to study stuttering treatment (Cordes, 1998). The variety of approaches used and behaviors measured as a part of "eclectic" therapies, makes the use of efficacy designs difficult (Yaruss, 1998). Thus, researchers have suggested the use of a treatment effectiveness approach (Langevin & Kully, 2003; Yaruss, 1998), especially when studying existing clinical programs. Effectiveness designs differ from efficacy designs in that the high level of control that is present in efficacy designs is relinquished in hopes of measuring beneficial treatment outcomes as they might occur under typical, clinical conditions (Stricker, 1997). The ability to generalize these findings to a clinical setting is strong. This approach allows the researcher to describe the feasibility of the therapy measured (Robey & Schultz, 1997) and how aspects of the therapy might be explored further (Stricker, 1997; Yaruss, 1998). Effectiveness designs have been applied in several studies of existing "eclectic" therapy programs (Boberg & Kully, 1994; Langevin & Kully, 2003; Yaruss, 1998). This type of approach was utilized in this study.

When designing treatment effectiveness or outcome based studies, it is important to clearly identify the basic criteria to describe the outcomes of treatment. For this study, the criteria were similar to the guidelines used in other studies that explored the outcomes of other therapy programs (Andrews, Guitar, & Howie, 1980; Bloodstein & Ratner, 2008; Langevin & Kully, 2003; St. Louis & Westbrook, 1987; Yaruss, 1998).

Criteria 1. The Characteristics of the Participants Must Be Described

For this study, the participants were 5 adults who attended the Intensive Stuttering Therapy for Adolescents and Adults during one year of the program. These participants were self-selected, meaning that they were the first five participants, and the only participants, that attended this offering of the program. Characteristics of the five participants are displayed in Table 1. The participants were between the ages of 18 and 23 (mean=20.6). One client was a high-school senior, three were college students, and the other participant was a recent college graduate who was working as a groundskeeper. All of the clients received therapy in the past, but none of them had been in therapy three months prior to attending the clinic. None had been involved in a therapy that incorporated an eclectic approach, like the one utilized in this clinic.

Table 1. Description of the five participants in this study.

Client	Age	Occupation	Severity	Past Therapy
Client #1	18	High School Student	Moderate	Yes
Client #2	23	College Student	Mild	Yes
Client #3	22	College Student	Severe	Yes
Client #4	23	Groundskeeper	Moderate	Yes
Client #5	18	College Student	Moderate	Yes

Criteria 2. The Nature of the Therapy Delivered Needs to be Described in Detail

The therapy program that was studied was Bowling Green State University's (BGSU's) Intensive Stuttering Clinic for Adolescents and Adults. This program was described briefly in the first part of this chapter. The use of an effectiveness design seemed appropriate for studying this program for several reasons. First, the clinic employs both fluency shaping and stuttering modification approaches. Second, the clinic did not operate within a "controlled" environment. That is to say that control was not used in the identification of participants and multiple clinicians were utilized to deliver the therapy. Third, the clinic was relatively new (first year of the program) and measuring issues related to feasibility and benefits of the entire program seemed to be an appropriate first step in studying the clinic. Finally, a combination of therapists (professionals and graduate students) delivered the therapy.

The duration of the entire clinic was 15 days. The five participants lived residentially on the BGSU campus while attending therapy. Sessions lasted from five to seven hours a day and included both group and individual sessions. The therapy was divided into three phases. The first phase of the program helped the participants increase their awareness of their stuttering behaviors. The clinicians guided the participants in identifying all the behaviors related to their stuttering, including disfluencies, secondary physical reactions, negative emotional reactions, and negative communication attitudes. This was essentially what Van Riper (1982) and Guitar (2006) described as the identification phase of stuttering modification therapy. In addition, the participants spent a significant amount of time learning about stuttering as a topic.

The second phase of the program guided the participants through a process of reducing the severity of their stuttering. To accomplish this, the participants were encouraged to stutter openly and honestly. In addition, the participants learned the difference between muscular tension and relaxation and applied this concept to their stuttering. Techniques such as voluntary stuttering (Van Riper, 1982) were utilized to assist participants in learning new ways to stutter easily and to reduce the anxiety related to their stuttering (Breitenfeldt & Lorenz, 1989; Sheehan, 1975). To further assist the participants in the desensitization process, they gave speeches and participated in a variety of conversations with unfamiliar listeners both inside and outside of the clinical setting.

The third phase of therapy focused the participants on developing techniques to modify their stuttering and to improve their fluency. To modify stuttering, pull-outs and cancellations were taught, first in controlled contexts (clinical setting) and then in real-life situations (e.g. talking to other participants, talking to strangers, phone conversations, giving speeches, etc.). The procedures taught were similar to those discussed in the literature (Breitenfeldt & Lorenz; 1989; Van Riper, 1982). The participants were also taught fluency shaping behaviors, specifically easy onsets (prolongations), deliberate phonation, airflow management, and reduced rate of speech. Initially, these behaviors were taught using delayed auditory feedback as suggested by Shames and Florence (1980). The participants used the techniques at very slow speech rates and gradually increased their speech rate to a more normal and comfortable rate. As with the modification techniques, these behaviors were first used in controlled settings and then in increasingly difficult settings. Each participant was encouraged to develop a combination of behaviors to assist them with communicating effectively.

The final phase of the therapy program was referred to as the maintenance phase of treatment. Throughout the clinic, the participants were engaged in discussions to help them develop an individual maintenance program following the intensive clinics, which might have included continued therapy. For two of the participants (participant #1 and #5), this maintenance included continued weekly therapy following the summer clinic. For two of the participants (participant #2 and #4), their continued therapy included short intensive refresher courses of treatment (ten hours of therapy) clinics held during two weekends following the clinic. One of the participants chose not to attend follow-up therapy (participant #3), primarily due to finances and distance from BGSU.

Criteria 3. The Outcome or Measures of Success Must be Clearly Defined, They Must be Measurable, and All Treatment Goals Must be Measured Appropriately

The first goal of the treatment program was to improve the participants' communication ability through the use of fluency shaping and stuttering modification techniques. The goals related to speech improvement were for each participant to reduce stuttering frequency, reduce stuttering severity, and increase the perceived naturalness of their speech, which were adapted from past studies exploring outcomes of programs combining fluency shaping and stuttering modification techniques (Boberg & Kully, 1994; Langevin & Kully, 2003; Yaruss, 1998). Prior to initiating treatment, each participant was involved in a standard diagnostic of stuttering behaviors. The measures taken during the initial diagnostic were completed at the end of treatment (day 15), during a six and 12 month follow-up periods. To evaluate changes in fluency and speech production, the percentage of stuttered syllables per 300 syllables was gathered during a reading and conversation sample. During the follow-up period, these measures were taken from tapes the clients submitted to the first author. The Stuttering Severity Instrument- 3 (SSI-3) (Riley, 1994) was used to evaluate stuttering severity. Finally, a seven point rating scale (1=unnatural to 7= natural) was used to evaluate the perceived changes in naturalness for each participant. This scale was similar to those suggested in the literature (e.g. Onslowe, Adams, & Ingham, 1992). These measures were completed by three independent judges trained in completing fluency analysis. Agreement indexes for the presence of stuttering behaviors were completed for each measure using procedures discussed in the literature (Cordes, 2000). For the identification of stuttered syllables, >90% interjudge agreement was found for each participant during each phase of treatment. The SSI-3 and the naturalness ratings made by the judges were highly correlated ($r>.90$). The first author completed intrajudge agreement for all measures, with >90% found for the measures of disfluency. High intrajudge agreement ($r>.90$) was also found for the SSI-3 and speech naturalness ratings.

The second goal of therapy was to assess changes in the participants' affective and cognitive reactions to their stuttering. Three scales were used and were similar to those scales reported for other outcome studies (Boberg & Kully, 1994; Langevin & Kully, 2003). The first measure was the *S-24 scale* (Andrews & Cutler, 1974), which assesses an individual's attitude and feelings toward interpersonal communication. The second scale was the *LCB* (Craig, et. al, 1984). The *LCB* is a 17-item Likert-type scale used to measure an individual's locus of control for behavior. The final scale was the *SP-LOC* (McDonough & Quesal, 1988). This eight-item scale was developed to determine an individual's speech locus of control is internal versus external. Finally, the *OASES* (Yaruss & Quesal, 2008) was used to measure the impact of stuttering on the person's life. This four section scale includes 100 questions that explore the speaker's experiences and perceptions of general information about stuttering, reactions to stuttering, communication in daily situations, and quality of life.

In addition, qualitative methodologies were used to measure the participants' perceptions of the benefits of treatment. To gather this data, each participant was engaged in a semi-structured interview (Patton, 2002) conducted during the initial diagnostic and at the end of treatment. During these interviews, the participants responded to questions about their perceptions of their own stuttering, how they felt about their stuttering, personal goals for treatment, and their perceptions of the benefits of therapy. This data was analyzed thematically, with important themes related to stuttering and recovery being the focus. These interviews were both video- and audio-taped and the following questions were used to guide the interviews:

1. Tell me about your speech.
2. Tell me about your stuttering.
3. Feelings, attitudes, behaviors.
4. How does your stuttering affect you?
5. What would you like to change about your self and your stuttering?
6. What would you like to (or have you) gotten out of therapy?
7. How has your speech and other aspects of your life changed as a part of therapy (only at the end of therapy)?

At six and 12 months, the participants completed written narratives regarding their progress following the therapy, their perceptions of therapy, and their perceptions of their speech. These narratives were analyzed thematically, using qualitative methods similar to those described in the literature (Patton, 2002).

Though reliability and validity are not identified as important components of qualitative designs, a related concept of credibility is necessary and was adhered to in this study. Credibility is a process by which researchers assure that the results obtained are accurate from the point of view of the participants, researchers, and the readers of the study. Credibility was established using procedures similar to those discussed by Patton (2002). The procedures are as follows:

1. Each semi-structured interview (beginning, middle, and end of treatment) was recorded (audio and video) and transcribed verbatim. Each written narrative obtained during follow-up was transcribed verbatim.
2. The primary interviewer was not the first author.
3. The transcripts for each participant were reviewed by the three reviewers independently. Two of the reviewers had a background in stuttering treatment and are PWS. The third was trained to do qualitative analysis, but had no background in stuttering. First, each reviewed the transcripts individually and developed their own understanding of the theme structures. Then, each interpretation was discussed until consensus on the major themes was established.
4. Finally, credibility was further ascertained by a process of member-checking (Patton, 2002). Member checking is an effective means for authenticating findings of qualitative studies (Patton, 2002). In this study, the first author shared the results of

the qualitative analysis with three of the participants and asked them to share their perceptions of the themes and whether these themes reflected their experience with the clinic. Each felt that the themes were a fair interpretation of their experience and perceptions of therapy.

Criteria 4. All the Changes in Treatment, Both Positive and Negative, Must be Measured, Analyzed, Compared, and Reported Clearly

All the outcome data gathered in this study, both qualitative and quantitative, was analyzed descriptively for each participant and for the entire group of participants who attended the program. From this data, the importance of each type of measurement was evaluated and both positive and negative changes were documented. Finally, the individual changes for each participant and the impact of certain phases of the clinic were identified.

RESULTS

Quantitative Data

Table 2 summarizes the outcomes related to the speech measures for each of the clients. Five of the six participants made dramatic changes in all aspects of their speech at the end of therapy. While participant #1 did not change the frequency of his stuttering, he did reduce the severity. In addition, he also improved his speech naturalness. All of the clients maintained these changes at six and 12 months. For all of the clients, it appears that the therapy program provided them the ability to produce speech that contained less stuttering behaviors with less severity. In addition, they were able to speak at faster rates of speech and each sounded more natural.

Table 3 summarizes the outcome data for the affective and cognitive questionnaires. For the *S-24* scale (Andrews & Cutler, 1974), each participant reported a lower score following therapy. This finding suggests that participants reported more positive attitudes towards communication following therapy. Three of the participants scored within the range expected for individuals who do not stutter. For the *LCB* scale (Craig, et. al, 1984), a lower score suggests a more internal locus of control. Each client scored in the range suggestive of an internal locus of control. It should be noted that only one of the participants presented a score indicative of an external locus of control at the beginning of therapy. Also, all clients reported improvements on the measure for *Speech Locus of Control* (McDonough & Quesal, 1988).

Table 4 provides outcome data related to the *OASES* (Yaruss & Quesal, 2008). The OASES measured the perceptions that each participant had related to the impact stuttering has on their lives. Each participant reported positive changes for each subscale and the total score. For participants 3 and 5, this change was less dramatic than the other three participants. Both of these participants anticipated that stuttering would continue to have a moderate effect on their life, while the other three participants reported that stuttering would have either a mild impact or a mild to moderate impact following therapy.

Table 2. Speech measures for the five participants.

Client	Speech Measures	Initial	Final	Six-Month	Twelve-Month
1	%SS for Reading/Conversation	4/11%	1%/11%	0%/8%	0/9%
	SSI#	29	10	13	12
	Speech Naturalness*	6	7	7	7
	Speech Rate Conversation (wpm)	71	208	201	207
2	%SS for Reading/Conversation	9%/13%	1%/7%	0/4%	0/5%
	SSI#	23	12	12	13
	Speech Naturalness*	6	7	7	7
	Speech Rate Conversation (wpm)	98	118	122	117
3	%SS for Reading/Conversation	47%55%	13%/21%	26%/26%	25%/22%
	SSI#	32	24	23	22
	Speech Naturalness*	3	4	4	5
	Speech Rate Conversation (wpm)	59	63	65	72
4	%SS for Reading/Conversation	1%/9%	0%/2%	0%/1%	0/1%
	SSI#	27	4	4	4
	Speech Naturalness*	6	7	7	7
	Speech Rate Conversation (wpm)	102	116	118	117
5	%SS for Reading/Conversation	1%/25%	0%/2%	0/2%	0/2%
	SSI#	29	11	--	--
	Speech Naturalness*	3	6	6	7
	Speech Rate Conversation (wpm)	67	117	111	112

Ranges for SSI-3 (Riley & Riley, 1994) are as follows:
10-17=Very mild
18-24=Mild
25-31=Moderate
32-36=Severe
37-46=Very Severe
* A naturalness score of 1=unnatural with a score of 7=natural

Table 3. Measures related to emotional and cognitive aspects of stuttering.

Participant	Speech Measures	Initial	Final
1	S-24 Scale#	19	6
	LCB*	38	22
	Speech Locus of Control~	6	4
2	S-24 Scale#	19	6
	LCB*	26	14
	Speech Locus of Control~	5	2
3	S-24 Scale#	19	12
	LCB*	10	18
	Speech Locus of Control~	7	7
4	S-24 Scale	7	5
	LCB*	23	15
	Speech Locus of Control~	5	4
5	S-24 Scale	18	12
	LCB*	21	22
	Speech Locus of Control~	7	3

#Higher score suggests a more negative attitudes. Mean for PWS=19.22; mean for PWDS=9.14.
*Scores higher than 29.8 are indicative of an external locus of control
~Higher score is indicative of a more external locus of control.

Qualitative Data

Narratives gathered during the interviews prior to and following therapy as well as the written questionnaires were analyzed qualitatively to identify important themes. These themes were those that reflected the participants' experiences with stuttering and their perceptions of therapy. At the beginning of therapy, the major themes that emerged from the narratives included reduced self-confidence, reduced self-esteem, and fears related to stuttering. These themes suggest that the participants were discussing the impact of stuttering and how stuttering made them feel. Examples of statements appear below:

P1: "I fear getting up in front of people that I don't know and people that don't know I have a stuttering problem. That's the worst."
P2: "It makes me feel inferior to others."
P3: "In school, I only have a few friends because of my stuttering. At my job place I don't need to talk much and that's good."
P4: "I can't communicate with people."
P5: "I really don't like talking on the phone and I really don't like talking to strangers. I really don't like to go into a room and introduce myself to people I don't know and tell them who I am."

Table 4. Summary of the OASES.

Client	Speech Measures	Initial	Final
1	Section I: General Information	3.85	1.5
	Section II: Reactions to Stuttering	3.80	1.63
	Section III: Comm. in Daily Situations	3.16	1.84
	Section IV: Quality of Life	3.72	1.36
	Total	3.63	1.59
2	Section I: General Information	3.00	1.45
	Section II: Reactions to Stuttering	3.13	1.43
	Section III: Comm. in Daily Situations	3.56	1.48
	Section IV: Quality of Life	2.72	1.16
	Total	3.11	1.38
3	Section I: General Information	2.80	2.25
	Section II: Reactions to Stuttering	2.33	1.83
	Section III: Comm. in Daily Situations	3.64	2.88
	Section IV: Quality of Life	3.32	2.80
	Total	3	2.42
4	Section I: General Information	3.15	1.70
	Section II: Reactions to Stuttering	2.93	1.73
	Section III: Comm. in Daily Situations	2.36	1.44
	Section IV: Quality of Life	2.08	1.12
	Total	2.63	1.50
5	Section I: General Information	3.10	2.15
	Section II: Reactions to Stuttering	3.46	2.87
	Section III: Comm. in Daily Situations	3.24	4.28
	Section IV: Quality of Life	3.12	1.76
	Total	3.25	2.80

Mild Impact=1.00-1.49
Mild/Moderate Impact= 1.50-2.24
Moderate Impact= 2.25-2.99
Moderate/Severe Impact= 3.00-3.74
Severe Impact= 3.75-5.00

Interestingly, it appears that these individuals chose to focus on issues related to their stuttering that were beyond simply issues with loss of speech fluency. Situational fears and talking with others, as well as effects of stuttering on self-esteem and feelings were discussed. Certainly, each individual had their own experiences with stuttering, but the shared impact of stuttering on specific aspects of each person's experience seemed to be shared by all participants.

At the end of treatment, the participants completed another interview where they were asked to respond to similar questions. Following therapy, the themes that arose reflected the speakers' increased self-confidence, self-esteem, feelings of control over their stuttering, awareness, and a more positive outlook toward communication. Some examples of these types of comments include:

P1: "I have more control over my speech. Early in therapy I had lots of blocks. I leaned that using easy onsets can help me reduce my blocks."
P3: "My attitude has changed from negative to positive."
P4: "I feel more confident talking to strangers and talking on the phone."
P5: "As each day goes on, the negative feelings get less and less, and the negative self-talk gets less and less, and so my attitude has definitely changed a lot. I am in control of my problem."

As with the initial interviews, the themes from the final narratives suggested that the participants were identifying issues related to the impact of stuttering on their lives, feelings, and emotions. Thus, their views of the outcomes of the therapy experience were related to changes that were much broader than simply a change in speech fluency. Of course, changes in speech, especially the amount of control they felt, were identified as important factors in therapy. These changes appear to suggest multiple benefits to the therapy program. Examples of these comments follow:

At six months and 12 months, the clients completed written narrative describing their progress since the end of treatment, their perceptions of therapy, and their speech. The themes that arose from these narratives included increased feelings of control, continued need to monitor and manage their speech, and continued use of therapy techniques. Examples of these comments at six months included:

P2: "My stuttering (when I do stutter) is much easier. Also, I'm not so nervous when I speak. I am going out more often and socializing with friends."
P3: "Sometimes I just let my stuttering happen."
P4: "In the past 6 months or so my rules [techniques] were a great help to me. I know they could have helped me even more if I had more time to practice."
P5: "I've been doing well! I am taking a public speaking class next semester. I went back to work and I felt more in control of my speech."

At 12 months, the participants reported similar themes in their narratives, along with reports of some increasing difficulties. Examples of these comments included:

P2: "Currently, my speech is still in control, but I still put effort into using my techniques."
P4: My speech is still rocky. A few days it will be great, then I'll hit a slump of about 1 month or more. I just have to keep working at it."
P5: "I do still stutter but hardly ever think about it anymore. I just do it."

From these comments during the follow-up narratives, it appears clear that the participants continued to utilize their skills learned in therapy and continued their process of attitude change. Each appeared to have accepted stuttering and was willing to engage in the process of working on their speech. In addition, they all appeared to have experienced some difficult situations, but were willing to work to continue to make positive changes. A long statement by P3 is a good summary of this process:

> P3: "Over the past 12 months, my speech had ups and downs. In other words, sometimes it has gotten better and other times it has gotten worse. . . . Almost everyday for the past few months I've been practicing for one hour with my father. So far, this has resulted in a major improvement of my speech. I am willing to keep working so I can continue to make the positive changes and use the skills I learned in the clinic."

In summary, the results of interview analyses suggest that the participants gained increased knowledge and understanding of stuttering, and expressed improved attitudes, confidence, and positive thoughts toward speaking situations. These changes appeared to be reflected in the six and 12 month follow-up narratives, though the participants expressed the need to continue to work on their speech.

Follow-up Therapy

An important consideration for this therapy program, and other intensive programs, is follow-up therapy. With this group of participants, all but the third client received follow-up therapy. Participant 5 lived several states away (New York) from BGSU (Ohio). So, attending therapy was not feasible. The client did not choose to use the phone for therapy or consults. Participant 1 received weekly therapy through his school district. His therapist was the first author and one of the graduate student clinician who participated in the clinic. Participants 2 and 4 attended two weekend follow-up clinics. Each of these clinics was 10 hours in duration. For these weekend follow-up clinics, the first author and one of the graduate student clinicians provided therapy. Finally, Participant 5 attended weekly therapy sessions at BGSU's Speech and Hearing Clinic. As with the other participants, the first author and a student clinician provided services.

CONCLUSION

Outcomes of Treatment

As with the earlier study exploring the benefits of this program (Gabel, et. al, 2008), the present study explored the benefits of therapy using a mixed methods, also known as mixed model, design. Though we cannot say whether the therapy had a direct cause effect relationship with the improvements made by the participants, the data does suggest that the therapy lead to a variety of benefits for the participants.

In this study, all of the participants showed positive changes in their speech. With the exception of participant 1, four of the clients showed improvement in all measures of speech. Though participant 1 did not show changes in frequency of stuttering, he did show a reduction in stuttering severity and speech naturalness. Only two of the participants displayed frequency of stuttering that was less than 3% syllables stuttered, which has been suggested as a goal in other therapy programs (Kully et. al, 2007; O'Brian, et. al, 2008). Each of these participants maintained their changes in speech production at six and 12 month follow-up periods.

It should be noted that the frequency and severity of stuttering for participant 3 at the end of the clinic and during follow-up were relatively high, compared to the other participants. As one might suspect, this might be related to the severity of stuttering that this participant displayed at the beginning of therapy. Though his final measures would still suggest a moderate to severe stuttering disorder, this is still an improvement from the beginning of treatment. These changes were maintained at six and 12 month follow-up.

As found in the other study of this program (Gabel, et. al, 2008), participants made improvements in their speech following therapy and maintained these changes during follow-up. As with the other study, these changes were maintained at six months. In the present study, these changes were maintained at both six and 12 months. Therefore, for the nine participants included in these two studies, it appears as if the therapy program is helpful in maintaining positive changes in speech production.

Similar to Gabel et. al (2008), the findings of this study suggest that participants made positive changes in the affective and cognitive behaviors related to their stuttering. This was most evident by improvement in the reports on the *S-24* (Andrews & Cutler, 1974), suggesting that the participants had improved their attitudes towards communication at the end of therapy. Three participants were actually reporting scores below the mean expected for people who do not stutter (PWDS). These findings are also similar to those reported from other intensive programs (Boberg & Kully, 1994; Kully, et. al, 2007; Langevin & Kully, 2003). Additionally, there were changes in responses on the LCB (Craig, et. al, 1984) and SP-LOC (McDonough & Quesal, 1988). Though these results were less dramatic, the participants reported an increased feeling of control following therapy during their interviews. These findings were similar to the results from Gabel et. al. Future studies exploring the benefits of this therapy may consider using other measures of affective and cognitive change. In other offerings of this program, the first author has used the *Self-Efficacy Scale for Adult Stutterers* (Ornstein and Manning, 1985). This scale measures the person's beliefs regarding their ability to approach certain situations and to be fluent, which would be a good measure of many of the goals of this program.

Unlike Gabel, et. al (2008), the current study utilized the *OASES* (Yaruss & Quesal, 2008) to measure the participants' perceived impact of stuttering on their lives. As with other measures, the participants reported a positive change for this measure following therapy. All of the participants perceived that stuttering would have less of an impact on their lives following therapy. Two of the participants reported that stuttering would continue to have a moderate effect on their lives following therapy. Thus, there was a general sense of improvement, but not an equal improvement across the five participants.

One of the weaknesses of this study was that the affective and cognitive measures were not repeated during the follow-up. This decision was primarily a financial one, since there was a very small budget allowed to gather follow-up measures. In future studies of this program, these measures will need to be completed to gain a better sense of maintenance of change following therapy. One way to do this is to use the internet to deliver the questionnaires to future participants, using available software. In this way, the measures could be completed at little cost and the use of the software would allow for easier scoring.

The qualitative results provided additional support for improved affective and cognitive changes following therapy, as well as additional data about the participants' experiences during and following therapy. Most of the changes reported were related to altered affective reactions to stuttering, such as improved self-esteem, self-confidence, outlook on communication, and increased awareness of their stuttering. These are all positive changes that were important goals for therapy and have been identified as important aspects of long-term change (Manning, 2001). It should be noted that though there are subtle difference between these themes and those identified by Gabel, et. al (2008). The findings of the previous study and the present one, suggest the utility of including qualitative methods to identify changes in therapy.

In addition, the participants reported an increase in feelings of control following therapy, as did the participants in Gabel et. al (2008). Developing a feeling of control has been identified as important in several therapy programs (Breitenfeldt & Lorenz, 1989; Kully, et. al, 2007; Van Riper, 1982). This feeling of control, though it might be thought of as a cognitive change, might also reflect the perceived ability that the client has related to their use of therapy skills, improved fluency, decreased severity of their stuttering, and improved affective responses to the problem. Control might be a more global concept that encompasses all of these changes. Conversely, control may be interpreted or experienced differently among different PWS. Future studies should explore this concept further to gain a better understanding of this important process.

In general, the results of this study and Gabel et. al (2008) support the need for future research on this type of therapy program. These studies, though lacking experimental control, describe the variety of benefits of this therapy program and the ability for a small number of participants to maintain changes following therapy. Future research will need to develop studies that incorporate larger groups of participants as well as control groups to provide a better sense of the efficacy of this program.

Future Directions for This Program

Though this program has shown some evidence of success, there are several additional issues related to feasibility that need to be discussed. Some of this information is evident from the results of this study and Gabel et. al (2008), however much of it is also evident from unpublished data. The first issue is related to the follow-up therapy. In this study and Gabel et. al, there was no way to control the type of follow-up therapy utilized. This is similar to the other 18-20 participants who have attended the program since its inception. Thus, one of the primary weaknesses identified in offering this program is the lack of structure to the follow-up component of therapy. There simply are not enough opportunities to monitor and provide support to our clients directly and a consistent basis following the intensive portion of therapy. We believe this contact is critical for the clients to have any long term success. Additionally, it has been nearly impossible to measure the long-term benefits, feasibility, or efficacy of this program without this type of contact. Following the intensive clinic in 2008, the authors began piloting the use of telepractice follow-up with computerized, video teleconferencing technology (using a Logitech QuickCam and WEBEX) for the clients who attended the intensive clinic. Similar approaches have been reported by other intensive programs (Kully, et. al, 2007; O'Brian et. al, 2008). Though it is too early to assess the benefits of this telepractice service, initial data suggests that all participants were able to access the service, complete weekly or bi-weekly therapy sessions, and continued to maintain and progress in their therapy. As an added benefit, the use of the telepractice model allows us to gather the necessary data to report the long-term outcomes of treatment. For this type of program, in which very few people attend who live within a short distance from BGSU, the use of telepractice may prove to be critical.

Another major issue is that this therapy program continues to be difficult for many individuals to attend. Each year, between 15 and 20 individuals have inquired and requested application information for attending the intensive program. Fewer than half of these individuals have been able to attend each year. The primary obstacles to attending the program appear to be finances and spending time away from work and school during the three week program. Not surprisingly, other intensive programs report similar difficulties, and have suggested avenues for reducing the length of these program, without compromising the therapy (Kully, et. al, 2007; O'Brian, et al., 2008). To overcome this issue, the intensive clinic will be offered as a larger program, which is named the *Multifaceted Therapy Program for Adolescents and Adults*. In this new program, the intensive portion will be offered over 50 hours during a nine day session. An additional 25 hours of therapy will be offered using telepractice. Thus, the program will still include 75 hours of therapy and incorporate all of the approaches and goals of the earlier three-week program. In essence, the shorter period will both reduce the financial costs (i.e., room and board) related to attending the program and allow clients to take less time away from work and other activities. These changes, along with the telepractice portion of the program, will allow more individuals to access this program.

REFERENCES

American Speech-Language-Hearing Association. (2004, October 13). *Report of the joint coordinating committee on evidence-based practice*. Retrieved August 26, 2008, from http://www.asha.org/NR/rdonlyres/B1DF75A7-83A0-4F78-8A09-4113139CE5CE/0/JCCEBPReport04.pdf

American Speech-Language-Heamring Association. (2005). *Evidence-Based Practice in Communication Disorders* [Position Statement]. Available from www.asha.org/policy.

Andrews, G. & Cutler, J. (1974). Stuttering therapy: The relation between changes in symptom level and attitudes. *Journal of Speech and Hearing Disorders, 39,* 312-319.

Andrews, G., Guitar, B. & Howie, P. M. (1980). Meta-analysis of the effects of stuttering treatment. *Journal of Speech & Hearing Disorders, 45*(3), 287-307.

Bloodstein, O. & Bernstein-Ratner, N. (2008). *A handbook on stuttering* (6th ed.). *Clifton Park*, NY: Delmar.

Boberg, E. & Kully, D. (1994). Long-term results of an intensive treatment program for adults and adolescents who stutter. *Journal of Speech and Hearing Research*, *37*, 1050-1059.

Breitenfeldt, D. & Lorenz, D. (1989). *Successful stuttering management program. Cheney*, WA: Easter Washington University School of Health Sciences.

Brisk, D. J., Healey, E. C. & Hux, K. A. (1997). Clinicians' training and confidence associated with treating school-age children who stutter: A national survey. *Language, Speech, and Hearing Services in Schools*, *28*, 164-176.

Cooper, E. B. (1993). Second Opinion. Chronic perseverative stuttering syndrome: A harmful or helpful construct. *American Journal of Speech-Language Pathology*, *2*, 11-15.

Cordes, A. K. (1998). Current status of the stuttering treatment literature. In A. K. Cordes & R. J. Ingham (EDs.), *Treatment efficacy for stuttering: A search for empirical bases* (pp. 117-144). San Diego, CA: Singular.

Cordes, A. K. (1998). Current status of the stuttering treatment literature. In Cordes, A. K. & Ingham, R. J. (EDs.), *Treatment efficacy for stuttering: A search for empirical bases* (pp. 117-144). *San Diego*, CA: Singular.

Cordes, A. K. (2000). Individual and consensus judgments of disfluency types in the speech of persons who stutter. *Journal of Speech, Language, and Hearing Research*, *43*, 951-964.

Craig, A., Franklin, J. & Andrews, G. (1984). A scale to measure locus of control of behaviour. *British Journal of Medical Psychology*, *57*, 173-180.

Crichton-Smith, I. (2002). Communicating in the real-world: Accounts from people who stammer. *Journal of Fluency Disorders, 27,* 333-352.

Gabel, R., Daniels, D. & Hughes, S. (2008). A Mixed-model Approach to Studying Treatment Outcomes. *Perspectives on Fluency and Fluency Disorders, 18*, 6-16.

Gregory, H. (2003). *Stuttering therapy: Rationale and procedures. Boston*, MA: Allyn & Bacon.

Guitar, B. (2006). *Stuttering: An integrated approach to its nature and treatment*, (3rd ed.). Baltimore: Williams and Wilkins.

Klompas, M. & Ross, E. (2004). Life experiences of people who stutter, and the perceived impact of stuttering on quality of life: Personal accounts of South African individuals. *Journal of Fluency Disorders, 29,* 275-305.

Kully, D., Langevin, M. & Lomheim, H. (2007). Intensive treatment of stuttering in adolescents and adults. In Conture, E. C. & R. F. Curlee (Eds.). *Stuttering and Related Fluency Disorders (3rd Edition),* (pp. 213-232).

Langevin, M. & Kully, D. (2003). Evidence-based treatment of stuttering: III. evidence-based practice in a clinical setting. *Journal of Fluency Disorders, 28*(3), 219-236.

Manning, W. H. (2001). *Clinical decision making in fluency disorders.* (2nd ed.) *San Diego*, CA: Singular-Thomson.

McDonough, A. & Quesal, B. (1988). Locus of control orientation of stutterers and nonstutterers. *Journal of Fluency Disorders, 13*, 97-106.

O'Brien, S., Packman, A. & Onslow, M. (2008). Telehealth delivery of the Camperdown program for adults who stutter: A Phase I Trial. *Journal of Speech, Language, and Hearing Research, 51(1)*, 184-195.

Onslow, M., Adams, R. & Ingham, R. (1992). Reliability of speech naturalness ratings of stuttered speech during treatment. *Journal of Speech and Hearing Research, 35*, 994-1001.

Ornstein, A. & Manning, W. (1985). Self-efficacy scaling by adult stutterers. *Journal of Communication Disorders*, *18*, 313-320.

Patton, M. Q. (2002). *Qualitative research and evaluation methods. Thousand Oaks*, CA: Sage Publications, Inc.

Robey, R. R. & Schultz, M. C. (1997). A model for conducting clinical-outcome research: An adaptation of the standard protocol for use in aphasiology. *Aphasiology*, *12*, 787-810.

Sheehan, J. (1975). Conflict theory of stuttering. In J. Eisenson (Ed.), *Stuttering: A second symposium. New York*, : Harper & Row.

St. Louis, K. & Durrenberger, C. (1993). What communication disorders do experienced clinicians prefer to manage? *ASHA,* Dec., 23-31.

St. Louis, K. O. & Westbrook, J. B. (1987). The effectiveness of treatment for stuttering. In Rustin, L. Purser, H. & Rowley, D. (EDs.), *Progress in the treatment of fluency disorders* (pp. 235-257). London: Whurr.

Stewart, T. & Richardson, G. (2004). A qualitative study of therapeutic effect from a user's perspective. *Journal of Fluency Disorders, 29,* 95-108.

Stricker, G. (1997). Are science and practice commensurable? *American Psychologist, 52*, 442-448.

Tellis, G., Bressler, L. & Emerick, K. (2008). An exploration of clinicians views about assessment and treatment of stuttering. *Perspectives on Fluency and Fluency Disorders*, *18*, 16-23.

Van Riper, C. (1982). *The nature of stuttering* (2nd ed.). *Englewood Cliffs*, NJ. :

Wingate, M. (1964). Recovery from stuttering. *Journal of Speech and Hearing Disorders*, *29*, 312-321.

Yaruss, J. S. (1998). Treatment outcomes in stuttering: Finding value in clinical data. In Cordes, A. K. & Ingham, R. J. (Eds.), *Treatment efficacy for stuttering: A search for an empirical bases* (pp. 213-242). *San Diego*, CA: Singular Publishing Group.

Yaruss, J. S. & Quesal, R. (2002). Academic and clinical education in fluency disorders: An update. *Journal of Fluency Disorders*, 27, 43-63.

Yaruss, S. J. (2007). Application of the ICF in fluency disorders. *Seminars in Speech and Language, 28(4),* 312-322.

In: Speech Disorders: Causes, Treatment and Social Effects ISBN: 978-1-60876-213-2
Editor: Alan E. Harrison, pp. 159-176

Chapter 7

IS PROSODY A DIAGNOSTIC AND COGNITIVE BELLWETHER OF AUTISM SPECTRUM DISORDERS?

Joshua John Diehl[1] and Lauren D. Berkovits[2]
[1]University of Notre Dame and Haskins Laboratories
[2]Yale Child Study Center

ABSTRACT

Atypicalities in prosody are a prominent characteristic of all autism spectrum disorders. Despite the centrality of prosody to the behavioral presentation of the disorder, our knowledge of the nature of these deficits is limited. In this chapter, current research on prosody production and comprehension in autism spectrum disorders is examined. Particular attention will be given to the utility of prosody as an early diagnostic marker, as a behavioral indicator of subtypes of the disorder, and as a bellwether for strengths and weaknesses in an individual's cognitive profile. Future directions of prosody research will also be discussed, including the importance of acoustic analysis of speech and other psycholinguistic paradigms. Finally, the clinical implications research on prosodic deficits in autism spectrum disorders will be addressed, including the value of prosody for identifying individual differences and the promise of computerized instant feedback technology for treatment.

INTRODUCTION

Autism is a neurodevelopmental disability for which social-communication deficits are central (American Psychiatric Association, 2000), particularly in the area of pragmatic language use (Arnold, Bennetto, & Diehl, 2009; Tager-Flusberg, Paul, & Lord, 2005; Young, Diehl, Morris, Hyman, & Bennetto, 2005). Atypicalities in prosody are a prominent characteristic of autism, and one of the most stigmatizing aspects of the disorder (Shriberg et al., 2001). Prosody production deficits persist even as other areas of language improve (McCann & Peppé, 2003), and continue to be a stigmatizing behavioral feature even in high-functioning individuals on the autism spectrum (Shriberg et al., 2001). Despite the centrality of prosody to the behavioral presentation of the disorder, our knowledge of the nature of these deficits is limited (McCann & Peppé, 2003). In this chapter, it is argued that prosody: 1) may be the earliest appearing diagnostic marker of the disorder, 2) might provide important clues to nosological issues, especially as they relate to the heterogeneity of the disorder and subtypes, and 3) could be an indicator of the strengths and weaknesses of an individual's general cognitive functioning. Current research on prosody production and comprehension in autism spectrum disorders will be examined within the framework of these three topics. Future directions of prosody research will also be discussed. In particular, the importance of using established psycholinguistic paradigms for prosody processing and production will be stressed, with an emphasis on measures that have been validated on normative samples. Finally, the treatment of prosodic deficits in autism spectrum disorders will be addressed, specifically highlighting recent advances in computerized instant feedback technology.

WHY PROSODY?

Many of the areas in which children with autism struggle the most are closely linked with prosodic aspects of language and communication. Affect states, intention, the structure of discourse, and irony (among others) are all communicated, in part, through prosody. Individuals with autism also characteristically struggle in understanding facial expressions and gestures, both of which are integrally linked to prosody in conversation. Moreover, prosody perception is the earliest known social and linguistic ability to develop (Werker, 2005), and could provide the earliest diagnostic indicator of the disorder. Therefore, it is important to understand fully what prosody represents in communication and to explore the ways in which it is disrupted in autism.

At its most basic level, prosody represents the pitch, rhythm, and melody of language. In fact, the word prosody is derived from the Greek root *audE* or *ode* (a song sung), and the prefix *pros* (in addition to). Thus, prosody (roughly translated) means "a song in addition to" the words of speech. Prosody is the basis for the phrasal and informational structure of an utterance through variations in pauses, stress, rhythm, and intonation. Subtle prosodic changes can indicate the correct interpretation of a syntactically ambiguous sentence (e.g., "He chased the girl on the tricycle"). Prosody also provides cues to discourse structure and the speaker's affect. A variation in the prosodic pattern of the phrase "You're coming with me" can change the speaker's intention from a demand to an inquiry. Similarly, the meaning of the phrase "I'm finished" can be altered to communicate the major affective states (e.g., happy, sad) or convey a complex mental state (e.g., sarcasm). Prosody can also be communicative when essentially presented in isolation. For example, "oh." and "oh!" convey different meanings. Generally, though, prosody must be integrated with lexical (segmental) information that may provide supplemental, neutral, or even contrasting information about utterance meaning or the intentions of the interlocutor. Thus, it has an integral relationship with both *what* is communicated and *how* it is communicated.

Prosody is important for linguistic and communicative development as well. It is thought that we are able to perceive prosodic patterns in utero, which makes it, one of the first measurable cognitive capacities. Infants are born with the ability to distinguish their mother's voice from other voices (Decasper & Fifer, 1980; Decasper & Spence, 1986; Kisilevsky et al.,

2003) and the patterns of their native language from other languages (Moon, Cooper, & Fifer, 1993). Before babies start to speak, they can differentially perceive the affective and syntactic prosodic nature of words (Grossmann, Striano, & Friederici, 2005; Nazzi, Nelson, Jusczyk, & Jusczyk, 2000). Prosody perception in infancy facilitates language acquisition (Jusczyk, 2003) and predicts future language abilities (Tsao, Liu, & Kuhl, 2004); therefore, it should not be surprising that prosodic patterns emerge in babbling before words (Snow & Balog, 2002). Recently, Snow (2006) showed that prosodic patterns assume an adult-like form by the age of 6 months, but then regress between 9-11 months, only to begin to reassume adult-like patterns around 18 months of age. This temporary regression is thought to be a reorganization of the linguistic system in which typical children transition from the passive acquisition of speech to intentional communication. Research has indicated that this developmental shift to intentional communication includes a differentiation of vocalizations during shared experience (speech directed at interlocutors) and vocalizations during manipulation of a toy (undirected sounds and speech) (Dodorico & Franco, 1991). Furthermore, during this time period, prosodic rules are learned (e.g., the relationship between rising intonation and asking a question), generalized, and integrated functionally with productive speech (e.g., "Ball?" and "Ball." would begin to have different meanings).

In sum, prosody represents one of the primary end-state behaviors of the social use of language. Prosody, both in perception and production, seems to be the earliest social and linguistic behavior to appear, possibly even before a child is born. Moreover, after bootstrapping early linguistic development, prosody becomes a vehicle for the communication of meaning, affect, intent, and the structure of discourse. Therefore, this faculty shows promise for understanding the cognitive environment of autism, and could potentially provide the earliest diagnostic indicator of the disorder.

Prosody and Autism

Individuals with autism exhibit marked atypicalities in expressive prosody (Tager-Flusberg et al., 2005). Unusual prosody is present in both high- and low-functioning individuals with autism. These impairments typically persist through adulthood, and can have a significant negative impact on a range of communicative functions (McCann & Peppé, 2003). Even in the earliest descriptions of autism spectrum disorders (ASDs), Hans Asperger noted:

"one can invariably pick up these kinds of abnormalities in the language of autistic individuals, and their recognition is, therefore, of particular diagnostic importance..." (Asperger, 1944; as translated by Frith, 1991, p. 71)

Asperger noted that the children with this disorder could sound too soft and far away, shrill, or sing-songy, and that their intonation did not always fall appropriately at the end of a declarative statement. In the same paper, Asperger noted that "we do not intellectually understand many of these qualities and can only feel them intuitively" (p. 70). Descriptions of prosody in autism have included words such as flat or monotonous, variable, sing-songy, and/or pedantic (Amoroso, 1992; Baltaxe, 1984; Fay & Schuler, 1980; Goldfarb, Braunstein, & Lorge, 1956; Provonost, Wakstein, & Wakstein, 1966; Wing, 1981). Deficits in prosodic production are included as a diagnostic characteristic of the disorder in the Autism Diagnostic

Interview, Revised (ADI-R; Rutter, Le Couteur, & Lord, 2003) and the Autism Diagnostic Observation Schedule (ADOS; Lord, Rutter, DiLavore, & Risi, 1999), which are the gold-standard diagnostic tools used with this population. The important commonality to be found in these descriptive accounts of prosodic expression does not lie in the *type* of prosody used (sing-songy versus monotone). Instead, the unifying feature is that there seems to be a *mismatch* between the words spoken, the context in which the words were spoken, and the prosody that was used by the speaker. Moreover, although the presentation of prosodic atypicalities is heterogeneous, their presence in ASDs is ubiquitous.

Despite the numerous descriptive accounts of prosodic impairments in autism, systematic research on prosodic abilities in individuals with autism has been limited until very recently, and the findings do not represent the pervasiveness of the deficits observed clinically. Before examining the research, though, several considerations must be taken into account. First, autism is considered by many to be a spectrum disorder with a wide array of functioning levels. Although all individuals on the spectrum share core deficits in social-communication, the presentation/severity of these impairments, as well as strengths and weaknesses in other areas, vary greatly throughout the spectrum. Studies may include participants of all functioning levels, or may characterize their sample as consisting of individuals with high-functioning autism (HFA) or low-functioning autism (LFA). Unfortunately, there are no set standards for what constitutes HFA or LFA. Most studies use a Standard Score cutoff of above 70 (or no more than two standard deviations below the mean) on either an IQ scale or subscale (Paul, Augustyn, Klin, & Volkmar, 2005; Rutherford, Baron-Cohen, & Wheelwright, 2002), although some use both a cognitive and a language measure (Diehl, Bennetto, Watson, Gunlogson, & McDonough, 2008; Diehl, Bennetto, & Young, 2006; Diehl, Watson, Bennetto, McDonough, & Gunlogson, 2009).

Second, there is some disagreement as to whether there are distinct subtypes, such as Asperger syndrome, or whether all individuals with the disorder are on the same continuum (Volkmar, Lord, Bailey, Schultz, & Klin, 2004). Although there are standard diagnostic subtypes (Autism, Asperger syndrome, Pervasive Developmental Disorder – Not Otherwise Specified, or PDD-NOS), research has shown that current definitions do not represent valid and reliable categorical distinctions (Howlin, 2003; Miller & Ozonoff, 2000). As such, some studies include all subtypes and refer to their sample as having autism spectrum disorders (ASDs); whereas others compare specific subtypes or examine only one subtype. The Asperger syndrome label is particularly problematic because there are as many as five different definitions outside of the DSM-IV that are used for research and clinical diagnosis (Volkmar et al., 2004).

Despite the heterogeneity of the population, the initial push in research has been to establish a profile of prosodic functioning in ASDs, both for production and comprehension. In production, studies that have examined profiles of functioning across different prosodic functions (e.g., communicating affect, structuring discourse, syntactic/grammatical structure) have produced some inconsistent results (Paul, Augustyn et al., 2005; Peppé, McCann, Gibbon, O'Hare, & Rutherford, 2007). Studies looking at specific functions in isolation have also produced conflicting findings (see McCann & Peppé, 2003, for review). Some new studies have begun to measure prosody production acoustically in order to examine an overall manner of speaking (e.g., over/under-exaggeration) in addition to the specific functions mentioned above. These studies have shown promise at isolating signature patterns (Diehl & Paul, 2008; Diehl, Watson et al., 2009; Hubbard & Trauner, 2007).

Still, probably the most important finding in prosody production studies are that all individuals with ASD seem to show impairment in at least one area (Peppé et al., 2007). This is true even though some individuals with ASD have deficits in a particular function or manner of prosodic use, while others have completely different deficits with a different function/manner. For example, Shriberg and colleagues (2001) observed that the percentage of individuals with ASD with impairments in a particular type of prosody (e.g., stress, phrasing) differed across types. Although our group has had consistent acoustic findings across samples (Diehl, Watson et al., 2009), the findings have never been consistent within a sample, meaning that acoustic analyses could differentiate a statistically significant portion, but not all, of participants with an ASD from typical controls. This heterogeneity in prosodic function is the most consistent finding across all studies in that studies have been able to make statistical, but not categorical, distinctions groups based on prosodic abilities.

There have been similar inconsistencies across studies examining prosody perception. One popular theory that has emerged from research is that children with ASD are impaired at processing emotions/mental states in the voice, and are not impaired at perceiving lexical or syntactic (often called grammatical) cues from prosody (e.g., as described in Paul, Augustyn et al., 2005, and others). There are several issues that directly question this theory. First, even in very well-designed, rigorous, and well-controlled studies that have produced replicable findings (e.g., Rutherford et al., 2002), there was considerable variance in performance in the ASD group. In these studies, not all participants could be differentiated from controls solely by their emotion/mental state processing abilities. Second, it is reasonable to claim that the emotion/mental state processing used in research (e.g., is this person surprised or sarcastic?) is not equitable in difficulty to the tasks used to measure grammatical prosody (e.g., emphasis of BLUE cow versus blue COW). Indeed, studies using psycholinguistic paradigms to investigate more difficult forms of grammatical prosody, such as that used to determine syntactic structure, have found group differences between ASDs and controls (Diehl et al., 2008; Diehl, Snedeker, & Paul, 2009). The same issue of task complexity applies to a more recent theory that children with ASDs have difficulty with sentence-level prosody (prosody that unfolds over the course of an utterance) and word-level prosody (Jarvinen-Pasley, Peppé, King-Smith, & Heaton, 2008). It is quite possible that individuals with ASD, particularly those in the age range popular for research studies of HFA (late childhood through adolescence) have achieved a certain level of prosodic competence, but have not yet attained more complex structures that are acquired at later developmental stages.

Two findings emerge from both the production and comprehension data. First, it is clear that individuals with ASDs perform much better in these experimental settings with predictable prosodic tasks (that are often too simple for the study participants) than they do when using prosody in the dynamic social world. Psycholinguistic paradigms are useful to some extent at closing this gap, because these paradigms often mimic real world situations in experimental settings (Trueswell & Tanenhaus, 2004; Watson, Gunlogson, & Tanenhaus, 2006). Second, although having a deficit in some facet of prosodic functioning is a characteristic of the disorder, it is unlikely that we will find any signature deficits in function or manner that cut across the entire spectrum of the population.

We propose a different research approach to understanding prosodic functioning in ASDs, one that takes advantage of the heterogeneity in the population, rather than being hindered by it. While prosodic heterogeneity (in both population and in symptomatology) is problematic for making group level generalizations and comparisons, it can be advantageous for early differential diagnosis, establishing categorical subtypes (if they exist), understanding divergent developmental trajectories, and finding reliable behavioral markers of underlying cognitive strengths and weaknesses. In the following sections, we re-examine the literature on prosodic functioning in autism from this perspective.

Prosody as a Diagnostic Bellwether of ASDs

The utility of prosody for the diagnosis and classification of ASDs will depend on several factors. First, do prosodic impairments align with other diagnostic impairments considered to be core deficits in ASDs? Second, do prosodic deficits cluster categorically in a way that could be useful for delineating subtypes? Third, do markers of early prosodic perception and production serve as valid, reliable, and early indicators of social deficits in ASDs? Additionally, do these behaviors provide clues to typical and atypical developmental trajectories for social communication?

Relationship of Prosody to Core Impairments in ASDs

Only a few studies have examined the relationship of prosodic impairments to other characteristic deficits of autism. One popular research design is to collect prosodic data, and then determine whether prosodic performance correlates with scores from a diagnostic instrument, such as the ADOS (Lord, Rutter, DiLavore, & Risi, 1999), which is a semi-structured play session, or the ADI-R (Rutter, Le Couteur, & Lord, 2003), which is a detailed parent interview. These instruments provide raw summary scores in the domains of social functioning, communicative functioning, and repetitive behaviors or stereotyped interests. Summary scores are collected from a number of items in each domain that can be scored on a scale of 0-2 (and sometimes 0-3). A score of zero generally means the absence of a behavior, a score of one means the behavior is present but not in a way that is consistent with an ASD, and a score of two or three represents the presence of behavior in a manner that is consistent with an ASD. Although using the ADOS and ADI as correlates of ASD behaviors has the benefit of using widely-known, gold standard diagnostic tools, children with ASDs regularly score within a restricted range on these measurements (by definition, because they need to meet diagnostic criteria). Therefore, the variability in these scores, which so often is linked to ASD severity in research, is statistically limited.

Despite these limitations, several studies have begun to link prosodic functioning, and prosody production in particular, to the domains of communication and socialization on diagnostic measures of ASDs. Paul and colleagues (Paul, Shriberg et al., 2005) used the Prosody-Voice Screening Profile to measure aspects of prosody production (Shriberg, Kwiatkowski, & Rasmussen, 1992) and found that the percentage of appropriate stress was negatively correlated with ADOS Communication. In other words, low levels of appropriate stress in individuals with HFA or Asperger syndrome were correlated with higher severity ratings on ADOS Communication. The study also found that children with a lower percentage of appropriate resonance were more likely to receive higher (meaning more impaired) ratings on the Socialization subscale of the Vineland Adaptive Behavior Scales (Sparrow, Balla, &

Cicchetti, 1984). Recently, our group used an acoustic analysis of intonation to measure prosody production in ASDs (Diehl, Watson et al., 2009). We found that individuals in our high-functioning ASD group were more likely than typically developing individuals matched on age, IQ, and language abilities to exhibit wider pitch ranges (as measured by standard deviation in fundamental frequency over the course of a narrative). Patterns of performance correlated with ADOS Communication scores in the ASD group. Put differently, children with ASD with more atypical pitch ranges tended to have behavior that was rated as more symptomatic of autism. Likewise, brain activity was linked to ADOS communication scores for children with ASD in a study that used prosody and context to generate ironic situations (Wang, Lee, Sigman, & Dapretto, 2006). It should be noted that a direct link between the observed brain activity/ADOS correlation and prosodic processing deficits was not explicitly made by the authors, who instead connected the finding to the ability to process mental states.

Few research studies have been able to conceptually relate the domain of stereotyped or repetitive behaviors to deficits the in language and communication functioning seen in ASDS, but prosody may provide the insight needed to make this link. For example, there is some initial evidence that, during communication, individuals with ASD show cognitive priming for the first type of prosody they hear in a conversational exchange, and may have trouble shifting interpretations as their interlocutor changes their intended meaning (Diehl, Snedeker et al., 2009). These findings are preliminary and the study did not include any neuropsychological measures of set-shifting or specific measures of restricted or repetitive behaviors. Still, this line of research is promising for linking deficits in these two separate domains.

In sum, only a limited number of studies have attempted to relate prosodic functioning to other core impairments in ASD, but these studies have repeatedly shown that the severity of prosodic impairments is related to the perception of severity of other deficits in language and communication as measured by standard diagnostic instruments. It should be noted that one study that looked at the integration of prosody and facial expressions (Magnée, de Gelder, van Engeland, & Kemner, 2007) did not find any correlation between integration abilities and ADOS/ADI or Vineland scores. Further research is needed to understand the extent of the relationship between prosody and ASD diagnosis, particularly whether the severity of prosody reflects true severity of the disorder or if it primarily influences the *perception* of deficit severity.

Prosody and Nosology

The idea that prosody could delineate subtypes of autism has received modest research interest. Specifically, it has been thought that individuals diagnosed with Asperger syndrome and verbal children with autism might exhibit different prosodic patterns. Fine and colleagues (1991) found that individuals with HFA were less likely to utilize "useful" intonation patterns (such as contrastive stress) than individuals with Asperger syndrome or outpatient controls, and were more likely to use stress patterns that did not convey additional information to the listener. Ghaziuddin and Gerstein (1996) used open-ended and semi-structured interviews to compare the prosodic patterns of the two groups. Individuals with Asperger syndrome were judged to have a more pedantic speech pattern (overly formal prosody, among other characteristics) than individuals with HFA. The authors noted the possibility that this behavior could supplement a parent's report of early language delay to make differential diagnoses, and could even supplant the need for retrospective, and therefore often imprecise, information. Similarly, a study by Paul and colleagues (2009) found that individuals with Asperger syndrome are more likely to exhibit inappropriately formal speech, and are also more likely to be rated as having unusual intonation. It has also been argued that individuals with Asperger syndrome might be better at understanding emotion in the voice than individuals with HFA (Mazefsky & Oswald, 2007), from which it follows that there would be differences in the production of affective prosody as well.

There are several problems with using prosodic performance to differentiate between Asperger syndrome and other ASDs. The studies reviewed here all used diagnostic criteria which have been shown to have little validity in distinguishing groups (Howlin, 2003; Miller & Ozonoff, 2000). Furthermore, qualitative descriptions, such as pedantic, formal, and unusual (among others), are subjective and therefore difficult to translate into formal acoustic criteria. We propose an alternative research method that uses prosodic behaviors to define subgroups rather than to validate existing criteria. Studies using this method should: 1) begin analyzing all individuals with ASDs as one group, 2) use acoustic properties to attempt to identify different prosodic production styles (or subgroups), and 3) identify other phenotypic traits that cluster with these subgroups.

Prosody as an Early Diagnostic Marker

Prosody has tremendous potential as an early diagnostic marker because it is one of the (if not *the*) earliest linguistic and social abilities to develop (Decasper & Fifer, 1980; Decasper & Spence, 1986; Kisilevsky et al., 2003; Moon et al., 1993), and because prosodic impairments appear to be present in individuals with ASD of all functioning levels and all developmental stages. It is feasible to think that a basic prosody processing deficit, or a more general sound or voice processing deficit (Dawson et al., 2004), could be an initial core deficit that launches individuals onto deviant linguistic/social developmental trajectories. It is more probable, however, that prosody serves as an alarm for early linguistic, social, and perhaps even cognitive deficits, because it is so intrinsically tied to all of these abilities at a very early stage.

There is some initial evidence that atypicalities in vocalizations and voice processing are a reliable indicator of ASDs very early in development. For perception, infants with ASD under the age of 1 were observed to orient to their name being called less frequently than infants who later showed mental retardation and typically developing infants during retrospective reviews of home videos (Osterling & Dawson, 1994; Osterling, Dawson, & Munson, 2002). Children with ASDs between the ages of three and five were more likely than typically developing children (one group matched on chronological age, the other on mental age) to prefer non-speech analogues over "motherese" type intonation patterns (Kuhl, Coffey-Corina, Padden, & Dawson, 2005).

For production, atypical prosody was one of nine items that was found to be useful in differentiating toddlers with ASDs from those with general developmental/language delays and those with typical development (Wetherby et al., 2004). Similarly, a second study found phonation (but not syllable production) to differentiate preverbal children with ASDs from children with general developmental disabilities (Sheinkopf, Mundy, Oller, & Steffens,

2000). Additionally, preliminary findings suggest that prosody production differences may be detectible acoustically through automatic acoustical analysis programs (Oller et al., 2009).

Even if early prosodic impairments are not found to be the core cause of the disorder, it would make sense that these deficits would be the first to emerge in a social-communication disorder such as autism. The studies reviewed here only begin to address the potential benefits of prosody perception and production in aiding early diagnosis. Currently, several research groups are studying the younger siblings of individuals with ASDs from birth in order to track the development of infants who are at a higher-risk for the development of an ASD. Because ASDs are not reliably diagnosed until after the first year of life, this approach is a more effective way of examining the broader autism phenotype from birth and tracking early markers and their relationship to typical and atypical developmental trajectories. When examining current research on the topic, it is apparent that social and linguistic abilities, particularly in prosody perception, appear at or before birth and have tremendous promise as useful early diagnostic markers.

Prosody as a Cognitive Bellwether of ASDs

Many of the cognitive deficits that are predicted to be a core deficit in ASDs are either communicated (in part), or can be exhibited through, prosodic behaviors. Cognitive theories of autism have been prominent in the past three decades of autism research (Volkmar et al., 2004). It has been suggested that individuals with autism have a core deficit in cognitive faculties such as Theory of Mind (Baron-Cohen, 1995), executive functioning (Pennington et al., 1997), central coherence (Happé, 1999), complex information processing (Minshew, Goldstein, & Siegel, 1997), and integration (Just, Cherkassky, Keller, Kana, & Minshew, 2007), among many others. Psycholinguistic studies have often used prosody to understand the relationship between language and cognition (Trueswell & Tanenhaus, 2004; Watson et al., 2006); therefore, it is understandable that prosody is one of the behaviors of choice for examining a putative core cognitive deficit in ASDs. A key feature of ASDs is that the profile of cognitive strengths and weaknesses can vary from individual to individual or between subgroups (Kuschner, Bennetto, & Yost, 2007; Ozonoff & Jensen, 1997; Volkmar et al., 2004). In this section, we review literature that uses prosody as a behavior to understand cognition. Then, we propose that prosody may be better suited as a bellwether of an individual's cognitive environment than as an indicator of a specific core deficit that would define groups of individuals on the spectrum.

Theory of Mind

One of the most extensively researched areas of prosodic functioning is the processing of mental states and intentions in the voice. These studies often use affective prosody processing as a proxy for Theory of Mind abilities. Theory of Mind is the ability to understand that others' thoughts, mental states, or intentions are different from one's own, and deficits in this area are thought to be a signature of ASDs (Baron-Cohen, 1995). Several studies have indicated deficits in processing affect in the voice (Kleinman, Marciano, & Ault, 2001;

Korpilahti et al., 2007; Rutherford et al., 2002). It has also been argued, though, that emotion/mental state processing differences disappear when groups are matched on language abilities (Hobson, Ouston, & Lee, 1988; Prior, Dahlstrom, & Squires, 1990; although see Rutherford et al., 2002). Data on the production of affect in the voice has been more equivocal (Hubbard & Trauner, 2007; Paul, Augustyn et al., 2005; Peppé et al., 2007), although this might be due to methodological limitations of measuring prosody in the voice.

It should be noted that not all individuals with ASDs exhibit impairment on Theory of Mind tasks, and those that do have deficits often exhibit a range of ability (Baron-Cohen, 1995). This is important because if it can be shown that processing affect or mental states in the voice is correlated with other Theory of Mind abilities, such as reading the mind in the eyes (Baron-Cohen, Wheelwright, Hill, Raste, & Plumb, 2001), then it could be inferred more directly that prosody processing can be an indicator of Theory of Mind abilities.

Executive Functioning

Another cognitive theory of ASDs involves a profile of strengths and weaknesses in executive functioning (Pennington et al., 1997). Two particular areas of difficulty for children with ASDs are planning and cognitive flexibility (Ozonoff & Jensen, 1997). Other than an early study linking pauses to cognitive load (Thurber & Tager-Flusberg, 1993), there has been scant evidence linking prosody processing to executive functioning. This is unfortunate because the pragmatics of conversation (turn-taking, formulating a response, interpreting context) all involve crucial cognitive functions such as planning, cognitive flexibility, and inhibition of a proponent response.

Two recent studies (Diehl et al., 2008; Diehl, Snedeker et al., 2009) presented individuals with high-functioning ASDs and typical controls with sentences with ambiguous semantic meanings, but with cues (prosodic or syntactic) to aid in sentence disambiguation. In both studies, individuals with ASD appeared to have difficulty switching interpretations between prosodic structures. For example, in Diehl, Snedeker, and Paul (2009), participants were presented four examples of one prosodic structure that indicated one behavior, and then halfway through the task the prosodic cue switched to indicate a different behavior. Individuals with ASD performed similarly to controls on the behavior elicited by the initial prosodic structure, but were not able to shift their interpretation when the prosodic cue changed. These two studies indicate that prosody processing in autism might be affected by executive functioning deficits.

Similar to Theory of Mind deficits, not all individuals with ASD show the same profile of executive functioning; therefore, prosody could be an indicator of an individual's neuropsychological strengths and weaknesses. To test this hypothesis, future research on prosody processing should attempt to link prosodic behaviors to measures of neuropsychological functioning that assess planning, cognitive flexibility, and inhibition of a preponent response. Second, prosody production behaviors, especially those related to aspects of pragmatic communication that are moderated through executive functioning (e.g., turn-taking), should also be studied for their relationship to measures of general executive functioning.

Intermodal Integration

Another area of impairment in ASDs for which prosody has been a key area of research is information integration. This theory is rooted in neuroimaging evidence that indicates under-connectivity between brain areas in individuals wit ASDs (Just et al., 2007). It has been argued that individuals with ASD have difficulty integrating information from different modalities, particularly between the auditory and visual domains (Silverman, 2007; Smith & Bennetto, 2007). Crucial to prosody processing and production are their integration with other aspects of speech, facial expressions, and gestures.

Individuals with ASDs have consistently shown deficits in the intermodal integration of faces and voices. In an early study of face-voice processing, it was found that individuals with autism had difficulty matching pictures of emotional faces to recordings of voices with the same emotion (Hobson et al., 1988). Later studies more complex methodologies to examine intermodal perception in ASDs (Haviland, Walker-Andrews, Huffman, Toci, & Alton, 1996; Loveland et al., 1995). Participants in these studies viewed a split screen of an individual talking, with each face displaying a different affect, and a listened to a prerecorded voice that expressed a type of affective prosody that matched one of the two faces. Children with ASDs were significantly worse at intermodal integration than controls with Down syndrome (Loveland et al., 1995) and typical development (Haviland et al., 1996). More recently, it was demonstrated that individuals with ASD have difficulty using faces to aid in the perception of a speaker when there is interfering background noise (Smith & Bennetto, 2007)

This line of research is especially important because prosody rarely occurs in isolation in areal world conversational exchange; instead, it is most often part of a complex and multimodal presentation. The series of studies described here argue persuasively for deficits in the intermodal integration of faces and voices. Still, future research should further address how well children with ASDs are able to utilize aspects of prosody, including visual prosody (e.g., head nodding with speech), in conjunction with other modalities of information in communication in addition to faces, such as gestures, posture, and context.

Prosody as an End-State Behavior for Cognition

Many of these studies, especially those related to Theory of Mind, show how prosody is assumed to be an indicator of internal cognitive abilities/disabilities. The over-arching theme in studies of ASDs, though, is that there is individual variation within the population in terms of the presence or severity of cognitive deficits. It is possible, then, that prosody could be better utilized as an indicator of an individual's specific cognitive strengths and weaknesses rather than as a tool for proving a hypothesis about a group of individuals with the disorder. For example, an individual with ASD who shows a limited range of affect in their voice, but uses prosody correctly as it relates to grammar, might have particular difficulty (as an individual) at processing emotion or understanding the mental states of others.

One argument against this proposal is that most research has shown that prosodic deficits in ASDs are not correlated with, and thus considered separate from, general cognitive functioning (Ghaziuddin & Gerstein, 1996; McCann, Peppé, Gibbon, O'Hare, & Rutherford, 2007; Paul, Augustyn et al., 2005; Sheinkopf et al., 2000) or general language functioning (Diehl et al., 2008; Rutherford et al., 2002). Nevertheless, a profile of strengths and weaknesses is a characteristic of ASDs, so correlating performance with a global measure of language and/or cognitive functioning might cancel out the relationship of prosody to specific cognitive functions within the global measure. Consequently, it will be important in future research to examine the relationship of prosodic performance to specific cognitive functions rather than summary scales.

In sum, prosody has been used as a marker for cognitive deficits in areas such as Theory of Mind and executive functioning, but it has also been argued that prosody functions separately from general language and cognitive abilities. A hallmark of an ASD, though, is that there are individual differences in the presence/absence of a cognitive deficit, its severity, and the overall profile of cognitive functioning. Accordingly, an important future direction of research will be to utilize prosody as an indicator of cognitive strengths and weaknesses in order to personalize treatment plans for the individual.

Treatment of Prosodic Deficits in Autism

There is a paucity of research on the assessment and treatment of prosodic deficits (Diehl & Paul, 2009), particularly in ASDs. This is striking, considering that prosody production deficits persist even as other areas of language improve (McCann & Peppé, 2003), and prosodic deficits remain a stigmatizing barrier to social acceptance for many otherwise high-functioning individuals with ASDs (Shriberg et al., 2001). Minimally, the prominence of deficits in this area of functioning should highlight the need for prosody to be a focus of treatment research and clinical intervention.

One promising area of intervention research is in the use of direct acoustic analysis and instant feedback for individual therapy (van Santen, Prud'hommeaux, & Black, in press). As we have shown, acoustic analysis of prosody production in ASDs has yielded differences that are missed by other areas of measurement (Diehl, Watson et al., 2009; Paul, Bianchi, Augustyn, Klin, & Volkmar, 2008). Preliminary results using this method have suggested that instant feedback is helpful, especially for young individuals with ASDs (Kim, Newland, Paul, Scassellati, & Diehl, 2008). This kind of treatment technique could be beneficial to all ages, and future studies should continue to explore the benefit of this approach for adolescents with ASD.

In this chapter, we have attempted to demonstrate the potential of using prosody to identify individual differences in cognitive functioning, and this could be particularly useful for intervention. If prosody is a behavioral measure of cognitive deficits that are otherwise obscure to gauge through observation, then prosody can be used during evaluation to identify these impairments, and individualized education plans and/or outpatient treatment plans can be structured to account for the child's individual profile of deficits. Furthermore, if prosodic deficits are an early diagnostic indicator of ASDs, and if early deficits can affect the trajectories of social-communicative development, then early intervention could have particularly powerful effects on an individual's progress in therapy.

Conclusion

Atypicalities in prosody production are a signature characteristic of ASDs, and only recently has there been a surge in interest in studying the nature of these deficits. Even though the presentation of prosodic production impairments is heterogeneous, their presence is ubiquitous. Studies on prosody processing and production have identified some patterns of impairment, but these impairments have not been able to adequately capture what is observed in clinical settings. One promising research methodology is the acoustic analysis of prosodic patterns because of its potential for instant and quantitative analysis in research and diagnosis and for instant feedback during treatment. Another useful approach is to adapt psycholinguistic paradigms, which are designed to mimic real world situations, are able to test the relationship between language and cognition, and often have already been validated on a normative sample.

In this chapter, we have argued that prosody is a behavioral bellwether of ASDs. It has potential for delineating subtypes of ASDs because of its relationship to many different functions that are impaired in the population. It shows promise as an early diagnostic indicator of the disorder because of prosody's crucial role in early social-communicative development. Additionally, different aspects of prosody are related to (or affected by) specific cognitive functions. Consequently, prosody could be useful as an indicator of individual differences in cognitive functioning.

In order for prosody to be useful as a behavioral bellwether of ASDs, there are several important research links that need to be made. Prosodic performance in infancy needs to be a major focus of research, especially as it relates to the utility of using early deviations in ability to predict later social-communicative functioning in this population. Moreover, prosodic deficits in ASD need to be linked to specific cognitive and neuropsychological functions in research. Most importantly, the assessment and treatment of prosodic impairments needs to become a bigger focus of research than it has been to date. Only when we have answered these research questions will we know the true value of prosody for understanding ASDs.

Author Note

Acknowledgments. This work was supported in part by an Alexander Brown and James Hudson Brown-Coxe Postdoctoral Fellowship through the Yale School of Medicine.

References

Amoroso, H. (1992). Disorders of vocal signaling in children. In H. Papousek, U. Jurgens, & M. Papousek, (Eds.), *Nonverbal Vocal Communication: Comparative and developmental approaches*, (pp. 192-204). Cambridge: Cambridge University Press.

Arnold, J. A., Bennetto, L. & Diehl, J. J. (2009). Reference production in young speakers with and without autism. *Cognition, 110*, 131-146.

Asperger, H. (1944). Die 'autistischen psychopathen' im kindesalter. *Archive fur Psychiatrie und Nervenkrankheiten, 117*, 76-136.

Association, A. P. (2000). *Diagnostic and statistical manual of mental disorders* (4th ed., text revision ed.). *Washington, D. C*, Author.

Baltaxe, C. A. M. (1984). Use of contrastive stress in normal, aphasic, and autistic children. *Journal of Speech and Hearing Research, 27*, 97-105.

Baron-Cohen, S. (1995). *Mind blindness. Cambridge*, MA: MIT Press.

Baron-Cohen, S., Wheelwright, S., Hill, J., Raste, Y. & Plumb, I. (2001). The Reading the Mind in the Eyes Test Revised Version: A study with normal adults, and adults with Asperger syndrome or high-functioning autism. *Journal of Child Psychology and Psychiatry and Allied Disciplines, 42*, 241-251.

Dawson, G., Toth, K., Abbott, R., Osterling, J., Munson, J., Estes, A., et al. (2004). Early social attention impairments in autism: Social orienting, joint attention, and attention to distress. *Developmental Psychology, 40*, 271-283.

Decasper, A. J. & Fifer, W. P. (1980). Of human bonding - newborns prefer their mothers' voices. *Science, 208*, 1174-1176.

Decasper, A. J. & Spence, M. J. (1986). Prenatal maternal speech influences newborns perception of speech sounds. *Infant Behavior and Development, 9*, 133-150.

Diehl, J. J., Bennetto, L., Watson, D., Gunlogson, C. & McDonough, J. (2008). Resolving ambiguity: A psycholinguistic approach to understanding prosody processing in high-functioning autism. *Brain and Language, 106*, 144-152.

Diehl, J. J., Bennetto, L. & Young, E. C. (2006). Story recall and narrative coherence of high-functioning children with autism spectrum disorders. *Journal of Abnormal Child Psychology, 34*, 87-102.

Diehl, J. J. & Paul, R. (2008). *Acoustic and perceptual measurements of prosody production errors on the PEPS-C by children with autism.* Paper presented at the International Meeting for Autism Research, *London*, UK.

Diehl, J. J. & Paul, R. (2009). The assessment of prosodic disorders and neurological theories of prosody. *International Journal of Speech-Language Pathology, 11, 287-292*.

Diehl, J. J., Snedeker, J. & Paul, R. (2009). *Eye-tracking as a measure of prosody processing in autism spectrum disorders.* Paper presented at the Biennial Meeting of the Society for Research in Child Development, Denver, CO.

Diehl, J. J., Watson, D., Bennetto, L., McDonough, J. & Gunlogson, C. (2009). An acoustic analysis of prosody in high-functioning autism. *Applied Psycholinguistics, 30*, 1-20.

Dodorico, L. & Franco, F. (1991). Selective production of vocalization types in different communication contexts. *Journal of Child Language, 18*, 475-499.

Fay, W. & Schuler, A. L. (1980). *Emerging language in autistic children.* Baltimore: *University Park Press*.

Fine, J., Bartolucci, G., Ginsberg, G. & Szatmari, P. (1991). The use of intonation to communicate in Pervasive Developmental Disorders. *Journal of Child Psychology and Psychiatry and Allied Disciplines, 32*(5), 771-782.

Frith, U. (1991). *Autism and Asperger Syndrome*. Cambridge: *Cambridge University Press*.

Ghaziuddin, M. & Gerstein, L. (1996). Pedantic speaking style differentiates Asperger syndrome from high-functioning autism. *Journal of Autism and Developmental Disorders, 26*, 585-595.

Goldfarb, W., Braunstein, P. & Lorge, I. (1956). A study of speech patterns in a group of schizophrenic children. *American Journal of Orthopsychiatry, 26*(544-555).

Grossmann, T., Striano, T. & Friederici, A. D. (2005). Infants' electric brain responses to emotional prosody. *Brain Imaging, 16*, 1825-1828.

Happé, F. (1999). Autism: Cognitive deficit or cognitive style? *Trends in Cognitive Sciences, 3*, 216-222.

Haviland, J. M., Walker-Andrews, A. S., Huffman, L. R., Toci, L. & Alton, K. (1996). Intermodal perception of emotional expressions by children with autism. *Journal of Developmental and Physical Disabilities, 8*, 77-88.

Hobson, R. P., Ouston, J. & Lee, A. (1988). Emotion recognition in autism - coordinating faces and voices. *Psychological Medicine, 18*, 911-923.

Howlin, P. (2003). Outcome in high-functioning adults with autism with and without early language delays: Implications for differentiation between autism and Asperger syndrome. *Journal of Autism and Developmental Disorders, 33*, 3-13.

Hubbard, K. & Trauner, D. A. (2007). Intonation and emotion in autistic spectrum disorders. *Journal of Psycholinguistic Research, 36*(2), 159-173.

Jarvinen-Pasley, A., Peppé, S., King-Smith, G. & Heaton, P. (2008). The relationship between form and function level receptive prosodic abilities in autism. *Journal of Autism and Developmental Disorders, 38*(7), 1328-1340.

Jusczyk, P. W. (2003). The role of speech perception capacities in early language acquisition. In M. B. M. Mack (Ed.), *Language: Multidisciplinary Perspectives*, (pp. 61-83). Mahwah, N. J. : Lawrence Erlbaum Associates.

Just, M. A., Cherkassky, V. L., Keller, T. A., Kana, R. K. & Minshew, N. J. (2007). Functional and anatomical cortical underconnectivity in autism: Evidence from an fMRI study of an executive function task and corpus callosum morphometry. *Cerebral Cortex, 17*, 951-961.

Kim, D., Newland, E., Paul, R., Scassellati, B. & Diehl, J. J. (2008). *A robotic therapist for affective prosody in high-functioning autistic children.* Paper presented at the International Meeting for Autism Research, *London*, U. K.

Kisilevsky, B. S., Hains, S. M. J., Lee, K., Xie, X., Huang, H., Ye, H. H., et al. (2003). Effects of experience on fetal voice recognition. *Psychological Science, 14*, 220-224.

Kleinman, J., Marciano, P. L. & Ault, R. L. (2001). Advanced theory of mind in high-functioning adults with autism. *Journal of Autism and Developmental Disorders, 31*, 29-36.

Korpilahti, P., Jansson-Verkasalo, E., Mattila, M. L., Kuusikko, S., Suominen, K. & Rytky, S., et al. (2007). Processing of affective speech prosody is impaired in Asperger syndrome. *Journal of Autism and Developmental Disorders, 37*(8), 1539-1549.

Kuhl, P. K., Coffey-Corina, S., Padden, D. & Dawson, G. (2005). Links between social and linguistic processing of speech in preschool children with autism: behavioral and electrophysiological measures. *Developmental Science, 8*, 1-12.

Kuschner, E. S., Bennetto, L. & Yost, K. (2007). Patterns of nonverbal cognitive functioning in young children with autism spectrum disorders. *Journal of Autism and Developmental Disorders, 37*, 795-807.

Lord, C., Rutter, M., DiLavore, P. C. & Risi, S. (1999). *Autism Diagnostic Observation Schedule. Los Angeles*, : Western Psychological Services.

Loveland, K. A., Tunali-Kotoski, B., Chen, R., Brelsford, K. A., Ortegon, J. & Pearson, D. A. (1995). Intermodal perception of affect in persons with autism or Down syndrome. *Development and Psychopathology, 7*, 409-418.

Magnée, M. J. C. M., de Gelder, B., van Engeland, H. & Kemner, C. (2007). Facial electromyographic responses to emotional information from faces and voices in individuals with pervasive developmental disorder. *Journal of Child Psychology and Psychiatry, 48(11)*, 1122-1130.

Mazefsky, C. A. & Oswald, D. P. (2007). Emotion perception in Asperger's syndrome and high-functioning autism: The importance of diagnostic criteria and cue intensity. *Journal of Autism and Developmental Disorders, 37*, 1086-1095.

McCann, J. & Peppé, S. (2003). Prosody in autism spectrum disorders: a critical review. *International Journal of Language & Communication Disorders, 38(4)*, 325-350.

McCann, J., Peppé, S., Gibbon, F. E., O'Hare, A. & Rutherford, M. (2007). Prosody and its relationship to language in school-aged children with high-functioning autism. *International Journal of Language & Communication Disorders, 42(6)*, 682-702.

Miller, J. N. & Ozonoff, S. (2000). The external validity of Asperger disorder: Lack of evidence from the domain of neuropsychology. *Journal of Abnormal Psychology, 109*, 227-238.

Minshew, J., Goldstein, G. & Siegel, D. (1997). Neuropsychologic functioning in autism: Profile of a complex informational processing disorder. *Journal of the International Neuropsychological Society, 3*, 303-316.

Moon, C., Cooper, R. P. & Fifer, W. P. (1993). Two-day olds prefer their native language. *Infant Behavior and Development, 16*, 495-500.

Nazzi, T., Nelson, D. G. K., Jusczyk, P. W. & Jusczyk, A. M. (2000). Six-month-olds' detection of clauses embedded in continuous speech: Effects of prosodic well-formedness. *Infancy, 1*, 123-147.

Oller, D. K., Gray, S. S., Richards, J. A., Gilkerson, J., Niyogi, P. & Warren, S. F. (2009). *Automated assessment of naturalistic recordings as a potential diagnostic tool for autism.* Paper presented at the Biennial Meeting of the Society for Research in Child Development, Denver, CO.

Osterling, J. & Dawson, G. (1994). Early recognition of children with autism: A study of first birthday home videotapes. *Journal of Autism and Developmental Disorders, 24*, 247-257.

Osterling, J., Dawson, G. & Munson, J. (2002). Early recognition of 1-year-old infants with autism spectrum disorder versus mental retardation. *Development and Psychopathology, 14*, 239-251.

Ozonoff, S. & Jensen, J. (1997). Brief report: Specific executive function profiles in three neurodevelopmental disorders. *Journal of Autism and Developmental Disorders, 29*, 171-177.

Paul, R., Augustyn, A., Klin, A. & Volkmar, F. R. (2005). Perception and production of prosody by speakers with autism spectrum disorders. *Journal of Autism and Developmental Disorders, 35(2)*, 205-220.

Paul, R., Bianchi, N., Augustyn, A., Klin, A. & Volkmar, F. R. (2008). Production of syllable stress in speakers with autism spectrum disorders. *Research in Autism Spectrum Disorders, 2(1)*, 110-124.

Paul, R., Orlovski, S. M., Marcinko, H. C., & Volkmar, F. (2009). Conversational Behaviors in Youth with High-functioning ASD and Asperger Syndrome. *Journal of Autism and Developmental Disorders, 39(1)*, 115-125.

Paul, R., Shriberg, L. D., McSweeny, J., Cicchetti, D., Klin, A. & Volkmar, F. (2005). Brief report: Relations between prosodic performance and communication and socialization ratings in high functioning speakers with autism spectrum disorders. *Journal of Autism and Developmental Disorders, 35(6)*, 861-869.

Pennington, B. F., Rogers, S. J., Bennetto, L., Griffith, E. M., Reed, D. T. & Shyu, V. (1997). Validity test of the executive dysfunction hypothesis of autism. In J. Russell (Ed.), *Autism as an executive disorder*, (pp. 143-178). Oxford: Oxford University Press.

Peppé, S., McCann, J., Gibbon, F., O'Hare, A. & Rutherford, M. (2007). Receptive and expressive prosodic ability in children with high-functioning autism. *Journal of Speech Language and Hearing Research, 50*, 1015-1028.

Prior, M., Dahlstrom, B. & Squires, T. L. (1990). Autistic children's knowledge of thinking and feeling states in other people. *Journal of Child Psychology and Psychiatry and Allied Disciplines, 31*, 587-601.

Provonost, W., Wakstein, M. & Wakstein, D. (1966). A longitudinal study of speech behaviors and language comprehension in fourteen children diagnosed as atypical or autistic. *Exceptional Children, 33*, 19-26.

Rutherford, M. D., Baron-Cohen, S. & Wheelwright, S. (2002). Reading the mind in the voice: A study with normal adults and adults with Asperger syndrome and high functioning autism. *Journal of Autism and Developmental Disorders, 32*, 189-194.

Rutter, M., Le Couteur, A. & Lord, C. (2003). *Autism Diagnostic Interview-Revised.* Los Angeles: *Western Psychological Services.*

Sheinkopf, S. J., Mundy, P., Oller, D. K. & Steffens, M. (2000). Vocal atypicalities of preverbal autistic children. *Journal of Autism and Developmental Disorders, 30*, 345-354.

Shriberg, L. D., Kwiatkowski, J. & Rasmussen, C. (1992). *The Prosody-Voice Screening Profile (PVSP). Tucson*, AZ: Communication Skill Builders.

Shriberg, L. D., Paul, R., McSweeny, J. L., Klin, A., Cohen, D. J. & Volkmar, F. R. (2001). Speech and prosody characteristics of adolescents and adults with high-functioning autism and Asperger Syndrome. *Journal of Speech Language and Hearing Research, 44(5)*, 1097-1115.

Silverman, L. B. (2007). *Gesture comprehension in high-functioning autism. University of Rochester*, Rochester, NY.

Smith, E. G. & Bennetto, L. (2007). Audiovisual speech integration and lipreading in autism. *Journal of Child Psychology and Psychiatry, 48*, 813-821.

Snow, D. (2006). Regression and reorganization of intonation between 6 and 23 months. *Child Development, 77*, 281-296.

Snow, D. & Balog, H. L. (2002). Do children produce the melody before the words? A review of developmental intonation research. *Lingua, 112*, 1025-1058.

Sparrow, S., Balla, D. & Cicchetti, D. (1984). *Vineland Adaptive Behavior Scales. Circle Pines*, MN: American Guidance Service.

Tager-Flusberg, H., Paul, R. & Lord, C. (2005). Language and communication in autism. In Volkmar, F. R., Paul, R., Klin, A. & Cohen, D. J., (Eds.), *Handbook of Autism and Pervasive Developmental Disorders: Assessment, interventions, and policy.* (2nd ed., pp. 335-364). *New York*, NY: John Wiley and Sons.

Thurber, C. & Tager-Flusberg, H. (1993). Pauses in the narratives produced by autistic, mentally-retarded, and normal children as an index of cognitive demand. *Journal of Autism and Developmental Disorders, 23*, 309-322.

Trueswell, J. & Tanenhaus, M. K. (2004). *Approaches to processing world-situated language: Bridging the product and action traditions. Cambridge*, MA: MIT Press.

Tsao, F. M., Liu, H. M. & Kuhl, P. K. (2004). Speech perception in infancy predicts language development in the second year of life: A longitudinal study. *Child Development, 75*, 1067-1084.

van Santen, J. P., Prud'hommeaux, E. T. & Black, L. M. (in press). Automated assessment of prosody production. *Speech Communication.*

Volkmar, F., Lord, C., Bailey, A., Schultz, R. T. & Klin, A. (2004). Autism and pervasive developmental disorders. *Journal of Child Psychology and Psychiatry, 45*, 135-170.

Wang, A. T., Lee, S. S., Sigman, M. & Dapretto, M. (2006). Neural basis of irony comprehension in children with autism: the role of prosody and context. *Brain, 129*, 932-943.

Watson, D. G., Gunlogson, C. A. & Tanenhaus, M. K. (2006). *Online methods for the investigation of prosody. New York*, : Walter de Gruyter.

Werker, J. F. (2005). *Understanding how infant speech perception sets the stage for language acquisition.* Paper presented at the Biennial meeting of the Society for Research in Child Development, *Atlanta*, GA.

Wetherby, A. M., Woods, J., Allen, L., Cleary, J., Dickinson, H. & Lord, C. (2004). Early indicators of autism spectrum disorders in the second year of life. *Journal of Autism and Developmental Disorders, 34*, 473-493.

Wing, L. (1981). Asperger's syndrome - A clinical account. *Psychological Medicine, 11*, 115-129.

Young, E. C., Diehl, J. J., Morris, D., Hyman, S. L. & Bennetto, L. (2005). The use of two language tests to distinguish pragmatic language problems in children with autism spectrum disorders. *Language, Speech, and Hearing Services in Schools, 36*, 62-72.

In: Speech Disorders: Causes, Treatment and Social Effects ISBN: 978-1-60876-213-2
Editor: Alan E. Harrison, pp. 177-196

Chapter 8

The Multi Dimensional Voice Program (MDVP) in Conjunction with Other Tests in the Evaluation of Speech and Voice Disorders: Our Experience

A. Salami, R. Mora, B. Crippa, M. Dellepiane, L. Guastini and B. Jankowska
ENT Department, University of Genoa, Italy

Abstract

The Multi Dimensional Voice Program (MDVP) is a powerful software tool for quantitative acoustic assessment of voice quality; it is capable of calculating 33 parameters and provides flexible routines for graphical representation of the results.

Also a user-upgradeable voice database allows automatic comparison of the current results with different nosological groups. In our experience fundamental frequency (Fo), Jitter percent, Shimmer, noise to harmonics ratio (NHR), voice turbulence index (VTI), soft phonation index (SPI), degree of voiceless (DUV), degree of voice breaks (DVB) and peak amplitude variation (vAm) are the parameters which give the most objective information about the presence of vocal modification. A multiple regression analysis of these nine acoustic measures may provide a quick and relatively sensitive method that may be clinically useful in measuring change of vocal quality and articulation. These data provide a more complete analysis in conjunction with other tests: the mirror-fogging test from Glatzel and the Gutzmann test (for testing nasality); the voice handicap index (a validated questionnaire measuring psychosocial handicapping effects of voice disorders); Van Borsel's study (to evaluate articulation).

We have applied this protocol in the analysis of speech and voice before and one month after different surgical techniques (tonsillectomy, adenotonsillectomy, uvulopalatoplasty, septoplasty, microlaryngoscopy, etc).

Our protocol of voice and speech analysis provide objective, documentable and measurable data of vocal function, and these measurements are clinically helpful for the comparison of the patients' voice with those of healthy speakers. These measures maybe very useful to evaluate the patient affected by pathology and to provide a more secure diagnosis. For these reasons, otorhinolaryngologist should evaluate patients also using the MDVP, in conjunction with other test, at the beginning of their "diagnostic challenge".

INTRODUCTION

Human voice consists of sound made by a human being using the vocal folds for talking, singing, laughing, crying, screaming, etc. Human voice is specifically that part of human sound production in which the vocal folds (vocal cords) are the primary noise source [1].

The sound of each individual's voice is entirely unique not only because of the actual shape and size of an individual's vocal cords (difference in vocal folds size between men and women means that they have differently pitched voices), but also due to the size and shape of the rest of that person's body [2].

Humans have vocal folds which can loosen, tighten, or change their thickness, and over which breath can be transferred at varying pressures. The shape of chest and neck, the position of the tongue, and the tightness of otherwise unrelated muscles can be altered. Any one of these actions results in a change in pitch, volume, timbre, or tone of the sound produced. Sound also resonates within different parts of the body, and an individual's size and bone structure can affect the sound produced by an individual [2].

Human speech involves not only species-specific anatomy. Speech also requires a brain that can "reiterate"—freely reorder a set of motor gestures to form a potentially infinite number of words and sentences [3].

The end points of the evolutionary process are clear: the chimpanzee lacks a supralaryngeal vocal tract capable of producing the "quantal" sounds which facilitate both speech production and perception and a brain that can reiterate the phonetic contrasts apparent in its fixed vocalizations [3].

The human voice is the most complex sound with which we routinely deal, and human speech is arguably unparalleled in nature. Nonetheless, our brains seem to effortlessly pull information from the speech stream, extracting the meaning of what we hear as well as information about the speaker, such as their mood and identity.

The voice and speech production can be subdivided into four parts: the lungs, the vocal folds, the articulators and the brain. The lung (the pump) must produce adequate airflow to vibrate vocal folds (air is the fuel of the voice). The vocal folds (vocal cords) are the vibrators, neuromuscular units that 'fine tune' pitch and tone. The articulators (vocal tract consisting of tongue, palate, cheek, lips, etc.) articulate and filter the sound [4]. The vocal folds, in combination with the articulators, are capable of producing highly intricate arrays of sound. The tone of voice may be modulated to suggest emotions such as anger, surprise, or happiness. Singers use the human voice as an instrument for creating music.

Traditionally, the left frontal and parietal lobes have been associated with language production while regions in the temporal lobe are seen as crucial for language comprehension. However, recent evidence suggests that the classical language areas constitute an integrated network where each area plays a crucial role both in speech production and perception [4].

Many voice disorders remain unidentified. Often, voice complaints are dismissed as "par for the course" for a cold, flu, or an allergy. Other times, voice complaints are not considered to be part of a voice disorder – especially if the complaints have been present for a long time or most of the patient's life.

A voice is termed "disordered" when the vocal quality of an individual is altered/changed in such a way that it is thought to be abnormal to the listener [5]. The onset and development of these disorders can be "sudden" or "slow." Examples of characteristics of sudden onset may be: trauma, infection, injurious inhalation, intubation, conversion reaction, or a severe allergic reaction [6]. Degenerative neurologic disease, musculo-skeletal tension, vocal abuse and misuse, growths of folds, gastro-esophageal reflux, and chronic allergies may characterize slow onset [6].

All disorders do not have known etiologies, and some may occur as a result of numerous etiologies. Very few disorders are attributed to one known cause.

There are many disorders which affect the human voice: when vocal injury is done, often an *otorhinolaryngologist* may be able to help, but the best treatment is the prevention of injuries through good vocal production [7].

The proposal of this chapter is an attempt to reach better agreement and uniformity concerning the methodology for functional assessment of pathologic voice and speech.

The purpose is to allow relevant comparisons with the literature when presenting/publishing the results of voice treatment, e.g. a phonosurgical technique,or a new/improved instrument or procedure for investigating the pathological voice and speech.

Meta-analyses of the results of voice treatments are generally limited and may even be impossible owing to the major diversity in the ways functional outcomes are assessed.

A multidimensional set of minimal basic measurements suitable for all "common" dysphonias is proposed. It includes different approaches: endoscopic assessment using nasolaryngofibroscopy, videostroboscopy (closure, regularity, mucosal wave and symmetry), acoustics analysis (fundamental frequency, Jitter percent, Shimmer, noise to harmonics ratio, voice turbulence index, soft phonation index, degree of voiceless, degree of voice breaks and peak amplitude variation), **speech analysis** (fundamental frequency), **nasality tests** (mirror-fogging test from Glatzel and the Gutzmann test), **evaluation of articulation** (Van Borsel's study), and **subjective rating by the patient** (voice handicap index).

The protocol is elaborated on the basis of an exhaustive review of the literature, of the experience of the ENT Department of the University of Genoa (Italy), Chairman Prof. A. Salami, and of the Specialization School in "Audiology and Phoniatry" of the University of Genoa (Italy), Chairman Prof. B. Jankowska.

Speech and Voice Production

In order to understand the nature of the speech and voice disorders it is necessary to first describe normal speech production.

The basis of voice production is controlled exhalation of air from the lungs which causes the vocal fold to vibrate and produce sound. The air stream is shaped into specific speech sound by the articulators. The tongue and the lips are the most evident articulators but also the soft palate plays an important role. In typical speech production the soft palate is lifted for a large part of the speaking time to close the opening between the oral and nasal cavities. A high intra-oral pressure is necessary to produce many of the speech sounds, which is achieved with lifted soft palate which forces the air stream exhaled from the lungs to take the route through the mouth only. When the soft palate (the velum) is lifted the walls of the pharynx move towards the soft palate, i.e. to achieve a compete closure. Velopharyngeal function is thus very important to speech.

We speak at a rate of 12-14 speech sounds each second which means that many small but swift movements are combined into complex movement patters every time an individual speaks. For each speech sound the articulators have to be changed according to place and manner of articulation for that particular sound.

If the movement of the velum and/or the pharyngeal walls is not sufficient for closure for a velopharyngeal impairment is evident which can result in hypernasal speech, audible nasal air emission/nasal turbulence, and weak pressure consonants.

Hypernasality is evident when the voice is characterized by excessive nasal resonance; the reason is that the velopharyngeal port is not closed during production of oral speech sounds and the sound resonates in both the oral and nasal cavities (other conditions, as enlarged tonsils, may cause hypernasality).

Hyponasality occurs when there is reduced nasal resonance, such as the sound of a blocked nose associated with a nasal congestion due to a common cold. Besides a cold, hyponasality may be due to an anatomical condition such as a deviation of nasal septum, etc.

PROTOCOL

The protocol, elaborated on the basis of an exhaustive review of the literature and on the clinical experience, is characterized by the following tests:

Mirror-Fogging Test

In the mirror-fogging test, the nasalization is assessed by evaluating the degree of condensation (0: no condensation; 4: severe condensation) on a cold mirror held 0.5 cm under the nose during phonation (subjects are asked to sustain the vowels “a” and “i” and the consonant “m”) [8,9].

Gutzmann Test

In the Gutzmann test, subjects are asked to produce a series of “a” and “i” sounds alternately with the nares held open and closed (a change in vowel quality when the subject produced the vowels with the nares closed is indicative of hypernasality, in which case a score of 1 was assigned; absence of change is assigned a score of 0) [8,9].

Voice Handicap Index

Before and 1 month after surgery, the voice handicap index (VHI) was performed. The VHI is a validated questionnaire measuring psychosocial handicapping effects of voice disorders (translated and validated in Italian) [10].

The VHI consists of 30 statements on voice-related aspects in daily life, with 5 response levels, scored 0–4 (0: good; 4: very bad). Summarizing the scores on the 30 statements leads to a total VHI score, ranging from 0 to 120. A higher score corresponds to a worse voice-related functional status [11].

Test of Van Borsel

To evaluate articulation, the speech samples were elicited by means of the picture-naming test, described in Van Borsel's study, before and 1 month after surgery [12].

This test requires subjects to name black-and-white drawings of common objects and actions and elicit a speech sample containing instance of all Italian simple speech sounds and most clusters in all possible syllable combinations.

The speech sample gathered consisted of 120 different words from which consonant production are compared with target productions and analyzed for errors at the segmental level.

Multidimensional Voice Program (MDVP)

Phonetically balanced sentences and sustained vowels "a", "e", "i" are carried out and digitalized with MDVP (Kay Elemetrics). Recordings are made in a quiet room using a microphone at a constant mouth-to-microphone distance (10 cm). The vocal samples have intensity between 55 and 65 dB and duration of at least 5 seconds. The oronasal sentences correspond to the English ''Rainbow'' passage, the oral sentences are similar to the ''Zoo'' passage, and the ratio of nasal consonants to the total number of consonants in the nasal text is 50.4% (55/109) [8].

The sentences were done by a certified speech pathologist (M.G.S.). *The specific sentences are presented in the Appendix.*

Patients are asked to repeat the same passages sentence by sentence. The MDVP system computes a set of 33 acoustic voice parameters in about 16 seconds and provides flexible routines for graphical representation of the results. Also, a user-upgradeable voice database allows automatic comparison of the current results with different nosological groups.

The following parameters are estimated: fundamental frequency (Fo); Jitter percent (Jitter); Shimmer; noise-to-harmonics ratio (NHR); voice turbulence index (VTI); soft phonation index (SPI); degree of voiceless (DUV); degree of voice breaks (DVB), and peak amplitude variation (vAm).

Fundamental frequency (Fo) is indicative of the vocal fold vibratory rate and reflects resonance characteristics, of the supralaryngeal vocal tract, related to tongue articulation and placement.

Jitter and Shimmer reflect the grade of hoarseness and roughness of the speech spectrum.

NHR measures the aperiodic noise present in the analyzed signal, while VTI is the ratio of spectral inharmonic energy to spectral harmonic energy.

SPI is the vocal fold adductory force; DUV measures the nonharmonics area, while DVB is the ratio of the total length of areas representing voice breaks to the time of the complete voiced sample.

vAm is the standard deviation of the period to period calculated peak to peak amplitude.

Perturbation measures (Jitter, Shimmer, NHR, VTI, SPI, DUV, DVB, and vAm) are obtained from the sustained vowels, whereas Fo is extracted from both balanced sentences and sustained vowels.

PERSONAL EXPERIENCES

We have applied our protocol in the analysis of speech and voice before and one month after different surgical techniques (tonsillectomy, adenotonsillectomy, uvulopalatoplasty, septoplasty, microlaryngoscopy, etc).

In our experience Fo, Jitter, Shimmer, NHR, VTI, SPI, DUV, DVB and vAm are the acoustic parameters which give the most objective information about the presence of vocal modification; ***a multiple regression analysis of these nine acoustic measures may provide a quick and relatively sensitive method that may be clinically useful in measuring change of vocal quality***.

These data provide a more complete analysis in conjunction with other tests: the mirror-fogging test from Glatzel and the Gutzmann test (for testing nasality); the voice handicap index (a validated questionnaire measuring psychosocial handicapping effects of voice disorders); Van Borsel's study (to evaluate articulation).

All the patients before and one month after surgery underwent all the previously tests. All the data, presented in this chapter, are related to adults male patients.

Statistical analysis was performed using t-test: probability values at less than 0.05 were regarded as significant; the results were reviewed and approved by the Institutional Review Board of the University of Genoa, Italy.

1. TONSILLECTOMY

There has been little interest in the role of tonsils in speech and voice, although the negative impact of enlarged tonsils vocal communication and nasooral resonance is well recognized. Enlarged tonsils with posterior placement of the upper poles into the oropharyngeal and nasopharyngeal airway, interposed between the velum and posterior pharyngeal wall, have been shown to cause hypernasal speech with incomplete velopharyngeal closure.

Unfortunately, otolarynologists who have no formal training in speech or resonance disorders may be not be able to qualitative analyze different speech characteristics in patients with enlarged tonsils: therefore they primarily use endoscopy for diagnosis.

Table 1.Mathematical mean (with normal ranges in parentheses) of the preoperative (A) and postoperative (B) vocal parameters (minimal, maximum and mean) in adults (males) underwent tonsillectomy: average of fundamental frequency (Fo), Jitter percent (Jitt), Shimmer, noise to harmonics ratio (NHR), voice turbulence index (VTI), soft phonation index (SPI), degree of voiceless (DUV), degree of voice breaks (DVB) and peak amplitude variation (vAm). P<0.05 represents the significant statistical analysis by comparing mean values of each preoperative and postoperative parameters.

		Fo (Hz)	JITTER (%)	SHIMMER (%)	NHR	VTI	SPI	DUV (%)	DVB (%)	vAm (%)
Minimal value	A	127 (104)	0,28 (0,39)	1,61 (1,79)	0,08 (0,12)	0,01 (0,02)	1,02 (4.16)	0 (0)	0 (0)	14,02 (4,34)
	B	92 (104)	0,10 (0,39)	1,32 (1,79)	0,05 (0,12)	0 (0,02)	1,75 (4.16)	0 (0)	0 (0)	5,02 (4,34)
Maximum value	A	188 (158)	2,97 (1,31)	8,87 (4,12)	0,64 (0,17)	0,88 (0,07)	44,88 (20,43)	2,69 (0)	3,82 (0)	44,18 (21,61)
	B	160 (158)	1,24 (1,31)	4,98 (4,12)	0,29 (0,17)	0,24 (0,07)	21,96 (20,43)	0 (0)	0 (0)	19,31 (21,61)
Mean value	A	133 (118)	1,75 (0,83)	5,77 (2,49)	0,40 (0,14)	0,38 (0,04)	22,05 (14,47)	0,41 (0)	0,44 (0)	24,11 (9,01)
	B	121 (118)	0,84 (0,83)	3,34 (2,49)	0,16 (0,14)	0,05 (0,04)	14,46 (14,47)	0 (0)	0 (0)	8,77 (9,01)
		P<0.05	P<0.05	P<0.05	P<0.05	P<0.05	P<0.05	P<0.05	P<0.05	P<0.05

Although tonsillectomy is therapeutic for chronic tonsillitis, this procedure has the potential to affect speech and vocal quality by altering the resonant characteristics of vocal tract and speech articulation. Until now, the effects of tonsillectomy on speech has been unclear, as has the appropriate choice of speech analysis methods. There are several quantitative studies on the effects of tonsillectomy on speech, but these studies mainly concentrate on the fundamental frequency, with contrasting results.

Our data showed an improvement in all tested parameters one month after tonsillectomy: the analysis of Fo, Jitter, Shimmer, NHR, VTI, SPI, DUV, DVB and vAm showed a significant postoperative ($P<0.05$) decrease; comparison with healthy adults highlighted a significant ($P<0.05$) postoperative normalization of Fo, Jitter, NHR, VTI, DUV, DVB and vAm. (Table 1)

Fo data showed a postoperative normalization in both the speech and vocal samples: in the speech samples the postoperative mean value fell from 131 Hz to 120 Hz, while in the healthy adults the mean value is 116 Hz.

Subjective decrease of hypernasality was noted in all the patients at their postoperative clinical controls (1 month after tonsillectomy): the mirror-fogging test presented a postoperative mean assessment of 1.5 (decreased from the preoperative mean value of 2.8), the Gutzmann test values fell from 1 before the treatment to 0 after it. VHI had a postoperative mean value of 22 (decreased from the preoperative mean value of 68). The results of the phonetic analysis showed that all the patients were capable of producing all Italian vowels and consonants pre and postoperatively. Before surgery, the phonetic analysis comparing consonant productions to target productions at the segmental level revealed difficulties in the articulation of several consonants: data are presented in table 2.

Since the normal resonance of speech relies on an unobstructed nasopharyngeal passage, any barrier, such as hypertrophied tonsils, causes change in resonance and thus speech quality. Very little has been published with regard to the role that tonsils play in either normal or disordered speech; although some authors report that hypertrophic tonsils could alter oropharyngeal resonance characteristics.

In our patients, enlarged tonsils were found to be in the nasopharynx and interposed between the velum and posterior pharyngeal wall. These large masses are known to obstruct sound transmission into both the oral and nasal cavities, causing an increase in nasal resonance: in several patients, speech became hypernasal when the tonsils became hypertrophic [13].

Hypertrophic tonsils in the oropharynx that extend upward into the nasopharynx cause velopharyngeal insufficiency, impending full palatal movement [13].

Many otolaryngologists and speech pathologists believe that tonsils and adenoids should never be removed in patients with hypernasal speech as adenotonsillectomy in patients with pre-existing velopharyngeal insufficiency is often observed to exacerbate hypernasality [14]. Our experience shows that this concern is unfounded, thus hypernasal speech is indeed not a contraindication for tonsillectomy.

With the understanding that closure of the nasopharynx is velar-adenoidal, tonsillectomy would not be expected to cause hypernasality, a hypothesis confirmed by our data.

Patients with hypernasality are often referred for pharyngeal flap surgery, a risky procedure which in patients with tonsillar hypertrophy can be fatal (obstructive sleep apnea is a well-recognized complication of pharyngeal flap surgery) [15]. Enlarged tonsils can result in an anterior tongue base position and a long soft palate. Furthermore, when the tonsils prolapse posteriorly during speech, they prevent the palate from fully approximating the posterior pharyngeal wall [16,17]. **For these reasons, our data indicate that tonsillectomy should be recommended prior to the more dangerous pharyngeal flap surgery**.

Fo showed significant change postoperatively, both in the vocal and speech samples: this observation indicates that tonsillectomy, although a procedure that doesn't affect the larynx, changes the structure of the vocal tract and thus the resonance of speech production (lowering the pitch of the voice often decreases the resonance and consequently can decrease the nasal resonance values), and is thus a surgery capable of improving speech quality [18].

The postoperative normalization and improvement of Jitter and Shimmer highlight improvement of the vocal quality, with the absence of a slight grade of hoarseness and roughness in the voices [19].

The postoperative normalization of Fo, Jitter, Shimmer and vAm show the regularization of loudness. Although sound originates at the laryngeal level, there are significant alterations and enhancement of the vocal output as a result of the transfer function in the supraglottic cavities. Large tonsillar tissue has a damping effect during the transfer function, causing a reduction in quality and precision of the output. These damping effects influence noise: NHR measures the aperiodic noise present in the analyzed signal, while VTI is the ratio of spectral inharmonic energy to spectral harmonic energy [20].

In patients with enlarged tonsils, the tonsillar tissue may cause important turbulent air passage, through the vocal resonator, and produces an augmentation of vocal tract inertance and resistance that can interfere with a speaker's ability to produce a regular voice. The augmentation of inertance causes skewing of the glottal flow, while a higher resistance produces a non linear pressure-flow relation in the glottis, resulting from air leakage through the glottis during phonation, caused by an incomplete closure of the glottis [21]. NHR and VTI postoperative normalization represents an altered dynamic in the structures of the resonator which implies postoperative changes of vocal tract structures and a greater acoustical quality of the voice, with less nasalized vowels.

The postoperative values of Jitter, VTI, SPI, DUV, and DVB highlight the regularization of the supraglottic flow with the reduction of vocal tract inertance and resistance, with resulting in less laryngeal adductory force necessary for phonation [22]. (Table 1)

Studies regarding articulation and deglutition suggest risk of articulation difficulties (more or less temporary) in patients with enlarged tonsils. When the tonsils occupy the pharyngeal airway, to maximize the oral airway, dropping of the mandible and tongue is frequently seen in patients as a compensatory mechanism. It is known that hypertrophied tonsils may alter facial growth by contributing to tongue and mandibular displacement. Patients with enlarged tonsils have a retroclined lower incisiors, protruded upper incisions and a shorter lower dental arch; furthermore they have retrognathic, posteriorly inclined mandibles, an anterior tongue base position, enlarged anterior facial height and enlarged skeletal open bite [23].

When enlarged tonsils alter the dimensions of the pharyngeal orifice and interfere with sound transmission, should be removed as first surgical option.

The postoperative normalization of nasalance highlights the absence of nasal air escape during speech, and the important role of enlarged tonsil in velopharyngeal closure. For all these reasons an objective speech analysis in all patients affected by tonsillar hypertrophy should be performed.

2. Uvulopalatopharyngolplasty

The surgical techniques used for snoring and obstructive sleep apnea syndrome (OSAS) treatment include partial/complete resection or tissue reduction of the oropharyngeal structures such as uvula, palatine tonsil, soft palate, lateral pharyngeal tissue and tongue base [24]. So it is predictable for these techniques to affect speech and vocal quality by altering the resonant characteristics of vocal tract and speech articulation [8].

We report changes in acoustic feature of speech and voice after UPPP in adults, with the Ultracision Harmonic Scalpel® (Ethicon Endo-Surgery, Cincinnati, U.S.A.). The HS is an ultrasonic cutting and coagulating surgical device. The equipment consists of a generator, an hand-piece, and specific inserts. *Among the available hand-pieces and inserts, a specific hand-piece and insert was preferred (*shaped like scissor) [25].

Table 2. Articulation outcome (%) before (T 1) and one month after tonsillectomy (T 2), in 40 adult male patients.

	Articulation outcome (%) T 1	Comments	Articulation outcome (%) T 2
/r/	85.0 (34/40) deviations 65.0 (26/40) derhotacized /r/ 15.0 (6/40) dentalized /r/ 12.5 (5/40) devoiced /r/	Production of a rolled sound without sufficient trill Production of the /r/ with the tongue tip between the incisors	100 normal (40/40)
/s/	47.5 (19/40) deviations 35.0 (14/40) sigmatismus simplex 15.0 (6/40) sigmatismus dentalis	Production of the /s/ sound without sufficient frication Production of the /s/ with the tongue tip between the incisors	100 normal (40/40)
/f/ /v/	12.5 (5/40) bilabial production		100 normal (40/40)
/l/ /d/ /n /t/	42.5 (17/40) dentalisation	Production of several alveolar sounds with the tongue tip between the incisor	100 normal (40/40)
/sch/	40.0 (16/40) articulation without sufficient frication		100 normal (40/40)
Devoicing	15.0 (6/40) devoicing of /b/ 42.5 (17/40) devoicing of /d/ 37.5 (15/40) devoicing of /g/ 35.0 (14/40)devoicing of /z/		100 normal (40/40)

The HS was used in all the surgical step: after tonsillectomy, two incisions, each of the same length, were made on each side of the lateral margin of the uvula, at the level of the posterior edge of the soft palate, with upward direction into the soft palate, to retract the tissue and diminish the thickness of the soft palate, according to the characteristics of the soft palate. After, an excision of the redundant mucosa of each posterior arch and subsequent creation of neouvula by a partial uvulectomy was done.

The patients enrolled presented a Friedman tongue position grade I, tonsil size 2-3, a body mass index <40 (kg/m^2) and apnea-hypopnea index >15 [26].

Table 3. Mathematical mean (with normal ranges in parentheses) of the preoperative (A) and postoperative (B) vocal parameters (minimal, maximum and mean) in adults (males) underwent uvulopalatopharyngoplasty: average of fundamental frequency (Fo), Jitter percent (Jitt), Shimmer, noise to harmonics ratio (NHR), voice turbulence index (VTI), soft phonation index (SPI), degree of voiceless (DUV), degree of voice breaks (DVB) and peak amplitude variation (vAm). P<0.05 represents the significant statistical analysis by comparing mean values of each preoperative and postoperative parameters.

		Fo (Hz)	JITTER (%)	SHIMMER (%)	NHR	VTI	SPI	DUV (%)	DVB (%)	vAm (%)
Minimal value	A	92 (104)	0,38 (0,39)	1,81 (1,79)	0,22 (0,12)	0,01 (0.02)	8,92 (4.16)	0,22 (0)	0,12 (0)	11,02 (4,34)
	B	112 (104)	0,32 (0,39)	1,72 (1,79)	0,10 (0,12)	0 (0.02)	5,15 (4,16)	0 (0)	0 (0)	4,82 (4,34)
Maximum value	A	120 (158)	6,47 (1,31)	7,87 (4,12)	0,84 (0,17)	0,83 (0,07)	34,88 (20,43)	2,59 (0)	2,82 (0)	34,18 (21,61)
	B	133 (158)	0,93 (1,31)	4,38 (4,12)	0,27 (0,17)	0,23 (0,07)	18,96 (20,43)	0 (0)	0 (0)	16,31 (21,61)
Mean value	A	97 (118)	2,75 (0,83)	4,77 (2.49)	0,43 (0,14)	0,38 (0,04)	21,75 (14,47)	0,81 (0)	1,02 (0)	19,11 (9,01)
	B	120 (118)	0,80 (0,83)	2,51 (2,49)	0,15 (0,14)	0,05 (0,04)	14,44 (14,47)	0 (0)	0 (0)	8,88 (9,01)
		P<0.05	P<0.05	P<0.05	P<0.05	P<0.05	P<0.05	P<0.05	P<0.05	P<0.05

Table 4. Mathematical mean (with normal ranges in parentheses) of the preoperative (A) and postoperative (B) vocal parameters (minimal, maximum and mean) in adults (males) underwent septoplasty: average of fundamental frequency (Fo), Jitter percent (Jitt), Shimmer, noise to harmonics ratio (NHR), voice turbulence index (VTI), soft phonation index (SPI), degree of voiceless (DUV), degree of voice breaks (DVB) and peak amplitude variation (vAm). P<0.05 represents the significant statistical analysis by comparing mean values of each preoperative and postoperative parameters.

		Fo (Hz)	JITTER (%)	SHIMMER (%)	NHR	VTI	SPI	DUV (%)	DVB (%)	vAm (%)
Minimal value	A	130 (104)	0,23 (0,39)	1,84 (1,79)	0,14 (0,12)	0,01 (0,02)	2,41 (4,16)	0,22 (0)	0,12 (0)	11,92 (4,34)
	B	92 (104)	0,12 (0,39)	1,44 (1,79)	0,06 (0,12)	0 (0,02)	2,15 (4,16)	0 (0)	0 (0)	4,92 (4,34)
Maximum value	A	177 (158)	9,47 (1,31)	8,57 (4,12)	0,83 (0,17)	0,85 (0,07)	31,88 (20,43)	2,54 (0)	2,81 (0)	39,68 (21,61)
	B	133 (158)	0,94 (1,31)	4,98 (4,12)	0,29 (0,17)	0,21 (0,07)	17,93 (20,43)	0 (0)	0 (0)	17,01 (21,61)
Mean value	A	140 (118)	3,11 (0,83)	5,77 (2,49)	0,45 (0,14)	0,42 (0,04)	20,75 (14,47)	0,97 (0)	0,96 (0)	21,11 (9,01)
	B	122 (118)	0,77 (0,83)	3,01 (2,49)	0,15 (0,14)	0,05 (0,04)	13,44 (14,47)	0 (0)	0 (0)	8,75 (9,01)
		P<0.05	P<0.05	P<0.05	P<0.05	P<0.05	P<0.05	P<0.05	P<0.05	P<0.05

Table 5. Mathematical mean (with normal ranges in parentheses) of the preoperative (A) and postoperative (B) vocal parameters (minimal, maximum and mean) in adults (males) underwent direct microlaryngoscopy: average of fundamental frequency (Fo), Jitter percent (Jitt), Shimmer, noise to harmonics ratio (NHR), voice turbulence index (VTI), soft phonation index (SPI), degree of voiceless (DUV), degree of voice breaks (DVB) and peak amplitude variation (vAm). P<0.05 represents the significant statistical analysis by comparing mean values of each preoperative and postoperative parameters.

		Fo (Hz)	JITTER (%)	SHIMMER (%)	NHR	VTI	SPI	DUV (%)	DVB (%)	vAm (%)
Minimal value	A	94 (104)	0,55 (0,39)	2,91 (1,79)	0,34 (0,12)	0,11 (0,02)	1,91 (4,16)	0,28 (0)	0,16 (0)	12,02 (4,34)
	B	98 (104)	0,11 (0,39)	1,64 (1,79)	0,06 (0,12)	0 (0,02)	1,55 (4,16)	0 (0)	0 (0)	5,23 (4,34)
Maximum value	A	127 (158)	2,47 (1,31)	12,57 (4,12)	1,53 (0,17)	0,88 (0,07)	34,88 (20,43)	2,89 (0)	2,93 (0)	38,26 (21,61)
	B	153 (158)	1,04 (1,31)	4,99 (4,12)	0,24 (0,17)	0,31 (0,07)	19,63 (20,43)	0 (0)	0 (0)	18,21 (21,61)
Mean value	A	108 (118)	1,61 (0,83)	6,01 (2,49)	0,65 (0,14)	0,52 (0,04)	26,81 (14,47)	1,07 (0)	1,10 (0)	19,11 (9,01)
	B	122 (118)	0,84 (0,83)	3,11 (2,49)	0,15 (0,14)	0,05 (0,04)	15,54 (14,47)	0 (0)	0 (0)	8,83 (9,01)
		P<0.05	P<0.05	P<0.05	P<0.05	P<0.05	P<0.05	P<0.05	P<0.05	P<0.05

After surgery, our data showed a significant improvement ($p<0.05$) in all tested acoustic parameters: comparison with healthy adults highlighted a significant ($p<0.05$) postoperative normalization of all the parameters. (Table 3)

Fo data showed a postoperative normalization in both the speech and vocal samples: in the speech samples the postoperative mean value fell from 93 Hz to 117 Hz, while in the healthy adults the mean value is 116 Hz.

An improvement of nasalance was noted in all the patients at their postoperative clinical control (six months after surgery): the mirror-fogging test presented a postoperative mean assessment of 2.0 (increased from the preoperative mean value of 1.4) and the Gutzmann test values fell from 1 before the treatment to 0 after it. VHI had a postoperative mean value of 35 (decreased from the preoperative mean value of 67). The results of the articulation analysis showed that all the patients were capable of producing all Italian vowels and consonants pre and postoperatively, without difficulties.

Velopharyngeal sphincter provides the closure of the nasopharyngeal hiatus and its responsible for the coupling between the oropharyngeal and the nasal cavities which act as resonators, during respiration, blowing, sucking, swallowing and speech. The postoperative data of the acoustic parameters highlight the postoperative regular sphincter action of the nasopharyngeal hiatus; the postoperative improvement of nasalance, caused by the excision of the redundant mucosa of each posterior arch, is showed by the postoperative data of the Glatzel and the Gutzmann tests.

All of our patients who underwent UPPP also received tonsillectomy: because tonsil may impend full palatal movement, the postoperative improvement of nasalance and of the acoustic parameters highlights the absence of nasal air escape during speech and the impact of tonsil in velopharyngeal closure [18].

Fo showed significant change postoperatively, both in the vocal and speech samples: this observation indicates that UPPP, although a procedure that doesn't affect the larynx, changes the structure of the vocal tract and thus the resonance of speech production, and is thus a surgery capable of improving speech quality [18]. The improvement of the nasalance, at the Glatzel and Gutzmann tests, confirms these observations.

Although sound originates at the laryngeal level, there are significant alterations and enhancement of the vocal output as a result of the transfer function in the supraglottic cavities: inadequate velopharyngeal function and redundant oropharyngeal mucosa have a damping effect during the transfer function, causing a reduction in quality and precision of the output.

These damping effects influence noise too: in patients with velopharyngeal inadequacy, redundant soft palate may cause important turbulent air passage, through the vocal resonator, and produces an augmentation of vocal tract inertance and resistance that can interfere with a speaker's ability to produce a regular voice. The postoperative values of Jitter, VTI, SPI, DUV, DVB and vAm represent the regularization of the supraglottic flow with the reduction of vocal tract inertance and resistance, with resulting in less laryngeal adductory force necessary for phonation [21,27].

Studies regarding articulation suggesting the possibility of postoperative articulation difficulties (more or less temporary) are rare: our experiences are in agree with these authors.

Patients perception of voice is an important treatment outcome measure, especially in the case of benign disease where the greatest impact is on quality of life. Our preoperative results indicate that patients with snoring and/or OSAS encounter the same degree of problems in daily life as other voice-impaired patients, and therefore require the maximum level of attention and care: for these reasons an objective speech and voice analysis should be performed in all these patients.

3. SEPTOPLASTY

The supraglottic larynx, pharynx, oral and nasal cavity, and sinus have been considered to act as a resonator to shape the sound quality. Therefore changes in nasal volumes may produce changes in nasal resonance. Changes in the structure of the vocal tract, after surgery, are assumed to cause changes in the acoustic features of voice [28].

Nasal cavity and resistance are primarily dependent upon the size and configuration of the internal nasal cavity. Approximately two thirds of the resistance occurs at the liminal valve, located at the junction of the upper lateral cartilage and nasal septum. Congenital structural craniofacial anomalies often are associated with maxillary growth deficit, as well as nasal deformities such as deviated septum, vomere spurs and alar collapse.

The anterior nasal obstruction increases the resistance to nasal airflow and sound transmission, by reducing nasal airway patency. The nasal obstruction due to septal deviation may create enough impedance as to reduce or even to prevent sound from entering the nasopharynx, even when the velopharyngeal port is open during speech. On the other hand, obstruction of the anterior nasal cavity may add acoustic aspects to the speech signal that result in "cul-de-sac" resonance [29].

Upper airway operations have the potential to affect vocal quality by altering the resonant characteristics of the vocal tract.

There has been little interest in the role of septoplasty on voice, although its impact on naso-oral resonance is well recognized. In the literature there aren't many studies about **septoplasty and changes in acoustic features of voice, furthermore these studies mainly concentrate on the fundamental frequency (Fo), with opposite results.**

Nasal obstruction causes an hyponasality, after surgery patients present a subjective normalization of hyponasality: the mirror-fogging test presented a postoperative mean assessment of 2.9 (increased from the preoperative mean value of 0.8), the Gutzmann test values changed from 0 before the treatment to 1 after it. VHI had a postoperative mean value of 25 (decreased from the preoperative mean value of 77). The acoustic parameters presented an improvement in all tested parameters one month after septoplasty. (Table 4)

Normal Fo was also shown in the balanced sentences (112 Hz vs 136 Hz) one month after surgery: this observation indicates that septoplasty, although a procedure that doesn't affect the larynx, changes the structure of the vocal tract and thus the resonance of voice production (lowering the pitch of the voice often decreases the resonance and consequently can decrease the nasal resonance values), and is thus a surgery capable of improving speech quality [18,27].

The postoperative values of Jitter, VTI, SPI, DUV, and DVB highlight the regularization of the supraglottic flow with the reduction of vocal tract inertance and resistance, with resulting in less laryngeal adductory force necessary for phonation [22].

All these data demonstrate that nasal obstruction plays a crucial role in the development of voice: patients, and particularly voice professionals, should be informed about the possible alterations in speech following major surgical interventions on nasal septum.

4. Microlaryngoscopy

We report our experiences on adults, males, with disphonia by vocal cord polyps, interesting one vocal fold. All the patients underwent direct microlaryngoscopy, in general anesthesia, with excision of the polyps.

One month after surgery, the mirror-fogging test presented a postoperative mean assessment of 2.3 (instead of a preoperative mean value of 1.4); the Gutzmann test was 0 before and after the treatment; the voice handicap index presented a postoperative mean value of 21 (instead of a preoperative mean value of 82) and the test from Van Borsel was normal.

In the patients with disphonia by vocal polyps, the analysis of Jitter, Shimmer, NHR, VTI, SPI, DUV, DVB and vAm showed a postsurgical decrease. Comparison with healthy adults highlighted a postsurgical normalization of Fo, Jitter, Shimmer, NHR, VTI, SPI, DUV and DVB. (Table 5)

The SPI, DUV and DVB preoperative values highlight the incomplete closure of the glottis. The preoperative values of VTI, SPI, DUV, DVB show that a stronger laryngeal adductory force. Their postoperative values highlight the regularization of the supraglottic flow with the reduction of vocal tract inertance and resistance.

Endolaryngeal microsurgery is functionally oriented, therefore, assessment of vocal function is important to evaluate the effect of the surgery on voice. We highlight the importance of objective evaluation of voice disorders, the MDVP method may be useful for analyzing abnormal vocal function and quantitatively evaluating the effects of surgical excision of vocal nodules and polyps: our results confirm a high degree of effectiveness of endolaryngeal microsurgery on vocal rehabilitation.

Conclusion

The consequences of voice disorders are potentially devastating to a patient's quality of life, several studies have shown that patients with speech disorders are often stereotyped as less intelligent, less pleasant and less attractive than people with normal speech; such perceptions can seriously affect the social life and self-esteem of these patients.

Our experience shows that the decision to perform ENT surgery depends on its potential effect on speech and voice too. Our results indicate that an objective evaluation of speech and voice helps the specialist in the management of the patients and avoids incorrect and potentially dangerous procedures.

The Multi-Dimensional Voice Program is a powerful software tool for quantitative acoustic assessment of voice quality; It is capable of calculating 33 parameters from a single vocalization. These acoustic analysis, which provide an extensive representation of vocal function, cannot be obtained from airway resistance or perceptual measures alone. Therefore, the precise knowledge of changes in these tested parameters provides a comprehensive and thus superior depiction of vocal function and aids in providing more objective predictions of the effects of surgery. According with other authors, articulation problems may affect acoustic properties of vocal fold: for this reason we consider important the analysis of the different acoustic measures (Fo, Jitter, Shimmer, NHR, VTI, SPI, DUV, DVB and vAm) in patients underwent surgery.

In our experience Fo, Jitter, Shimmer, NHR, VTI, SPI, DUV, DVB and vAm are the parameters which give the most objective information about the presence of vocal modification; *a multiple regression analysis of these eight acoustic measures in conjunction with the other tests present in our protocol* (the mirror-fogging test from Glatzel, the Gutzmann test, the voice handicap index and the Van Borsel's study) *may provide a quick and relatively sensitive method that may be clinically useful in measuring change of vocal and speech quality.*

APPENDIX: BALANCED SENTENCES

The oronasal sentences below contain a mixture of nasal and non-nasal sounds in the approximate proportion found in everyday Italian speech (11.6% nasal consonants). The oral sentences below exclude nasal consonants and are designed to detect hypernasality. The nasal sentences are loaded with nasal consonants and are designed to detect hypo nasality.

All the adults are instructed to repeat each passage with a comfortable vocal pitch and loudness. If a subject made an error, the passage was repeated.

Oronasal Sentences

Si presume che in caso di omonimia gli interessati producano la documentazione necessaria a disambiguare la situazione.

Il colloquio di lavoro al quale mi sono recato ieri non credo che porterà significativi sviluppi alla mia carriera lavorativa.

Oral Sentences

La strada è stata asfaltata ieri dagli operai dopo quel periodo così protratto di piogge e forti acquazzoni.

Se corri veloce alla chiesa che è di lato alla piazza puoi vedere la sorella di Dario che oggi si sposa.

Vorrei ripetere il viaggio che ho fatto a febbraio sulla costa del Libano al più presto per rivedere i posti più suggestivi.

Nasal Sentences

Mi sembra di mentire mutando sempre la mia impressione in merito al mantenimento di Manuela con il mansionario di smistare le missive importanti.

Nino Musante è un importante componente della Commissione impegnata al mantenimento del monumento di marmo messo nel Museo di Musica di Milano.

References

[1] Titze, IR. The human instrument. *Sci.Am,* 2008, 298, 94-101.
[2] Hunter EJ; Titze, IR. Overlap of Hearing and Voicing Ranges in Singing. J Singing, 2004, 61, 387-392.
[3] Leff, AP; Schofield, TM; Stephan, KE; Crinion, JT; Friston, KJ; Price, CJ. The cortical dynamics of intelligible speech. J Neurosci, 2008, 28, 13209-15.
[4] Fridriksson, J; Moss, J; Davis, B; Baylis, GC; Bonilha, L; Rorden, C. Motor speech perception modulates the cortical language areas. *Neuroimage,* 2008, 41, 605-13.
[5] Scott, S; Robinson, K; Wilson, JA; MacKenzie, K. Patient-reported problems associated with dysphonia. *Clin Otolaryngol,* 1997, 22, 37-40.
[6] Andrew, EM; Gray, NS; Snowden, RJ. The relationship between trauma and beliefs about hearing voices: a study of psychiatric and non-psychiatric voice hearers. Psychol Med, 2008, 38, 1409-17.
[7] Finck, C. Vocal fold structure and speech pathologies. Rev Laryngol Otol Rhinol, 2005, 126, 295-300.
[8] Van Lierde, KM; Van Borsel, J; Moerman, M; Cauwenberge, P. Nasalance, nasality, voice, and articulation after uvulopalatopharyngoplasty. *Laryngoscope*, 2002, 112, 873-878.
[9] Van Lierde, KM; Claeys, S; De Bodt, M; Baudonck, N; De Ley, S; Marks, LA; Van Borsel, J. Vocal quality characteristics in children with cleft palate: a multiparameter approach. *J Voice*, 2004, 18, 354-362.
[10] Schindler, A; Capaccio, P; Maruzzi, P; Ginocchio, D; Bottero, A; Ottaviani, F. Preliminary considerations on the application of the Voice Handicap Index to pediatric population. *Acta Otolaryngol Ital*, 2007, 27, 22-26.
[11] Maertens, K; de Jong, FI. (2007). The voice handicap index as a tool for assessment of the biopsychosocial impact of voice problems. *B-ENT*, 2007, 3, 61-66.
[12] Van Borsel, J. Articulation in Down's syndrome adolescents and adults. *Eur J Disord Commun*, 1996, 31, 415-444.
[13] Kummer, AW; Billmire, DA; Myer, CM. 3rd. Hypertrophic tonsils: the effect on resonance and velopharyngeal closure. *Otolaryngol Head Neck Surg*, 1996, 115, 319-23.
[14] Van Borsel, J. Articulation in Down's syndrome adolescents and adults. *Eur J Disord Commun,* 1996, 31, 415-444.
[15] Canady, JW; Cable, BB; Karnell, MP; Karnell, LH. Pharyngeal flap surgery: protocols, complications, and outcomes at the University of Iowa. *Otolaryngol Head Neck Surg*, 2003, 129, 321-6.
[16] Kawashima, S; Peltomäki, T; Sakata, H; Mori, K; Happonen, RP; Rönning, O. Craniofacial morphology in preschool children with sleep-related breathing disorder and hypertrophy of tonsils. *Acta Paediatr*, 2002, 91, 71-7.
[17] MacKenzie-Stepner, K; Witzel, MA; Stringer, DA; Laskin, R. Velopharyngeal insufficiency due to hypertrophic tonsils. A report of two cases. *Int J Pediatr Otorhinolaryngol*, 1987, 14, 57-63.
[18] Mora, R; Crippa, B; Dellepiane, M; Jankowska, B. Effects of adenotonsillectomy on speech spectrum in children. *Int J Pediatr Otorhinolaryngol*, 2007, 71, 1299-304.

[19] Smith, J; Rey, G; Dickens, P; Fletcher, N; Hollemberg, L; Wolfe, J. Vocal tract resonances and the sound of the Australian didjeridu (yidaki). III. Determinants of playing quality. *J Acoust Soc Am*, 2007, 121, 547-58.

[20] Bhuta, T; Patrick, L; Garnett, JD. Perceptual evaluation of voice quality and its correlation with acoustic measurements. *J Voice,* 2004, 18, 299-304.

[21] Shadle, CH; Barney, A; Davies, POAL. Fluid flow in a dynamic mechanical model of the vocal fold and tract. II. Implications for speech production studies. *The Journal of the Acoustical Society of America,* 1999, 105, 456-466.

[22] Svancara, P; Horacek, J; Vokral, J; Cerny, L. Computational modelling of effect of tonsillectomy on voice production. *Logoped Phoniatr Vocol*, 2006, 31, 117-25.

[23] Behlfelt, K. Enlarged tonsils and the effect of tonsillectomy. Characteristics of the dentition and facial skeleton. Posture of the head, hyoid bone and tongue. Mode of breathing. *Swed Dent J Suppl,* 1990, 72, 1-35.

[24] Birkent, H; Soken, H; Akcam, T; Karahatay, S; Gerek, M. The effect of radiofrequency volumetric tissue reduction of soft palate on voice. *Eur Arch Otorhinolaryngol*, 2008, 265, 195-8.

[25] Salami, A; Dellepiane, M; Bavazzano, M; Crippa, B; Mora, F; Mora, R. New trends in head and neck surgery: A prospective evaluation of the Harmonic Scalpel®. *Med Sci Monit*, 2008, 14, PI1-5.

[26] Friedman, M; Ibrahim, H; Bass, L. Clinical staging for sleep-disordered breathing. *Otolaryngol Head Neck Surg*, 2002, 127, 13-21.

[27] Salami, A; Jankowska, B; Dellepiane, M; Crippa, B; Mora, R. The impact of tonsillectomy with or without adenoidectomy on speech and voice. *Int J Pediatr Otorhinolaryngol*, 2008, 72, 1377-84.

[28] Dang, J; Honda, K. (1994). Morphological and acoustical analysis of the nasal and paranasal sinuses. *J Acoust Soc Am,* 96, 2088-100.

[29] Watterson, T; Lewis, KE; Deutsch, C. Nasalance and nasality in low pressure and high pressure speech. *Cleft Palate Craniofac J*, 1998, 35, 293-98.

In: Speech Disorders: Causes, Treatment and Social Effects
Editor: Alan E. Harrison, pp. 197-219
ISBN: 978-1-60876-213-2

Chapter 9

LEARNING DISABILITIES AND MATHEMATICS IN HIGHER EDUCATION

***Brian Watson*[1*] *and Stuart Rowlands*[2]**
[1]Centre for Teaching Mathematics, University of Plymouth, UK
[2]Centre for Teaching Mathematics, University of Plymouth, UK

ABSTRACT

During the second half of the 20th century the proportion of the United Kingdom population attending higher education increased from around 5% to more than 40%. It should not be surprising that the Higher Education learning environment has become more diverse as we move towards the government target of 50% of the population.

There is a growing awareness of the numbers of students who are diagnosed as dyslexic and perhaps to a lesser extent, students who may be dyscalculic.

Dyslexia is essentially a deficit in working memory. In the same way that sight impairment or hearing impairment may be mild or severe, dyslexia may also be mild or severe.

Sight, hearing, and working memory are clearly factors which affect learning, but consideration of a single factor cannot give a reliable assessment of a person's ability, intelligence or potential.

The term 'constructive alignment' (John Biggs 2003) is used to describe the desired harmony between the student and all of the elements which make up the learning environment. The assertion is that greater harmony will facilitate greater learning.

Disciplines such as psychology, sciences and social sciences, have significant mathematical and/or statistical concepts embedded in them. It is common for students to find themselves undertaking projects which involve the collection and analysis of data. Individual students might have returned to full time education after a number of years; they might not have a formal mathematics qualification and be a little surprised and daunted by the mathematics involved. In such situations any learning disability compounds the principal problem that the student is attempting to apply relatively

[*] Author for correspondence bwatson@plymouth.ac.uk

complex statistical/mathematical analysis without having a good understanding of the necessary underpinning concepts, such as ratio, proportion and probability.

The study of mathematics requires assimilation of a hierarchy of concepts. Without an understanding of lower concepts on which the higher concepts are built, study of the higher concepts can be frustrating and unproductive.

We need to develop our student support facilities so that students can be shown the necessary hierarchy of mathematical concepts and can assimilate them at their own pace. This will be of benefit to students with and without learning difficulties.

INTRODUCTION

An increasing number of students entering Higher Education (HE) in the United Kingdom (UK) have learning disabilities (Grant 2002). Two reports (Cockcroft 1982; Smith 2004) on the state of mathematics in the UK education system indicate that, for a variety of reasons, mathematics continues to be perceived as a difficult subject to learn, and that there is a shortage of suitably qualified mathematics teachers.

The main part of this paper concerns our observations of difficulties which dyslexic students have with mathematics. With references to the works of Tall and Vinner (1981) and Skemp (1993) we attempt to link students' difficulties to specific concepts.

Widening Participation

Between 1971 and 2001 the number of undergraduate enrolments in UK institutions of higher education increased by approximately 170% (DfES 2001). Over the same period the total population of the United Kingdom changed by only a few percent (ONS 2001). In 2003, 43 percent of 18-to-30 year olds were participating in higher education in England and Wales (DfES 2003a), and it is the policy of the UK Government to increase this figure towards 50 per cent by the year 2010 (DfES 2003b). In the first half of the 20th century there was a steady increase in the numbers participating in higher education (Robbins 1963, p15 table 3). Figure 1, below, shows the numbers of full time students in higher education for the whole of the 20th century. It has been compiled from data from the Robbins report (Robbins 1963, p15 table 3) and data from the Department for Education and Skills (DfES 2001).

Widening Participation, an ongoing government initiative, actively encourages students from socio-economic backgrounds which traditionally would not provide entrants to HE, to enter HE.

Grant (2002, p 3) draws attention to the significant increase, between 1997 and 1999, in the number of graduates with declared disabilities, which he states was proportionally greater than the overall increase in the number of graduates. He recognises the need for accurate diagnosis of disabilities in order that resources can be appropriately and effectively targeted.

> "A misleading or incomplete diagnosis can result in a student being disadvantaged or advantaged." Grant (2002, p 12)

This can be an emotive issue, not least because of the significant Disabled Student's Allowance (DSA) available to those diagnosed as having recognised disabilities.

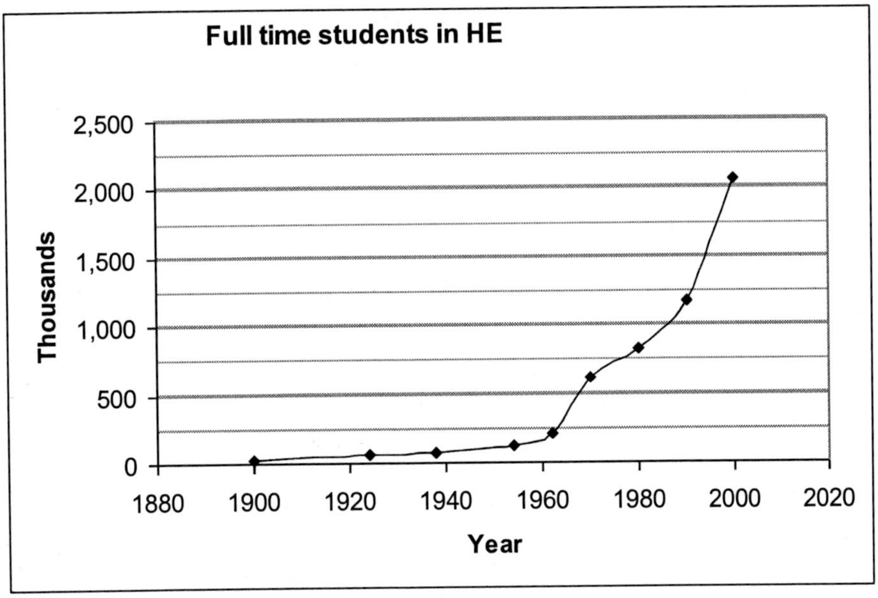

Figure 1. Growth in number of students in Higher Education

Grant (2002) further makes the point that university admissions policies should be based on academic criteria. He suggests that some HE institutions might be admitting students "for whom HE is not a viable option."

> "It is inevitable that while a widening access policy will result, rightly, in more students with disabilities entering and succeeding in higher education, it is also inevitable that more students will be admitted who lack the intellectual ability to succeed in higher education." (Grant 2002, p28)

In the United Kingdom, the majority of students with disabilities who seek advice are dyslexic. (Grant 2002, p3)

Dyslexia

Mortimer (2003, chapter 3) provides a helpful insight and summary into the nature of dyslexia and the difficulties in finding a precise definition. The prevalence of descriptions that focus on deficits in information processing is acknowledged.

McLoughlin et al (1994) find this focus to be useful and state

> "As a direct consequence of an inefficiency in working memory a dyslexic person will have more difficulty acquiring certain skills than a non-dyslexic of similar intelligence. Most notably, dyslexics take longer to develop literacy skills, and expend more time and energy in the process, than non-dyslexics. Less prominent features of dyslexia are difficulties with remembering fact, figures, sequences of instructions, messages, names and almost anything that places a heavy demand on working memory. Many dyslexics lack organisational skills; they are, because of a

poor concept of time, frequently late for meetings and appointments. They can also have trouble following and keeping track of what is said in a conversation, lecture or interview. All of these difficulties arise as a direct result of their constitutional defect in working memory and are, therefore, *primary* symptoms." (McLoughlin et al 1994)

Memory Acquisition and Retrieval

During a mathematical investigation with three year-5 pupils (age 9-10 years) the following question arose. Two is multiplied by a number and the result is one. What is the number? The three pupils looked puzzled. After a few moments one of them suddenly, with obvious delight announced the answer, a half. The others were surprised, and mildly disappointed with themselves, at how obvious it was once it was pointed out. Clearly they recognised the answer and arguably, the answer was somewhere within their brains. How does the brain search for answers?

Aristotle recognised three principles for information entering the brain; contiguity, frequency and similarity (Gluck et al 2008). Skemp (1993, chapter 2) uses the term 'schema' to describe mental structures of concepts. Gluck et al (2008) describe neural networks, their activation and interaction in response to visual and audio stimulus. Neural circuits are active when information is sent to the brain, for example when we see or hear, and when information is retrieved from the brain, for example to produce speech or movement. It is not possible to associate particular neurons with particular knowledge. There is evidence, however, that activation of one neuron can become a trigger to activate other neurons. The strength of the trigger can become stronger or weaker. The number of neurons which become active together can increase or decrease.

"Learning requires physical changes in neural circuits. Neurons can physically change in many ways, and many of these changes can affect their firing behavior. The most prominent and easily observable changes involve changes in the neurons' shape, size an number of connections to other neurons." (Gluck et al 2008)

There appears to be similarity between the idea of a schema and the idea of a neural network.

Hierarchical Nature of Mathematics

Butterworth (1999, p 298) states

"School maths is like a house of cards: the cards on the bottom layer must be firmly and accurately constructed if they are to support the next layer up. If a lower layer is shaky, the house will eventually fall down. .... The gap between the concepts currently being taught and the pupil's understanding will get wider and wider."

Tall and Vinner (1981) agree with Butterworth that mathematics is usually regarded as a subject in which concepts can be defined precisely and accurately to provide a firm foundation for mathematical theory. They observe, however,

> "The human brain is not a purely logical entity. The complex manner in which it functions is often at variance with the logic of mathematics. (Tall and Vinner 1981, p151)

Tall and Vinner (1981) use the term ***concept image*** to describe "the total cognitive structure that is associated with the concept." The concept image can be built up over a number of years through various experiences and stimuli. It includes mental pictures and processes. (Tall and Vinner 1981, p 151)

Skemp (1993, chapter 2) uses the term 'schema' to describe a mental structure of concepts. Higher level concepts are built onto and are thus dependent on lower level concepts. A concept at one level may support more than one concept at a higher level. Hence, the interrelation between concepts is complex. The assimilation of a new experience or new knowledge to an existing schema is referred to as 'schematic' learning. The counterpart of schematic learning is rote learning, where new knowledge is not related to existing schema. Skemp (1993, chapter 2) shows that much longer retention results from schematic learning than from rote learning, and refers to greater 'cognitive strain' being caused by rote learning. If 'cognitive strain' implies intense use of working memory then it is readily appreciated that rote learning will be especially unsuitable for dyslexics because the principle characteristic of dyslexia is a deficit in working memory. It is not suggested, however, that there are no circumstances under which rote learning can be appropriate.

Concepts and Conflicts

Tall and Vinner (1981) give examples where students' concept images are in conflict with mathematical concept definitions. Although students were aware of, and had used the mathematical definitions, the strength of their (deficient) concept images caused them to make incorrect conclusions in some situations.

One of the concepts investigated by Tall and Vinner (1981) was the concept of **continuity** of mathematical functions. **Continuity** is a fairly common word in the English language. One does not have to be a mathematician to have a concept of what the word means and to use the word meaningfully in communication with others. Within the context of mathematical functions, however, the distinction between continuous and non-continuous is subtle and comes from a precise definition of the concept, rather than the simple appearance of the graph of the function. Confusingly, some mathematically discontinuous functions have graphs which coincidentally match a simple concept image of discontinuity, but this is not always the case. It is observed that

> "The mental pictures which served the students well at an earlier stage may now become an impediment." (Tall and Vinner 1981, p 169)

Skemp says the same thing in different words.

> "A schema can be as powerful a hindrance as help if it happens to be an unsuitable schema." (Skemp 1993, p41)

Tall and Vinner's (1981) account seems to support Skemp's principle that

"Concepts of a higher order than those which people already have cannot be communicated to them by a definition, but only by arranging for them to encounter a suitable collection of examples." (Skemp 1993, p 30)

Common Cognitive Paths (CCP)

Vinner and Hershkowitz (1983) give examples of a common cognitive path (CCP) relevant to geometry. A **cognitive path** is essentially is a series of hierarchical images which form part of a concept image. If a person's concept image includes one of these hierarchical images then it will also include all the images subordinate to this image. By inference, if one of these hierarchical images is absent then higher images will also be absent. A **common cognitive path** is a cognitive path which is common to large number of people. Vinner and Hershkowitz detected CCPs empirically. We ponder whether it is possible to develop theoretical cognitive paths which would inform pedagogy. The hierarchical nature of mathematics is already recognised and is taken into account in the design and delivery mathematics curricula. The use and development of common cognitive paths is unlikely to change radically curriculum design, but it might usefully inform the pedagogy behind the delivery of the curriculum.

Figure 11 to Figure 13 show an initial attempt to construct theoretical cognitive paths.

Observations of Student Learning

These observations have been compiled from notes made during support sessions over a period of four years until now, 2009. Most of these support sessions have been with individual university students who have been allocated mathematics study skills support because of a learning disability – principally dyslexia. Other observations have been made during mathematics support 'drop in' sessions which are open to all students in the university, and some examples are taken from answers to written mathematics class-tests.

The order in which the observations are presented is not the order in which they occurred. We have tried to relate these observations to theoretical concept images and cognitive paths.

Fundamental Number

Student A, a mature student who had successfully run her own business for a number of years, was diagnosed as dyslexic when she enrolled on a degree course. Aware that maths had always been a problem for her she sought support as soon as possible. She is very clear about what makes sense to her and what doesn't, and shows determination to succeed.

At our first meeting she was asked to calculate 2 + 3 x 4. She gave the answer as 20. This student left school probably before the introduction of the mnemonic, BODMAS (Brackets Order Division Multiplication Addition Subtraction). This response, however, is not uncommon among first year students who are familiar with the mnemonic, which casts doubt on the usefulness of the mnemonic. (Readers may like to conduct a brief survey among their own students by asking them to perform the calculation).

Her new (non-scientific) calculator did, in fact, produce the answer 20. To her, the rule that multiplication takes precedence over addition seemed arbitrary and she wanted to know why.

If we define multiplication as repeated addition, then it's precedence over addition is natural. This was demonstrated using software shown in Figure 3.

If, in the original calculation, we replace "3 x 4" by "3 + 3 + 3+ 3", then there can be only one answer.

The demonstration can also show why multiplication is commutative (3 x 4 = 4 x 3; Figure 3 and Figure 4), although the simple statement that the order of the two numbers doesn't matter is probably more informative than the term, 'commutative'.

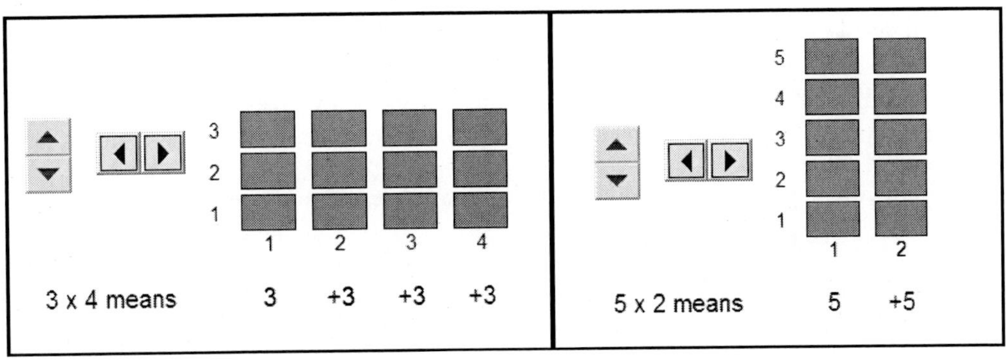

Figure 3. Multiplication as repeated addition

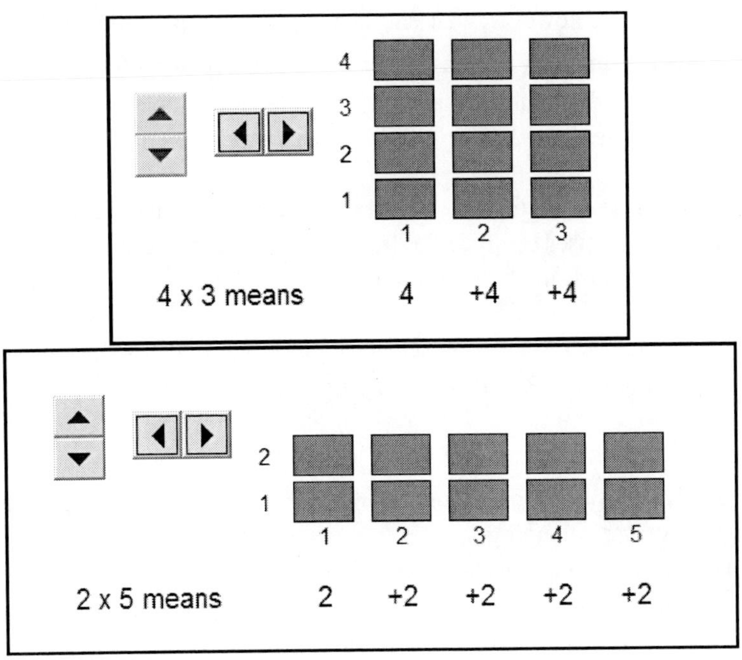

Figure 4. Commutative law (compare to Figure 3)

The student was very happy with this explanation. It was a revelation, and most importantly, it made sense. This is an example of schematic learning rather than rote learning of the rule that multiplication takes precedence over addition.

A number of dyslexic students have made comments to the effect that once they understand something they can remember it. ('*Once I get it, I'm OK*' is the type of phrase often used.). The works (Tall et al 1981; Skemp 1993; Butterworth 1999) cited in the previous section, Hierarchical nature of mathematics, explain why this is not surprising.

Fractions

What appears to be deficient or even missing for many students is a concept of fraction. In fact, many adult students from across the university who 'drop in' to the mathematics help centre will openly declare that they do not understand, or they 'can't do' fractions.

Student B, a 3rd year student of architecture, diagnosed as dyslexic after enrolling in university a number of years after leaving school, was truly amazed that the line in a fraction just meant divide. e.g. $\frac{3}{8}$ means 3 divided by 8. She expressed surprise that it was as simple as that.

We had started the session by looking at simple equations. She said that she had *"switched off"* from maths since the age of five years, but felt that she had to confront her mathematical limitations. She said that she couldn't see the purpose of algebra – replacing numbers by letters.

It soon became clear, however, that she had a good grasp on the concept of algebraic manipulation. Solving equations such as, $2x + 3 = 11$, presented no difficulty. She was not comfortable, however, with non integer answers. This led us to look at fractions.

At the end of the session, having used the software shown in Figure 5 she seemed relieved and enlightened.

Figure 5 shows a screen capture of software which demonstrates addition and subtraction of common fractions. The user can type the fractions onto the screen. The solution is revealed by using the controls towards the bottom of the screen.

Student C, enrolled on a foundation science course, was diagnosed as dyslexic and found mathematics very challenging. Referring to Figure 5 Student C stated, *"The diagram's really helpful."*

Student D, also enrolled on a foundation science course and diagnosed as dyslexic, found mathematics very challenging.

After we had used the fractions software (Figure 5) Student D seemed comfortable with the addition of fractions. She seemed keen to try the exercises in a textbook which she was using (Teach Yourself Maths) and use the software to check her answers.

Student E, also diagnosed as dyslexic stated with reference to the software (Figure 5), *"I've always struggled with fractions. Seeing that I don't know why I struggled."*

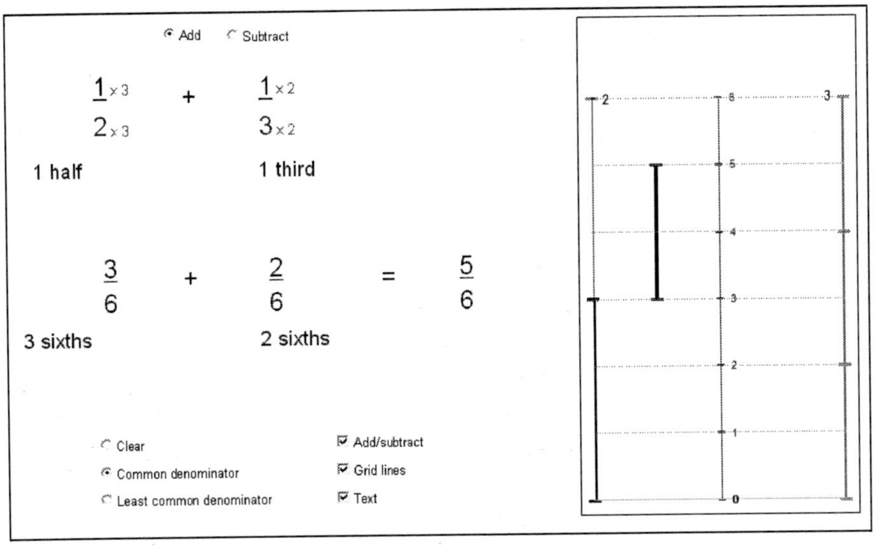

Figure 5. software for demonstrating addition and subtraction of fractions

The text, 'half', 'third' and 'sixths', seemed to help to emphasise addition of similar objects, and discourage the error of adding the denominators.

Student F was diagnosed as dyslexic and also was very challenged by mathematics. He wanted to understand decimals. Told that 0.1 was the same as $\frac{1}{10}$, he said he had never been aware of this, or that 0.01 was the same as $\frac{1}{100}$. He was not comfortable with common fractions and was surprised that $3 \div 8$ means the same as $\frac{3}{8}$. He was happy with the explanation that both of these mean 3 objects divided into 8 parts, or 3 objects (e.g. cakes) shared by eight people. He said he had been looking for another meaning for "three eighths", and couldn't understand what it meant. As his initial query focused on decimals, we looked at the example, $3 \div 12$. The illustration shown in Figure 6 was drawn on paper. This seemed to make sense to him.

ALGEBRAIC MANIPULATION

Denominators

Transposition of formulae is a topic which arises regularly. A particular difficulty seems to occur when a variable which is initially a denominator (or a term in a denominator) has to become the subject. We suspect that this difficulty might arise from a deficient concept image of division. Often students will solve the problem correctly if the numbers involved, including the answer, are integers.

$$\text{e.g. } 6 = \frac{18}{A}$$

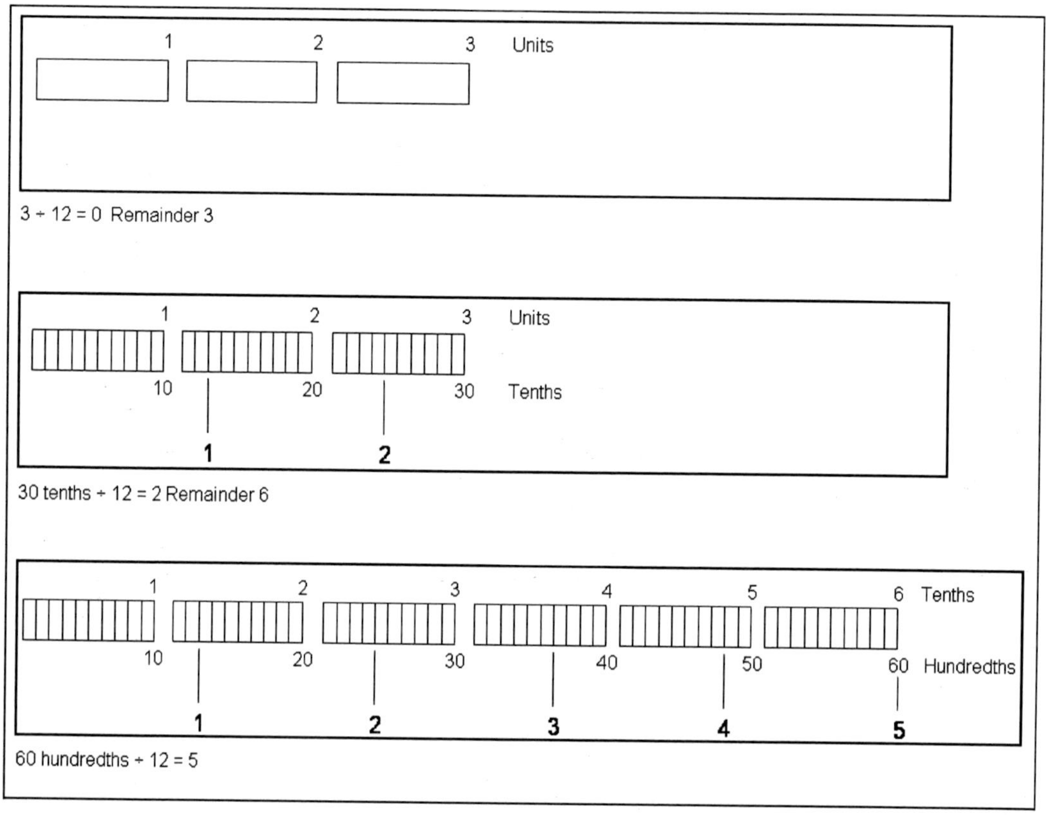

Figure 6. Illustration of 3 ÷ 12 = 0.25

The top diagram in Figure 6 illustrates, 3 ÷ 12 = 0 Remainder 3
The middle diagram in Figure 6 illustrates, 30 tenths ÷ 12 = 2 tenths, Remainder 6 tenths
The bottom diagram in Figure 6 illustrates, 60 hundredths ÷ 12 = 5 hundredths
Algebraic manipulation

Asked how they solved this problem, students have given answers such as having to **find a number that goes into 18 six times**. Even if they cannot readily recite multiplication tables they may be observed to count on their fingers. Given an equation to solve such as $4.7 = \frac{19.2}{A}$, they are unsure how to proceed. Their concept image of division seems to be limited to integers.

First year geology students take an in-class test in mathematics. In one question they are given 10 linear equations to solve. We have noticed that some students may be applying unreliable concept images. Extracts from test papers of two students are shown in Figure 7 and Figure 8. The complete questions are not shown, only the relevant lines of the students' answers.

Figure 7 illustrates that this student might be applying a rule to always divide the number on the right by the number on the left.

Figure 8 illustrates that this student might be applying a rule to always divide the greater number by the lesser number.

a)	b)
$10 = 11x$	$10x = 41$
$x = \frac{11}{10}$	$x = \frac{41}{10}$
Incorrect	Correct

Figure 7. Deficient concept image – always divide by number on left.

a)	b)
$14 = 8x$	$4 = 10x$
$x = 1\cdot 75$	$x = 2\cdot 5$
Correct	Incorrect

Figure 8. Deficient concept image – always divide by lesser number.

Student G is in year 11 (15/16 years old) of school. The author was providing extra tuition in mathematics in preparation for the national examination, General Certificate of Secondary Education (GCSE).

The student knew of trigonometry and had met the terms, sine, tangent, cosine, opposite, adjacent and hypotenuse but wasn't really familiar with the topic. He was unable to attempt a problem involving a scalene triangle. The solution required the use of the sine rule.

We used a software demonstration for tangent and showed that the size of an angle can be fixed/specified by the lengths of the adjacent and opposite sides. He was very comfortable with the principle that the angle could be specified in terms of the ratio of two sides; Tan(θ) = Opposite/Adjacent.

We now looked at problems involving tangent in right angled triangles. He was encouraged to write down the defining equation, Tan(θ) = P/A as the first line of each solution. 'P' is used for oPposite side to avoid confusion with zero.

He was confident in calculating θ given A and P e.g.

$$\tan(\theta) = \frac{P}{A} = \frac{40}{65}$$

$$\theta = \tan^{-1}\left(\frac{40}{65}\right) = 31.6^o$$

The above type of problem requires direct substitution of values in the equation.

He was also confident in solving problems of the following type, writing.

$$\tan(\theta) = \frac{P}{A}$$

$$\tan(20) = \frac{P}{15}$$

$$P = 15\tan(20) = 5 \cdot 6$$

This requires substitution of values and one step of transposition.
Given the problem

$$\tan(65) = \frac{36}{A}$$

He gave the solution as

$$A = 36\tan(65)$$

He wasn't confident about this and asked if this is 'what you do'.
His two solutions were rewritten side by side and he was asked to compare them.

$$\tan(20) = \frac{P}{15} \qquad\qquad \tan(65) = \frac{36}{A}$$

$$P = 15\tan(20) \qquad\qquad A = 36\tan(65)$$

He was asked whether it was reasonable that the second lines should have the same form (unknown = known x known) when the first lines had different forms (known = unknown/known and known = known/unknown)

He could sense that this wasn't right but wasn't sure how to resolve the problem.

He was now asked to solve the equation

$$4 = \frac{12}{A}$$

He immediately gave the correct answer, 3. Asked how he did it, he replied with confidence, 12 divided by 4.

The two problems were now written side by side

$$4 = \frac{12}{A} \qquad\qquad \tan(65) = \frac{36}{A}$$

With reasonable confidence he stated that the answer would be 36 divided by tan(65).

At an earlier point in the session the student had asked if sine and cosine were used in a similar way to tangent. This suggests that he had or was developing an appropriate concept image of trigonometry. His difficulty lay, not in trigonometry, but in the rearrangement of the equation. His concept image of solving equations seemed to exclude division, with the consequence that whenever an equation involved one unknown variable and two numbers, he was liable to calculate the answer as the product of the two numbers.

Visual Impact

At a support session, a dyslexic business studies student expressed concern that he could not follow the mathematical reasoning of a note he had taken during a business studies lecture.

He had recorded that, given

$$\frac{F_0}{S_0}=\frac{1+i_\$}{1+i_£}$$

it follows that

$$\frac{F_0-S_0}{S_0}=\frac{i_\$-i_£}{1+i_£}$$

Although it was not absolutely essential for him to prove the statement in order to make use of it, he did not feel comfortable in just accepting it. Prior to the support session he had attempted unsuccessfully to prove the statement for himself. His workings were algebraically correct. He did not appear to have any problem with the concept(s) of algebraic manipulation, but he baulked at expressions such as

$$\frac{(1+i_\$)}{(1+i_£)}-\frac{(1+i_£)}{(1+i_£)}$$

(This expression arises by subtracting 1 from the right hand side of the original equation).

Without difficulty he was able to simplify the expression, $\frac{4}{a+2}+\frac{2}{a+2}$

Then, by seeing the two examples side by side as shown in Figure 9, he was able to see the relevant similarity that in each example, the terms have a common denominator. The fact that one example involved addition and the other involved subtraction, did not distract him.

$\dfrac{4}{a+2}+\dfrac{2}{a+2}$	$\dfrac{(1+i_{\$})}{(1+i_{£})}-\dfrac{(1+i_{£})}{(1+i_{£})}$
$=\dfrac{4+2}{a+2}$	$=\dfrac{(1+i_{\$})-(1+i_{£})}{(1+i_{£})}$

Figure 9. Similar algebraic manipulations

We suggest that the example on the right hand side of Figure 9 appears to be more complicated, and thus more daunting, than the example on the left. It is possible that the visual impact of the example on the right masks the simplicity of the algebra required to simplify the expression. Skemp (1993, p 28) refers to the idea of *noise* which can impede recognition of a concept. *Noise* is data that is not relevant to a particular communication. What is *noise* in one context may not be *noise* in another context. What constitutes noise is open to individual interpretation. In the example on the right hand side of Figure 9, most of the brackets are, in a mathematical sense, superfluous. They could be considered as an unnecessary distraction – noise. Alternatively, it could be argued that the brackets give structure to the expression by grouping terms which can be manipulated as a single entity. There are also arguments for and against the use of subscripts.

Symbol Conventions and Layout

Sometimes students acquire rigid associations between specific symbols and methods. For example, in differential calculus it is common to use the symbol $\boldsymbol{u}$ for the chain rule, and the symbols $\boldsymbol{u}$ and $\boldsymbol{v}$ for the product rule. This can cause confusion when the chain rule has to be used within the product rule.

Consider differentiation of the following function.

$$y=\ln\left(x^2\right)(1-x)^{\frac{1}{2}}$$

Employing the product rule we let

$$y=uv$$

Where

$$u=\ln\left(x^2\right)$$

$$v=(1-x)^{\frac{1}{2}}$$

Employing the chain rule to differentiate $\boldsymbol{v}$ we now let

$$v = u^{\frac{1}{2}} \qquad \text{Where} \quad u = (1 - x)$$

The symbol u has now been used twice, giving scope for confusion. Many students will, in fact use the symbol twice and keep the two uses separate in their own minds. Indeed, we would expect that in due course, students would be able to use the chain rule to differentiate $v = (1 - x)^{\frac{1}{2}}$ without having to write down the intermediate variable.

It may seem obvious to the initiated that different symbols have to be introduced, but some students are hesitant to do this until they have been told that it is permissible to do so.

For dyslexic students, the layout of the working can be critical in assisting them or hindering them. There will always be individual preferences about what constitutes clarity and so we cannot be prescriptive. A general guideline is to make objects (e.g. terms in expressions) large enough, and with sufficient space between them so that they can be individually identified. Indentation and clear space between lines can be used as means of making each step of the process identifiable and explicit.

Statistics

Student H, diagnosed as dyslexic, was struggling with a foundation year statistics module. Asked what she understood by 'standard deviation' she attempted to describe how to calculate standard deviation. Her notes described standard deviation as a measure of dispersion. Asked for the meaning of the word, dispersion, she wasn't sure. Her response to examples such as dispersing a crowd, or dispersing an oil slick indicated that she did have a concept image of dispersion, even though it may have been weak and/or limited. It appeared that the dominant, or perhaps the only feature in this student's concept image of standard deviation, was a complicated calculation. Her concept image of standard deviation had nothing in common with her concept image of dispersion.

Software, shown in Figure 10 and Figure 11, was used to show how the standard deviation is a measure of the spread, or dispersion, of the data.

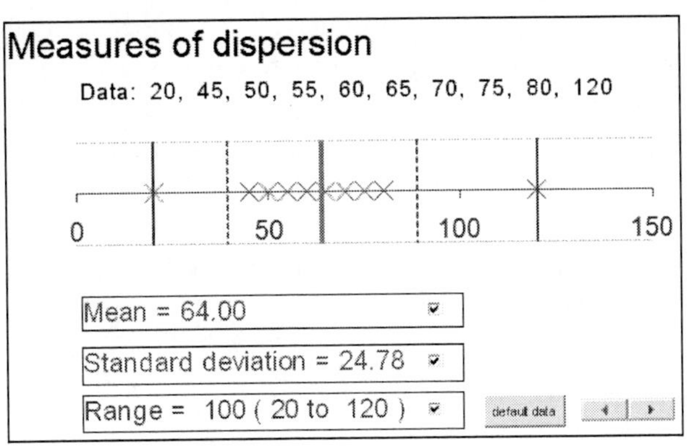

Figure 10. Standard deviation 1

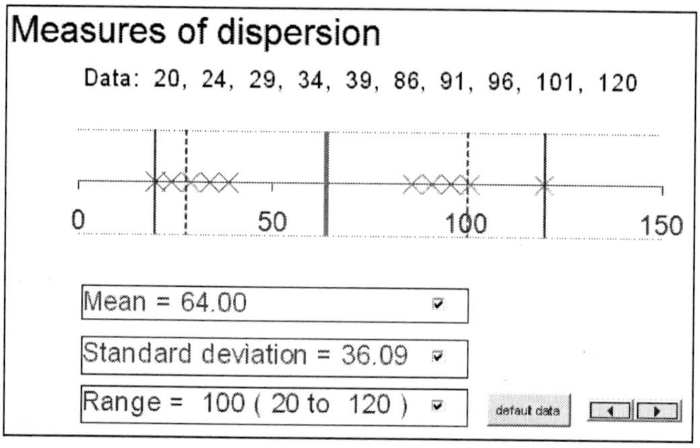

Figure 11. Standard deviation 2

The software allows the data points to be spread or bunched, such that the minimum, mean and maximum are always respectively, 20, 64 and 120. Figure 10 and Figure 11 show that, as a measure of spread, standard deviation is more representative than range.

The calculation of standard deviation was treated separately, using another pictorial presentation. At the end of the one-to-one support session Student A was very happy with what had been covered. She seemed relieved that she could make sense of the topic. She did, however express concern about the rate at which her course was progressing. Grant (2002, p 6) refers to the speed of information processing. Because of their deficit in working memory, dyslexics generally process information more slowly than non-dyslexics.

Hierarchy of Mathematical Concepts

In this section we have attempted to identify a hierarchy of fundamental mathematical concepts which can be used by students to audit their fundamental mathematical knowledge.

Figure 11 shows a hierarchy of fundamental number concepts.

A vital aspect of concept formation, which is difficult to illustrate in a static diagram, is that concept formation is dynamic. Figure 11 shows the concept of addition emerging from the concept of counting. As the concepts of negative numbers and fractions emerge, the concept of addition has to develop to include negative numbers and fractions. Similarly, the concepts of multiplication, division and indices will have to develop. In general, new concepts can require reappraisal and/or extension of existing concepts.

Figure 13 shows the concept of 'Using formulae' to be dependent on the fundamental number concepts shown in Figure 11.

Figure 13 shows the concept of 'Solving equations' to be dependent on the fundamental number concepts shown in Figure 11.

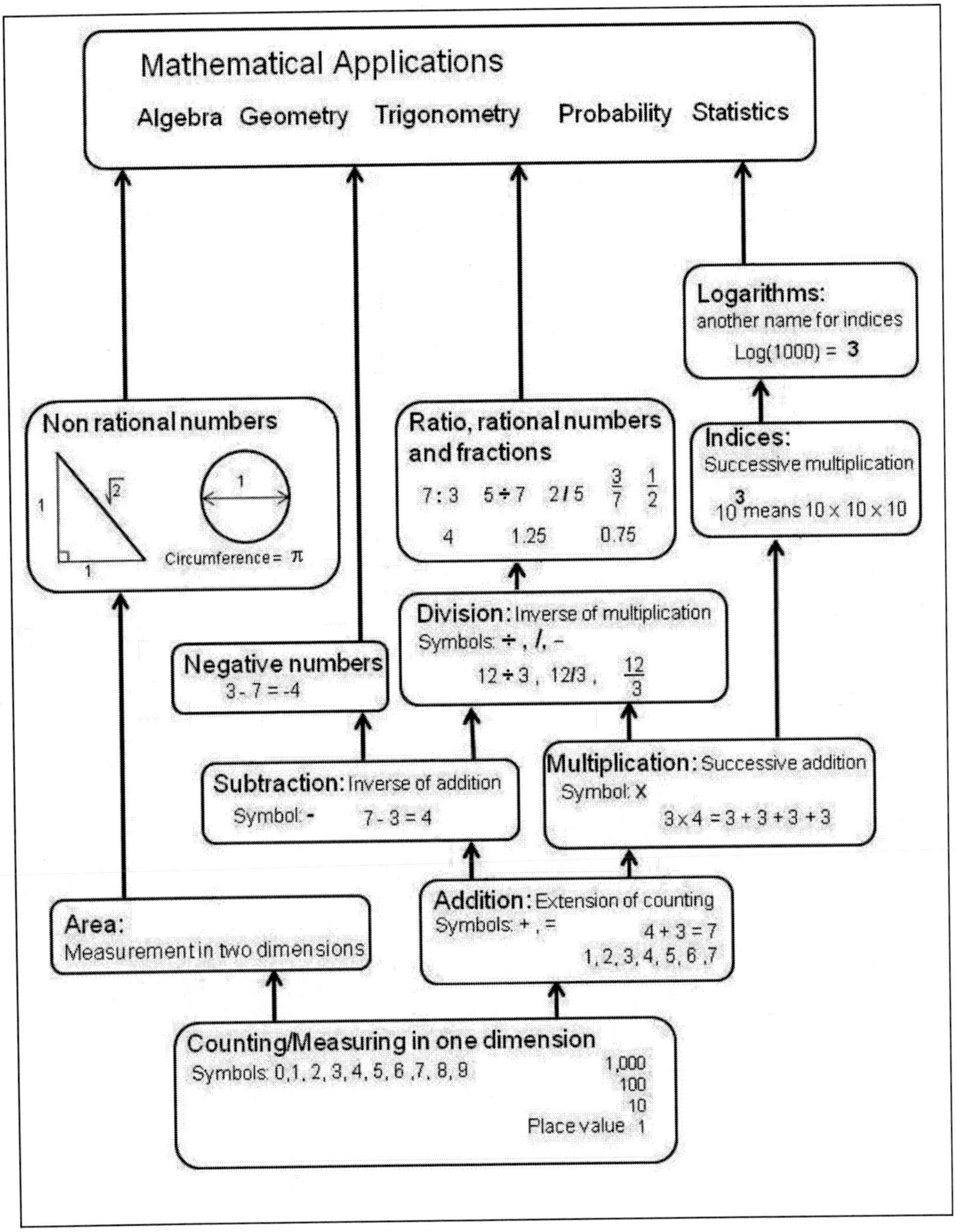

Figure 11. Hierarchy of number concepts

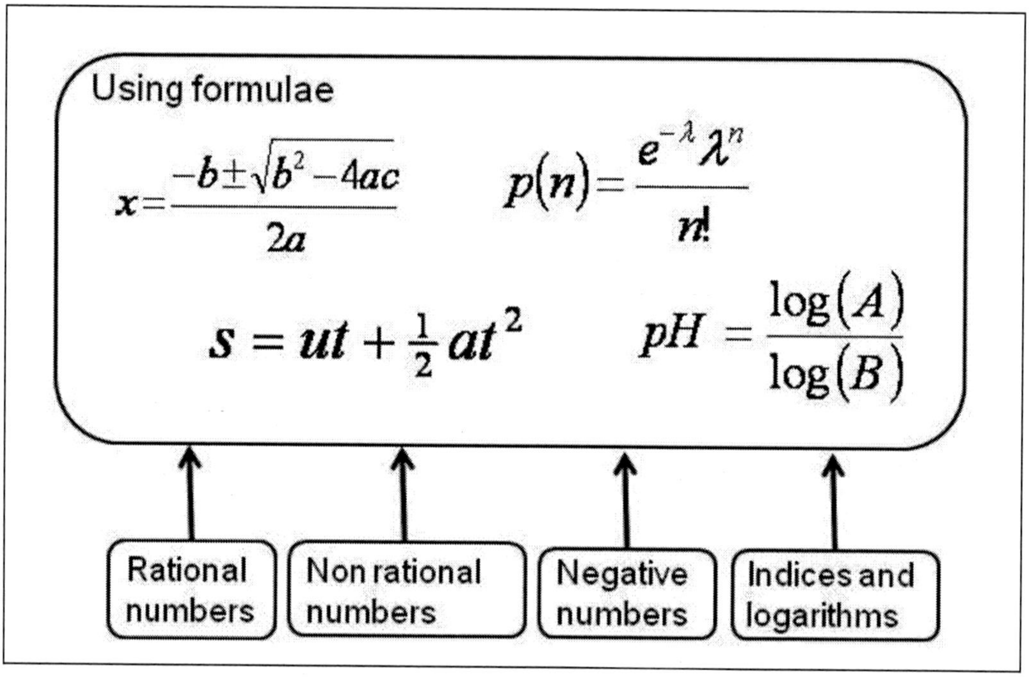

Figure 132. Concepts supporting the concept of 'using formulae'

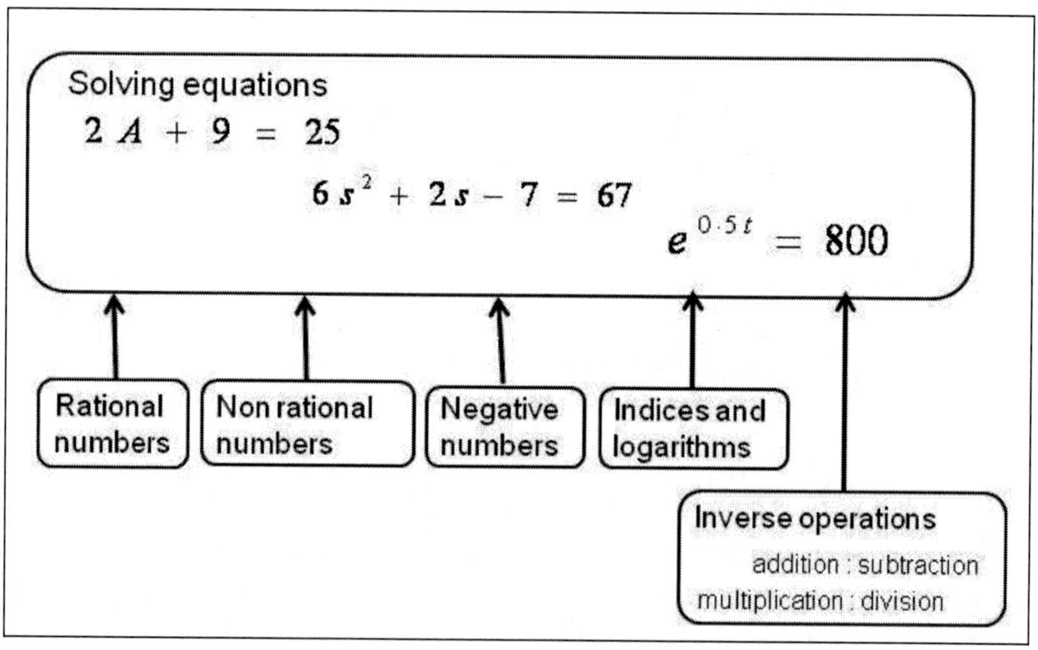

Figure 13. Concepts supporting the concept of 'solving equations'

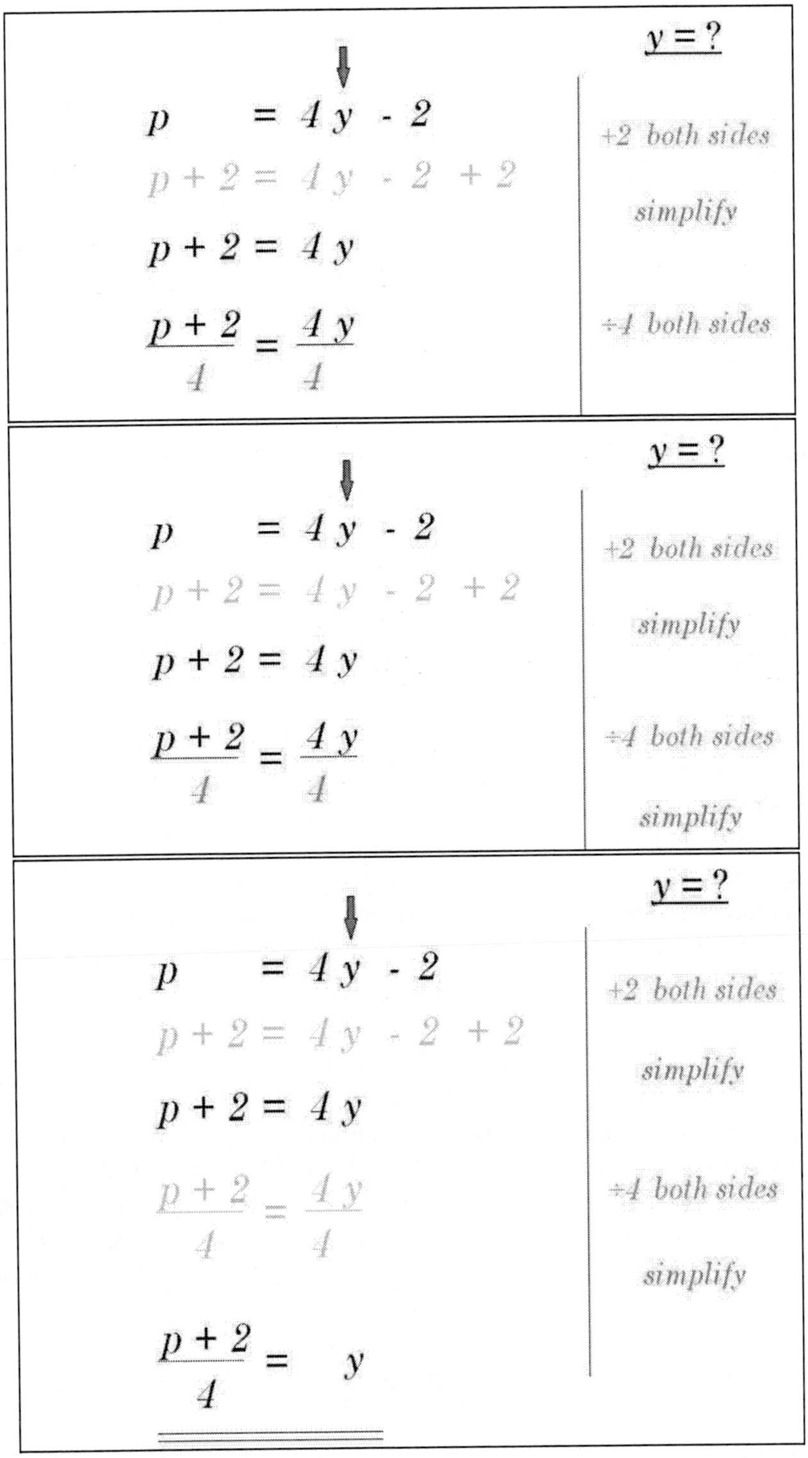

Figure 154. Differentiated pedagogy

Differentiated Pedagogy

In courses where a high formal mathematics qualification is not an entry requirement it is not uncommon for first year groups to be polarised in terms of their mathematical proficiency. This can be a problem for teachers delivering modules with mathematical content, or mathematics modules related to the major subject area.

A steady incline, or ramp, provides access for wheel chair users but does not inhibit walkers, joggers or runners. The principle of differentiated pedagogy is to engage within the same group at the same time, learners with different levels of proficiency. We describe particular instances of the application of the principle, in a particular context.

The material described below is used in our two-week Mathematics Summer School. The broad purpose of the summer School is to prepare students for entry to the Foundation Pathways in Technology (FPT) course at the University of Plymouth. The FPT programme provides an alternative pathway into Higher Education for students who do not have the necessary A level qualifications.

Figure 154 shows the final three slides of slide show demonstrating the transposition of a formula.

For some students intermediate steps in Figure 154 need not be explicit: they do not need to see them in writing. Seeing these steps in writing, however, is not a disadvantage to such students. Promptness of presentation ensures that for such students a minimum amount of time is spent on activity which is unnecessary for them, but which is helpful for others.

It is good pedagogy to explain even the apparently simplest and most obvious terminology. For example, 'the side opposite to the angle we are talking about is called the opposite side.' 'The side adjacent to the angle we are talking about is called the adjacent side. Adjacent means beside or next to.' Some students may be unfamiliar with the words 'adjacent' and/or other words, such as 'dispersion' and 'distribution', which others may regard as being of common usage.

CONCLUSION

Dyslexia is probably the most widely recognised learning disability, but this does not mean that it is widely understood. Grant (2002, p34) corrects some of the commonly held misconceptions, one being that dyslexia is a difficulty affecting only reading and spelling. Dyslexia is a deficit in working memory. Like other disabilities, such as sight and hearing impairments, the deficit can be mild or severe. It's effect on learning varies from one person to another.

Butterworth and Yeo (2004, p1), and Hannell (2005, chapter 1) describe dyscalculia and quote the definition from the United Kingdom Department for Education and Skills (DfES)

> "...a condition that affects the ability to acquire arithmetic skill. Dyscalculic learners may have difficulty understanding simple number concepts, lack an intuitive grasp of number, and have problems learning number facts and procedures..."

Butterworth and Yeo (2004, p2) point out that this definition of dyscalculia is not universally accepted and that there is no agreed criteria for diagnosis. Hannell (2005) cites an estimate that 5% to 8% of school pupils are dyscalculic.

Grant (2002, p 27/28) expresses serious concern that inexpert diagnosis of learning disabilities and their implications for the individual, combined with a policy of widening participation can result in admissions practice with insufficient focus on academic aptitude and potential.

Smith (2004) suggests that new approaches to pedagogy and the employment of ICT should be guiding principles in the construction of possible future pathways for mathematics in schools. Tomlinson (2004, p92-94), concerned that "too many young people are turned off learning and fail to achieve between 14 and 19 [years of age]", devotes a chapter to proposals intended to make education more relevant and appealing to this group. Higher education too is intended to respond to the needs of a wider section of the population.

> "As more people from non-traditional backgrounds go into higher education we must make sure that they are well-served when they get there. (DfES 2003, p63)"

Tomlinson (2004, p96) asserts that actively involving individuals in discussion on the effectiveness the teaching/learning process is not only appropriate but is also conducive to the development of wider attributes and skills. Learners are best served by consulting them.

Smith (2004, p96) puts forward the idea that education needs to be adapted to the needs, if not of the individual learner, then of a range of learners with differing characteristics.

This resonates with the concept of constructive alignment. Interactions, between the student, the teacher and the environment in which the learning takes place, all have a bearing on learning outcomes. Student achievement is maximised when all three of these factors are working in harmony with each other. This harmony is defined as constructive alignment (Biggs 2003).

It is feasible and desirable that as more people with learning disabilities enter main-stream higher education, accommodation of their disabilities will also become main-stream and will not require separate funding. There will almost certainly always be exceptions where special provision has to be made. It is a question of where the line is drawn to define disabled. How impaired does a person's sight have to be before they are diagnosed as 'sight impaired'?

As mathematical concepts are embedded in most HE studies it is imperative that deficient concepts images are identified and corrected. It is also important that new concepts are introduced in a way that relates them to supporting concepts.

There are some measures that can be taken to help develop appropriate concept images. Visual representation seems to be a powerful medium for many dyslexics.

An aspect of what Biggs (2003) calls constructive alignment is making students aware of the inherent mathematical content of the courses when they enrol. The mathematical content of degree courses and its relevance need to be openly identified. It is not satisfactory that higher education students merely acquire knowledge of how to perform statistical tests. It is often the case, however, that students do not see the relevance of the underlying concepts until they need to perform a relatively complex statistical analysis. This is often in the final stages a project which has a deadline, at which point they are less receptive to the acquisition of new concepts and more concerned with processes.

In our experience, adults are not averse to the idea of 'starting from square one'. In a sympathetic environment they are not embarrassed to reveal their perceived failings in mathematics. They want to be helped and welcome the opportunity to go over mathematics and number skills which were first introduced in primary schools. In practice, however, it can be difficult to find time for consolidation, especially when course deadlines have to be met. If the purpose of HE is to engage students in higher level cognitive skills (e.g. analysing, theorising, applying) then finding time to consolidate learning, to reinforce correct concept images and exorcise incorrect concept images, is necessary.

It would be helpful to students entering Universities to have a clear picture of the mathematical demands of their course.

In the preceding text we have put forward a hierarchy of mathematical concepts. With knowledge of this hierarchy and of cognitive paths students might be able to audit their own mathematical concepts and with tutorial support address any weaknesses.

Although our research is not extensive enough to quantify the problem, we suspect that many difficulties which HE students have with mathematics may originate from an inadequate concept image of division; what it means to divide one number by another.

Butterworth (p 302) wrote

> "Many people think they are bad at maths, and they are, but they are not dyscalculic. Usually they have been badly taught, or had unfortunate experiences that reduced zeal to zero." (Butterworth 1999)

Today there are still people entering higher education who acknowledge that they are 'bad at maths.'

The support we provide for students should enable them assimilate mathematical concepts and become confident in using mathematics in their chosen academic discipline. For some students this will mean revisiting fundamental concepts of number. Measures which facilitate schematic learning, allowing students to build appropriate schema or concept images, will be of benefit to students with and without learning difficulties.

REFERENCES

Biggs, J. (2003). *Teaching for Quality Learning at University*. Maidenhead, Open University Press.

Butterworth, B. (1999). *The Mathematical Brain*, Macmillan.

Butterworth, B. & Yeo, D. (2004). *Dyscalculia Guidance*. London, nferNelson.

Cockcroft, W. H. (1982). *Mathematics Counts*. London, Her Majesty's Stationery Office.

McLoughlin, D., Fitzgibbon, G. & Young, V. (1994). *Adult Dyslexia: Assessment, Counselling and Training. London*, Whurr.

DfES. (2001). Students in higher education: by type of course and gender: Social Trends 32. Retrieved 28 May, 2009, from http://www.statistics.gov.uk/STATBASE/ssdataset.asp?vlnk=5027

DfES (2003a). *The future of higher education.*

DfES. (2003b). *Widening participation in higher education*, UK Government.

Gluck, M. A., Mercado, E. & Myers, E. M. (2008). *Learning and Memory, From Brain to Behaviour*. New York

Grant, D. (2002). *The Dyslexias and Diagnosis Issues in Higher Education. Lincoln*, National Association of Disability Officers.

Hannell, G. (2005). *Dyscalculia action plans for successful learning in mathematics. Abingdon*, David Fulton.

Mortimore, T. (2003). *Dyslexia: and Leaning Style, A Practitioner's Handbook*. London.

ONS. (2001). Population: age, sex and legal marital status. Retrieved, 28 May, 2009, from http://www.statistics.gov.uk/statbase/Expodata/Spreadsheets/D9657.xls

Robbins, (1963). *Higher Education*. London, United Kingdom Government: 1-335.

Skemp, R. R. (1993). *The Psychology of Learning Mathematics*. Middlesex, Penguin.

Smith, A. (2004). *Making Mathematrics Count. London*, The Stationery Office Ltd.

Tall, D. & Vinner, S. (1981). Concept Image and concept Definition in Mathematics with particular reference to limits and continuity. Educational Studies in Mathematics *12*, 151-169.

Tomlinson, M. (2004). 14-19 *Curriculum and Qualifications Reform. London*, HM Government: 1-116.

Vinner, S. (1981). Concept definition, concept image and the notion of function. *International Journal of Mathematical Education in Science and Technology*, *14(3)*, 293-305.

Vinner, S. & Hershkowitz, R. (1983). On concept formation Zetrablatt Fur Didaktik. *Der Mathematik*, *83(1)*, 20-25.

In: Speech Disorders: Causes, Treatment and Social Effects ISBN: 978-1-60876-213-2
Editor: Alan E. Harrison, pp. 221-236

Chapter 10

SPEECH EVALUATION AND SPEECH REHABILITATION AFTER ORAL AND OROPHARYNGEAL CANCER TREATMENT

Viviane de Carvalho-Teles[1] and Ingrid Gielow[2]
[1]Instituto do Câncer Arnaldo Vieira de Carvalho, São Paulo, Brazil
[2]Federal University of São Paulo, São Paulo, Brazil.

ABSTRACT

The intra-oral structures are essential for the chewing, swallowing, speech and vocal production functions, effects in these functions, as well as the aesthetic, social and emotional aspects related to oral cancers, do affect these patients. These effects are caused both by the tumor, and by its treatment (surgery, radiotherapy and/or chemotherapy). There are few studies with the use of objective or subjective instruments to evaluate the resulting speech and voice, still scarcer are the studies that discuss the speech-therapy strategies and their results for these oncology patients. Objective: Review and present both the voice and speech evaluation instruments, and the therapy strategies used for the improvement of the oral communication of oral cavity and oropharynx cancer patients. Method: Perform a literature review between 1967 and 2009 with the Medline describer (speech OR voice OR therapy) AND (oral cancer OR oropharynx cancer), with the exclusion of the papers that present results without formal evaluation instruments and case studies. Results: Eighty four studies were found meeting the criteria established. Thirty-four studies used quality of life protocols for functional evaluation and in 50 studies there was the citation of the utilization of some type of voice or speech evaluation clinical observations to describe function. Speech therapy procedures and their strategies/results concerning speech and voice were found in only 5 studies. Conclusions: Perceptive-auditory evaluation was the most used, with speech intelligibility as the most analyzed parameter. But studies concerning the speech-therapy treatment of these patients are still scarce, and their results seem to be influenced by the size of the samples, by the number of speech-therapy sessions, and by the eventual effects of the variety of the exercises performed.

INTRODUCTION

The incidence of oral and oropharynx cancers is growing all over the world [1-3]. The intra-oral structures are fundamental for the chewing, swallowing, speech and vocal production functions. Effects in these functions, as well as aesthetic and emotional impacts, may occur due to the presence of the tumor and/or its treatment (surgery, radio-therapy and/or chemotherapy).

The impact on the oral communication of these patients may occur due to the reduction in the intelligibility of the speech caused by articulation, resonance or pronunciation alterations. Notwithstanding, there are few studies on this theme using subjective or objective tools to evaluate speech and voice [4-6]..Moreover, there is no uniformity concerning the methodologies used for these evaluations [7].

This is also the problem with the studies on the speech-therapy for rehabilitation of oral communication of these patients. Speech-therapy after ablative surgeries of the oral cavity and oro-pharynx is mentioned as one of the necessities to improve quality of life [8,9]. However, there are few studies that present the strategies and the functional results after speech-therapy related specifically to voice and speech. Due to the great impact that these patients feel concerning swallowing, and because this function is connected to survival [10], most of the studies deal with swallowing [11-13]. But oral communication rehabilitation is fundamental to restore independence as a speaker to the patient, as well as to improve his/her family relationships and to resume social and professional contacts [14].

Thus, the objective of the present work is to review and present the voice and speech evaluation tools, as well as the therapeutic strategies used for the improvement of the oral and oropharynx cancer patients oral communication.

Method

A literature review using the Medline data bank between 1967 and January 2009 was performed with the describers (speech OR voice) AND (oral cancer OR oropharynx cancer) AND (treatment OR rehabilitation). Excluded were the papers with only one clinical case, and the ones without a population study (such as reviews of surgical and/or prosthetic techniques), or which presented only functional results without evaluation criteria. The most relevant studies are presented in tables, and their results are discussed.

Results

Eighty four studies were found meeting the criteria established. Among them, there were 34 in which quality of life protocols for functional evaluation were employed, and the most used questionnaires were EORTC, Washington and Glasglow. In 50 studies the utilization of some type of voice or speech evaluation was cited. The number of patients varied between 5 and 293 patients (48.9 ± 61.1). The most frequent tumor sites were the oral cavity associated with the oropharynx (18), followed by the oral cavity (16). In 45 studies the most prescribed oncologic treatment was surgery, with or without adjuvant radiotherapy.

In 29 of the 50 studies speech articulation analysis was used to verify the functionality of a specific type of surgical and/or a prosthetic reconstruction. The most frequent reconstructions were on the oral tongue and/or on its base (10 studies), followed by the jaw and oral cavity associated with the oropharynx (5 studies each); there were 4 studies about lip reconstruction, and the reconstruction of the soft and hard palates was cited in 3 studies. Swallowing was evaluated in 35 of the 50 studies, but these results are outside the scope of this work. In 6 studies, besides subjective and/or objective evaluations, an auto-evaluation of the speech and/or the swallowing was performed by the patients.

In most of the studies (35), the functional evaluation was performed after the oncological treatment, with intervals that varied from 1 to 48 months. These evaluations were made from 2 to 4 times in 10 studies, with 1, 3, 6 and 12 months intervals being the most used. In 13 studies the functional characteristics were evaluated both before and after oncological treatment, as opposed to in only 2 where they were evaluated only beforehand.

In 48 studies a perceptive-auditory evaluation of speech and/or voice and/or resonance was carried out and, among them, only 5 studies were directed to voice and/or resonance analysis.

An objective speech articulation evaluation was used in 6 studies, considering the frequency of vowel formants of glossectomized patients (2), the voice resonance of patients with connection between the oral and the nasal cavities (2), and the application of computer programs for voice recognition (2).

Both studies concerning the vowel formants used spectrographic acoustic analysis with linear predictive coding to determine the formants F1, F2 and F3, having as speech material either /i/, or all the oral vowels of the language of the patients [15,16]. Objective evaluation of resonance was performed on the nasalance produced using sentences with voiced and voiceless consonants [17].

The main speech materials used in the 50 studies were: vowels (2), monosyllables (2), words (4), sentences (5), standardized speech articulation tests (9), and spontaneous talks (17). In 20 studies, most of them considering the effectiveness of the surgical reconstruction retails, the standardized speech materials were not used. Intelligibility of the speech was evaluated by the physicians or by the patients solely through informal conversation. Perceptive-auditory evaluation was carried out by speech-therapists (23 studies), linguists (1), phoniatricians (1) and physicians (6), while for the 19 remaining studies, which mostly concerned surgical reconstructions, the evaluator was not identified.

Speech intelligibility was classified using: standardized scales with 3 to 10 exposure levels (in 11 studies), percent of spontaneous speech intelligibility (17), and percent of correctly identified words (16). In most of the surgical reconstruction studies speech intelligibility was determined through non-standardized scales, usually with 3 or 4 levels: excellent, good, regular, and poor.

Table 1 shows 9 studies that were selected because they involve a greater number of patients and use a standardized evaluation protocol [5, 15, 16, 18-23].

Besides the studies on Table 1, the multi-centers study presented by Perry et al. [24] is noted, because it considers 293 head and neck surgery patients that were taken care of by speech-therapists between April 1997 and April 1999; 99 of them had laryngectomies or pharyngolaryngectomies, and 85 had oral cancer. Among these latter patients (oral cancer) the ones with T3 or T4 tumors who, thus, were submitted to more aggressive or extensive treatments, presented worse functional results than the T1 and T2 tumors patients. The T3 and

T4 patients had more statistically significant problems involving the saliva and husky voices when compared with T1 and T2 ones. Considering the patients with new oral cancers (59), 28 of them were treated only with surgery, 28 with surgery followed by radiotherapy, and 3 with radio and chemotherapy.

Concerning speech impairment, intelligibility and speech disability, 3 and 12 months after the procedures, the patients submitted to surgery followed by radiotherapy presented statistically significant worse functional results than the ones submitted only to surgery. Unfortunately, it is not mentioned if the patients underwent speech-therapy, the number of sessions or the specific exercises that were carried out.

Speech therapy procedures and their strategies/results concerning speech and voice were found (described) in only 5 studies, which are presented below.

Four of these studies [25-28] were carried out by American multi-center groups, and thus used similar methodologies.

Pauloski et al [25] evaluated the speech and swallowing functions of 16 patients (11 men and 5 women) aged 58±12 (range 30 to 71) years with anterior tongue and floor of the mouth resection, which were reconstructed with distal flap closure. The speech and swallowing data were collected before surgery and on the first and third months after surgery. The speech materials recorded were 6 to 7 minutes of spontaneous conversation, which were judged by novice listeners and through the Fisher Logemann Test of Articulation Competence, a standardized articulation test evaluated by a Speech Therapist. Seven of the 16 patients were submitted to 6±4 speech therapy sessions (range 1 to 10), with a duration of 36±22 and a range of 120 minutes; 83% of the treatments were effected during the first after-surgery month. The speech treatment of six of the patients emphasized articulation exercises: five patients worked on the improvement of the contact of the tip of the tongue with the hard palate, four exercised the contact of the middle of the tongue with the hard palate, and six patients worked the contact of the base of the tongue with the soft palate; two patients were also oriented concerning the compensatory articulation with the pharynx, glottal stops and fricatives. The intelligibility of spontaneous speech of the 16 patients was 77% before surgery, and fell to about 50% after surgery, thus showing the absence of improvement three months after surgery. Similarly, the percentage of consonants perfectly perceived fell from 84% to 47% (49%) during the first (third) month after surgery. The absence of improvement at the third month was attributed to the radiotherapy that finished two weeks before the last evaluation, to the few patients submitted to speech therapy and/or to the small number of speech therapy sessions.

A second study by the same researchers [26] evaluated the speech and swallowing of 11 patients submitted to resections greater than 1 cm at the tongue base, tonsil, and faucial arch, with the mandible resected on the side of the tumor and reconstruction by primary closure. The speech of all patients was recorded before surgery, and one and three months after surgery, with the inclusion of 6 to 7 minutes samples of spontaneous speech, and the sentence version of the Fisher Logemann Test of Articulation Competence. Nine patients were submitted to speech therapy, with six receiving swallowing rehabilitation, and only three getting swallowing and speech rehabilitations. There were 4±1 (range 1 to 11) speech therapy sessions, with a duration of 38±11 (range 8 to 195) minutes. The speech treatment objective was to improve the contact between the tongue and the palate, aiming at the alveolar and velar stops of plosive sounds. The intelligibility of the spontaneous speech for all patients fell from 86% before surgery to 72% (80%) during the first (third) month after surgery. The intelligibility percentage of consonants was practically normal before surgery, but one and three months after surgery the patients presented very low levels for these speech materials, mainly for lingual stops, fricatives and affricatives, which were less intelligible during the third month, although the one to three month differences were not statistically significant.

Paulosky et al [27] aimed to determine the improvement of speech and swallowing for 28 men and 10 women between one and eleven months after mouth cavity surgery, using a standardized protocol before surgery and at 1, 3, 6 and 12 months after surgery, with the same methodology of the two previous studies. The results showed that there was functional improvement between 1 and 12 months after surgery, as the speech and swallowing levels at 1 and 3 months were similar to the ones at 12 months after surgery. This lack of improvement was attributed to the small number of speech therapy sessions attended by the patients. In addition, several functional variables deteriorated at the sixth month probably due to radiotherapy after-effects.

Logemann et al [28] evaluated 102 patients in a pilot investigation of a large study on the effects of oral cancer resection and speech and swallowing procedures. All patients received speech therapy, and were assessed prior to treatment, and one and 3 months post-treatment. They were given instruction on how to perform range of motion (ROM) exercises for the lips, tongue, jaw, and larynx, as well as therapies to improve the placement of the tongue and lips to produce speech sounds. The ROM exercises involved extending the structure in the target direction as far as possible, holding the extended posture for 1 to 2 seconds, and then releasing it. This sequence was repeated 10 times in each session. The motion range of the laryngeal elevation involved sliding up the musical scale as high as possible into the falsetto range, and then holding the highest note produced for several seconds. For laryngeal adduction, the motion range included exercises to move the arytenoid cartilages, such as repeating the vowel "a" using a hard attack, taking a breath and then holding it with effort, cough, clear the throat, and so on. In contrast, the exercises to improve coordination involved chewing, manipulating something such as chewing gum or a button in the mouth from side to side, as well as teaching the placement of the tongue to produce particular speech sounds. The patients were instructed to do the set of exercises from 5 up to 10 minutes, 10 times each day, if possible. They had one to two follow-up sessions to check their performance of the exercises. All measurements of speech intelligibility and consonant production of the patients that performed ROM exercises were statistically more significant than those of the ones that did not do these exercises.

Fúria et al [29] evaluated the speech intelligibility before and after speech therapy of 27 patients (24 men and 3 women) between ages of 34 and 77 (mean 56.5 years) that underwent glossectomy. They were divided into three groups according to the extent of the tongue resection: 1- total (6 patients), 2- sub-total (9) and 3- partial (12). The objective of the perceptive-auditory evaluation was to verify the speech intelligibility, determined by three speech therapists, of the following speech materials that were recorded before and after the speech therapy: seven sustained oral vowels, vowel in a syllable, sequence of vowel-consonant-vowel (VCV) and connected speech, that is, a story after its visual presentation on cards. The intelligibility of the spontaneous speech (sequence story) was scored in consensus from 1 to 4. A 16 session program was proposed to all patients, and the average attended by groups 1 and 3 was 10, and for group 2 it was 12. It was intended to maximize the use of the remaining structures, mainly the residual motion of the tongue, and to develop compensatory articulation adaptations. The steps were the following: differentiation of isolated vowels and vowels with bilabial phonemes; phonemic review to maximize adaptation and compensatory movements (articulation contacts and/or mobility of remaining structures) to reduce distortion and substitute articulation; modification of supra-segmentary functions pause (distinctive value), duration, intensity, and intonation (ascendant and descendent curves, high and low pitch); reduction of speech rate (words per minute); pneumo-phono-articulatory coordination; speech and saliva coordination; over-articulation exercises; yawning and chewing; and support of auditory feedback. The average intelligibility of spontaneous speech improved significantly for groups 1 (3.33 to 2.50) and 2 (2.78 to 1.65). Group 1 improved vowels, VCV, and spontaneous speech; group 2 improved syllable, VCV, and spontaneous speech. Group 3 demonstrated better intelligibility in the pre-therapy phase, but the improvement after therapy was not significant, possibly due to the small and heterogeneous sample.

Comment

The impact on the speech and voice of patients after oncologic treatment of tumors of the oral cavity and oropharynx has been well established in the literature [29]. However, not all studies adopt standardized protocols for the evaluation of speech articulation, thus preferring the use of generic terms to qualify it. This complicates comparisons with other studies and, even, observation of the clinical evolution of a patient [25]. According to Logemann et al [26], the knowledge of the types of functional changes that occur after head and neck surgeries may be useful both for pre-surgery guidance, and for the planning and establishment of more effective procedures for the rehabilitation after a certain surgery.

The literature review shows that many studies adopted some type of formal evaluation that could more properly qualify the functional changes after the oncological treatment of oral cavity and oro-pharynx tumors. Thirty-four studies used quality of life protocols to evaluate the speech, voice and swallowing of the affected population. During the last two decades, the valorization of and preoccupation with the quality of life (QOL), and not only the survival of the patients, have led to the creation of several standardized protocols on QOL such as EORTC and Washington. QOL was defined as the perceived discrepancy between the actual status and the ideal standards of the patients [30]. These protocols are important to compare the functional results obtained by the multidisciplinary team with the satisfaction of the patient with the same items. In this way the team may know if the procedure used, both for the treatment and for the rehabilitation of the patient, is sufficient or has benefited him according to his expectations. This may lead to the remodeling of established strategies and procedures to serve patients of the same surgery type, considering their emotional, social and educational profiles. Also, the speech therapist may better direct his work when it is possible to improve the oral function that disturbs the patient, as well as making him accept his possible limitations.

The number of oral cavity or oro-pharynx tumor patients in the fifty studies that evaluated voice or speech was highly variable, which causes difficulty to homogenize groups. This is also due to the great number of structures of the oral cavity and oro-pharynx, in possibly different clinical stages and, consequently, leading to distinct treatments [28]. In the studies considered in the present work, most of the tumors were treated through surgery that may or not have been associated with radiotherapy.

Table 1. Studies with standardized evaluation protocol of speech and/or voice and/or resonance.

Paper	Patients	Surgery	Perceptual evaluation	Objective evaluation	Results
Carvalho -Teles et al [15]	36	Total glossectomy (14) Total glossectomy and partial mandibulectomy (12) Hemiglossectomy (6) Subtotal glossectomy plus radiotherapy plus augmentation prosthesis for at least 3 months (4)	Spontaneous speech intelligibility: assessed by expert listeners using a 4-category scale Number of correctly identified syllables with/without prosthesis	Formants spectrographic frequency assessment Seven sustained oral vowels in Brazilian Portuguese for at least 4s	Improvement: - Spontaneous speech intelligibility - Number of correctly identified syllables with the use of the prosthesis . - Mean F2 and F3 values were obtained for all vowels and the F1 values for the vowels /o,ó,u/.
Kazi et al[16]	26 control group (30)	Parcial glossectomy	No	F1, F2 and F3 determinations. Sustained vowel /i/ for at least 5 s	Mean F1 were raised, while mean F2 and F3 scores were reduced in partial glossectomy patients when compared with normal control.
Stecewicz et al [18]	112	Surgery plus radiotherapy Tumor site: Oral cavity	Speech articulation quality was evaluated audio-visually:. Syllables and words with phonemes of the contemporary Polish language (according to Roclawski).		Frequency and quality of abnormal phonation and the presence of characteristic compensatory mechanisms depended on the extent of post-operative deficits and functional efficiency of adjacent structures. Correlation between the quality of pronunciation and efficiency of swallowing was statistically significant.

Table 1. (Continued)

Paper	Patients	Surgery	Perceptual evaluation	Objective evaluation	Results
Markkanen-Leppa¨nen et al [5]	44	Surgery plus micro-vascular free tissue transfer plus radiotherapy. Tumor site: Oral cavity (28) Oral pharynx (13) Hypopharynx (3)	No	1.Nasalance: sentences with voiceless plosive consonants or voiced consonants 2. Measuring aeromechanically the velopharyngeal orifice area during speech plus the nasal cross-sectional area and nasal resistance. Evaluation before surgery, and 6 weeks, 3, 6 and 12 months thereafter.	After the surgery: The oral cavity patients showed adequate velopharyngeal closure and nasalance. Six months after surgery the velopharynx orifice size was significantly greater in the oropharyngeal Cancer patients than in the oral cavity ones.
Rogers et al, 2002 [19]	130	Surgery with/without radiotherapy Tumor site: Oral cavity Oral pharynx	Eleven clinical examination : Lip competence, tongue movement, oral mucosa, dental state, mouth opening, speech, drooling, diet, appearance, oral sensation and motion. Intelligibility Scale: 0- Unintelligible 1- Most words unintelligible 2- Few words unintelligible 3- Normal Evaluation:before operation, 6 and 12 months afterwards.		Speech Results: Pre-treatment: 2.90 6 months after treatment: 2.64 12 months after treatment: 2.77

Table 1. (Continued)

Paper	Patients	Surgery	Perceptual evaluation	Objective evaluation	Results
McKinstry, Perry[20]	20	Chemo and/or radiotherapy Oropharynx (11) Larynx (7) Hypopharynx (1)	% of words intelligible in an audiotape-recorded free speech/conversation task. plus Subscales of the Frenchay Dysarthria Assessment: 1. intelligibility of words, sentences ,conversation 2. respiration in speech; 3. lip spread, seal, alternate motion and in speech 4. soft palate maintenance and soft palate in speech; laryngeal time, pitch, volume and in speech; 5. tongue movements and in speech Clinical assessment by the researcher, and a self-assessment made by the patient. Evaluation: before treatment		Impairment in both speech intelligibility and in almost all aspects of speech. The site of the cancer vs the type of impairment experienced with respect to the speech function. Not all motor speech characteristics correlated with overall speech intelligibility and, lastly, self-report and clinical assessment were significantly correlated with respect to motor speech characteristics, but they differed slightly in the assessment of speech intelligibility.

Table 1. (Continued)

Paper	Patients	Surgery	Perceptual evaluation	Objective evaluation	Results
McConnel et al[21]	54	Oral tongue and/or tongue base surgery plus with/without radiotherapy. Three sets of patient pairs: 9 primary closure vs 9 distal-flap reconstruction. 9 primary closure vs 9 free-flap reconstruction. 9 distal-flap reconstruction vs 9 free flaps.	% Conversational speech intelligibility: recording of a 6- to 7-minute conversational speech sample % Sentence-articulation test : Fisher-Logemann Test of Articulation Competence. Speech Data were evaluated by Speech-language pathologists		Speech Intelligibility %: Primary closure 90.0 vs distal-flap closure 52.0*. Primary closure 72.0 vs free-flap closure 55.0**. Distal-flap closure 48.0. vs free-flap closure 49.0**. Correct consonant** % Primary closure 75.0 vs distal-flap closure 58.0. Primary closure 59.0 vs free-flap closure 49.0. Primary closure 75.0 vs distal-flap closure 58.0. Distal-flap closure 49.0. vs free-flap closure 59.0. * statistically different ** statistically not different

Table 1. (Continued)

Paper	Patients	Surgery	Perceptual evaluation	Objective evaluation	Results
Pauloski et [22]	142	Surgery plus Chemo and/or radiotherapy Tumor site: oral and oropharyngeal cancer	% Conversational speech intelligibility: recording of a 6- to 7-minute conversational speech sample % percent correct consonant phonemes : Fisher-Logemann Test of Articulation Competence. Speech evaluation: 3 months after treatment.		The worst speech function was associated with larger amounts of resected tissue. Measures of conversational understandability and % correct consonant phonemes were related to the extent of the oral tongue resection, floor of the mouth resection, soft palate resection, and total volume of tissue resected. The combination of: closure type, % oral tongue resected, - % soft palate resected had the strongest relationship with the overall speech function f
Bundgaard et al [23]	81	Surgery plus Chemo and/or radiotherapy Tumor site: intra-oral squamous cell carcinoma	Speech Intelligibility Scale: 7- No sound errors are noticed 6- Sound errors are occasionally noticed 5- Speech is intelligible but with many errors 4-Speech is intelligible only with careful listening 3-Speech intelligibility is difficult 2- Speech is usually unintelligible 1- Speech is unintelligible Evaluation: 28 months after surgery		Speech Intelligibility Scale Results Surgery (n = 17): 6.8 Radiotherapy (n = 13): 6.9 Combined therapy (n = 13): 6.4 Recurrence (n = 13): 5.2 Mucosal,surface cheek (n = 13) 6,3 Tongue (n= 12): 6.2 Mand. alveolus (n=4): 5.8 Retromolar area (n=4):6.5 Floor of mouth (n = 10):6.3

Reflecting the advance of the surgical techniques and a greater concern with the QOL of the patients with oral cavity and oropharynx tumors, more than half of the studies verified the functional impact (on speech, voice or swallowing) of a specific type of surgical reconstruction. According to Duflo et al [31] this therapeutic procedure may be considered as an integral part of the treatment and rehabilitation of head and neck cancer. However, most of the studies did not use standardized protocols for the speech articulation evaluation. As expected, swallowing, which is a neuro-vegetative function connected to survival was evaluated in 72% of the studies. Prosthetic reconstruction, associated or not to the surgical one, was the object of some studies [15,32,33].

The interval between the oncological treatment and the evaluation of the speech and voice, as well as the number of evaluations after surgery also varied among the 35 studies that considered them. Besides the difference of the time of application of the protocols among the different institutions, this may also reflect the weight given at each of them to these evaluations, as well as the adjustment of the multidisciplinary team.

Few studies compared the speech articulation aspects before and after the oncological treatment, or accompanied the time-longitudinal evolution of the patients after this treatment. The first type of study may show how these aspects are influenced by the treatment or the tumor. The second one determines: the sequels remain along time; the factors that contribute for the maintenance or the deterioration of post-oncological treatment sequels; the therapies (surgery, radiotherapy or chemotherapy) that cause greater impacts on the oral communication, and the power of the speech therapy to minimize these sequels.

The perceptual-auditory evaluation was the most used speech and voice analysis type used in the studies, as was also found by Mlynarek et al [7]. Even with the advent of objective voice and speech measures, which help and give foundation for the perceptual-auditory evaluation, it still remains above any acoustic voice and speech analysis [34]. The association among different methods of subjective and objective evaluations should be stimulated because it favors both a more global view of the speech and voice of the patients, and provides more clues about the changes of these functions [7].

Speech intelligibility was the most analyzed parameter among the studies. This was expected, because the oncological treatment of the oral cavity and oro-pharynx tumors causes important damages in the speech articulators [5]. Spontaneous conversation was the speech material most used to evaluate speech intelligibility, probably because it most accurately reflects the impact on the oral communication of the patients after the oncological treatment [25]. This type of material, due to its numerous contextual clues, may favor the increase of the spontaneous conversation intelligibility of these patients [35].

Speech intelligibility has been classically evaluated through scales with different levels. But, unfortunately, these scales vary widely, which makes the comparison among the studies that evaluate this parameter impossible. Some scales present up to 10 levels, thus increasing the confusion and variability of this evaluation among the judges, while others offer only three choices, thus limiting the possibility of intermediate levels. Probably to avoid this type of problem, the majority (33) of the studies used the percentage of spontaneous speech intelligibility, or the percentage of correctly identified words to evaluate the impact of this parameter. This method is intended to reduce the subjectivity of the analysis and permits a greater comparability among the studies.

Even as the vocal tract is also modified by the treatments above mentioned, studies concerning speech resonance and the formants of the vowels are still scarce [15,16].

Vocal evaluation per se was effected in only two studies, in which the vocal quality was considered normal after the oncological treatment of the patients. This was the case in the Markkanen-Leppänen [17] study because most of the patients had T2 tumors, which usually imply more conservative surgeries, with a reconstruction with a micro-surgical retail, thus resulting in a better functioning of the remaining structures [36]. However, the advanced T3 and T4 tumors, which require more aggressive oncological treatments, may evolve with vocal alterations such as the hoarseness observed by Perry et al [24] and Stecewicz et al [18]. Further, these patients may present saliva and food stases in the oropharynx and in the laryngeal vestibular, which may compromise the vocal quality and the resonance of these patients. Mády et al [37] cite that the surgery to extract a primary tumor of the oral cavity or the oro-pharynx may affect the supra and infra-hyoid muscles, and thus may specifically cause changes in F0 and the intonation, plus reduction of the voice modulation.

A speech therapist was responsible for judging the speech, voice or resonance in less than half of the studies that included the perceptual-auditory evaluation in their methodology; in the remaining studies, there was no reference to who evaluated these parameters, once more demonstrating the lack of standardization in these analyses, and hence inspiring doubts about their results.

Speech rehabilitation is fundamental for the re-establishing of patients' inter-personal communication, which is effected traditionally through speech therapy[28,38]; according to Markkanen-Leppänen et al [5] it is recommended even if important articulation alterations are not present. Despite this recognition, only 5 studies mentioned or presented strategies and results concerning the speech of the patients after the speech therapy intervention. Three of these studies were presented by the same research group [25-27], and less than half of the patients involved were submitted to speech therapy, with a low average number of sessions. These studies showed that the intelligibility of consonants deteriorated drastically after surgery. It did not recover even after one year, and the authors attributed this to the small number of speech therapy sessions and radio-therapy. However, these results do not nullify the role of speech therapy, and as the impacts of the surgery on speech, voice and resonance are very important, they signal that more efforts and time should be invested to achieve the rehabilitation of these functions. Probably other aspects, besides articulation, should be worked out, due to the permanent alteration caused to the vocal tract. So, compensatory strategies should be found for resonance, vocal projection, pitch and loudness, among others. The results of these studies may be used to alert the health caretaker and the patient about the impacts of radiotherapy on oral communication. Radiotherapy may postpone or slow down the clinical evolution of the speech therapy, and Markkanen-Leppa¨nen [5] and Logemann et al [26] mention that patients may develop xerostomy with consequent speech damages. The remaining structures must stay lubricated with saliva to achieve the maximum range of movement. Carvalho-Teles et al [39] noted that maxillectomized patients with a maxilla obturating prosthesis that were submitted to radiotherapy presented a lower intelligibility level when compared with the same type of patients without radiotherapy. To minimize the effects of radiotherapy, strategies such as taking small gulps of water over short intervals, or using artificial saliva, should be used not only during eating, but also when speaking.

The studies of Logmann et al [28] and Fúria et al [29] presented better results concerning speech-therapy treatments probably because of their great number of patients, with longer treatment times, thus permitting the employment of more therapeutic strategies, such as: isotonic and isometric exercises (ROM) involving all remaining structures; articulation exercises; supra-segmentary modifications; and pneumo-phono-articulatory coordination (related to the correct use of the pauses). Further, their patients were monitored during the whole treatment, which probably allowed doing changes and interventions when needed, thus improving the performance of each patient. Also, the frequency of the exercises probably improved the results, as the patients were oriented to exercise every day, several times.

Thus, as may be seen in this review, a great number of studies are still needed to demonstrate the effectiveness of speech-therapy for the rehabilitation of head and neck cancer patients. Notwithstanding, the number of these studies seems to be decreasing. They are not easy to carry out, due to factors such as, among others: the medium and longtime follow-up, which may lead to the patient's abandonment of the treatment; reduced survival; tumor recidivism; and acute and late radiotherapy consequences. Even so, more studies should be carried out, perhaps as cooperative multi-center efforts, aiming at not only post-surgery functional results, but also at post-speech-therapy results.

Conclusion

Considering the studies analyzed, there is a great variety of methodologies applied for the evaluation of the voice and speech of patients after oral cavity and oropharynx tumor treatment. Perceptive-auditory evaluation was the most used, with speech intelligibility as the most analyzed parameter. But studies concerning the speech-therapy treatment of these patients are still scarce, and their results seem to be influenced by the size of the samples, by the number of speech-therapy sessions, and by the eventual effects of the variety of the exercises performed. Thus, additional speech-therapy studies, using standardized protocols and possibly as cooperative multi-center efforts, are still needed for this group of patients.

References

[1] Kingsley, K; O'Malley, S; Ditmyer, M; Chino, M. Analysis of oral cancer epidemiology in the US reveals state-specific trends: implications for oral cancer prevention. *BMC Public Health*, 2008, 8, 87.

[2] Conway, DI; Stockton, DL; Warnakulasuriya, KA; Ogden, G; Macpherson, LM. Incidence of oral and oropharyngeal cancer in United Kingdom (1990-1999) recent trends and regional variation. *Oral Oncol*, 2006, 42(6), 586-92.

[3] Durazzo, MD; et. al. Clinical and epidemiological features of oral cancer in a medical school teaching hospital from 1994 to 2002: increasing incidence in women, predominance of advanced local disease, and low incidence of neck metastases. *Clinics*, 2005, 60(4), 293-298.

[4] Kazi, R. et al. Analysis of formant frequencies in patients with oral or oropharyngeal cancers treated by glossectomy. *Int J Lang Commun Disord*, 2007, 42(5), 521-32.

[5] Markkanen-Leppänen, M; Isotalo, E; Mäkitie, AA; Asko-Seljavaara, S; Pessi, T; Suominen, E; Haapanen, ML. Changes in articulatory proficiency following microvascular reconstruction in oral or oropharyngeal cancer. *Oral Oncol*, 2006, 42(6), 646-52.

[6] Nicoletti, G; Soutar, DS; Jackson, MS; Wrench, AA; Robertson, G; Robertson, C. Objective assessment of speech after surgical treatment for oral cancer: experience from 196 selected cases. *Plast Reconstr Surg*., 2004, 113(1), 114-25.

[7] Mlynarek, AM; et. al. Methods of functional outcomes assessment following treatment of oral and oropharyngeal cancer: review of the literature. *J Otolaryngol Head Neck Surg*, 2008, 37(1), 2-10.

[8] Goldstein, NE; Genden, E; Morrison, RS. Palliative care for patients with head and neck cancer: I would like a quick return to a normal lifestyle. *JAMA*, 2008, 299(15), 1818-25.

[9] Zarek, A. Psychological responses of patients after partial or total glossectomy due to carcinoma of the oral cavity. *Ann Acad Med Stetin*, 2006, 52 Suppl 3, 113-7.

[10] Mészáros, K; Remenár, E; Kásler, M. Swallowing and speech treatment in rehabilitation for head and neck cancer. *Magy Onkol*, 2008, 52(3), 293-7.

[11] O'Connell, DA; et al. Swallowing function in patients with base of tongue cancers treated with primary surgery and reconstructed with a modified radial forearm free flap. *Arch Otolaryngol Head Neck Surg*, 2008, 134(8), 857-64.

[12] Logemann, JA. The Role of Exercise Programs for Dysphagia Patients. Dysphagia 2005, 20, 139-140.

[13] Caliceti, U; Piccin, O; Macrì, G; Brusor, S. Recovery of swallowing function following surgery for advanced buccopharyngeal carcinoma. *Acta Otorhinolaryngologica Italica*, 2007, 27, 277-280.

[14] Rieger, J; Dickson, N; Lemire, R; Bloom, K; Wolfaardt, J; Wolfaardt, U; Seikaly, H. Social perception of speech in individuals with oropharyngeal reconstruction. *J Psychosoc Oncol*, 2006, 24(4), 33-51.

[15] Carvalho-Teles, V; Sennes, LU; Gielow, I. Arch Otolaryngol Head Neck Surg. 2008, 134(10), 1066-1070.

[16] Kazi, R; et al. Analysis of formant frequencies in patients with oral or oropharyngeal cancers treated by glossectomy. *Int J Lang Commun Disord*, 2007, 42(5), 521-32.

[17] Markkanen-Leppänen, M; Isotalo, E; Mäkitie, AA; Suominen, E; Asko-Seljavaara, S; Haapanen, ML. Speech aerodynamics and nasalance in oral cancer patients treated with microvascular transfers. *J Craniofac Surg*., 2005, 16(6), 990-5, discussion 996.

[18] Stecewicz, M; Wysocki, R; Halczy-Kowalik, L. Pronunciation and swallowing in patients with tongue deficits following resection of oral cavity tumor. *Ann Acad Med Stetin*, 2006, 52 Suppl 3, 97-106.

[19] Rogers, SN; Lowe, D; Patel, M; Brown, JS; Vaughan, ED. Clinical function after primary surgery for oral and oropharyngeal cancer: an 11-item examination. *Br J Oral Maxillofac Surg*., 2002, 40(1), 1-10.

[20] McKinstry, A; Perry, A. Evaluation of speech in people with head and neck cancer: a pilot study. *Int J Lang Commun Disord*., 2003, 38(1), 31-46.

[21] McConnel, FM; et al. Functional results of primary closure vs flaps in oropharyngeal reconstruction: a prospective study of speech and swallowing. *Arch Otolaryngol Head Neck Surg*., 1998, 124(6), 625-30.

[22] Pauloski, BR; et al. Surgical variables affecting speech in treated patients with oral and oropharyngeal cancer. *Laryngoscope*, 1998, 108(6), 908-16.

[23] Bundgaard, T; Tandrup, O; Elbrond, O. A functional evaluation of patients treated for oral cancer. A prospective study. *Int J Oral Maxillofac Surg*., 1993, 22(1), 28-34.

[24] Perry, AR; Shaw, MA; Cotton, S. An evaluation of functional outcomes (speech, swallowing) in patients attending speech pathology after head and neck cancer treatment(s): results and analysis at 12 months post-intervention. *J Laryngol Otol.*, 2003, 117(5), 368-81.

[25] Pauloski, BR; et. al. Speech and swallowing function after anterior tongue and floor of mouth resection with distal flap reconstruction. *J Speech Hear Res.*, 1993, 36(2), 267-76.

[26] Logemann, JA; et. al. Speech and swallow function after tonsil/base of tongue resection with primary closure. *J Speech Hear Res.*, 1993, 36(5), 918-26.

[27] Pauloski, BR; et al, Speech and swallowing function after oral and oropharyngeal resections: one-year follow-up. *Head Neck*, 1994, 16(4), 313-22.

[28] Logemann, JA; Pauloski, BR; Rademaker, AW; Colangelo, LA. Speech and swallowing rehabilitation for head and neck cancer patients. *Oncology*, 1997, 11(5), 651-6, 659, discussion 659, 663-4.

[29] Fúria, CLB; Kowalski, LO; Latorre, MRDO; Carrara-de-Angelis, E; Martins, NM; Barros APB; Ribeiro, KCB. Speech Intelligibility after glossectomy and speech rehabilitation. *Arch of Otolaringology Head and Neck*, 2001, 127(7), 272-80.

[30] Pepijn, A; et. al. Quality of life and functional status in patients with cancerof the oral cavity and oropharynx: *pretreatment values of a prospective studyEur Arch Otorhinolaryngol*, 2007, 264, 651-657.

[31] Duflo, S; Lief, F; Paris, J; Giovanni, A; Thibeault, S; Zanaret, M. Microvascular radial forearm fasciocutaneous free flap in reconstruction. *Eur J Surg Oncol.*, 2005, 31(7), 784-91.

[32] Bernhart, BJ; Huryn, JM; Disa, J; Shah, JP; Zlotolow, IM. Hard palate resection, microvascular reconstruction, and prosthetic restoration: a 14-year retrospective analysis. *Head Neck*, 2003, 25(8), 671-80.

[33] Robbins, KT; Bowman, JB; Jacob, RF. Postglossectomy Deglutitory and Articulatory Rehabilitation with palatal augmentation prostheses. *Arch of Otolaringology Head and Neck*, 1987, 113, 1214-8.

[34] Behlau, MS. A voz do especialista. São Paulo: *Revinter*, 2001.

[35] Uwiera, T; Seikaly, H; Rieger, J; Chau, J; Harris, JR. Functional outcomes after hemiglossectomy and reconstruction with a radial forearm free flap. *J Otolaryngol*, 2004, 33(6), 356-9.

[36] Chien, CY; Su, CY; Hwang, CF; Chuang, HC; Jeng, SF; Chen, YC. Ablation of advanced tongue or base of tongue cancer and reconstruction with free flap: functional outcomes. *Eur J Surg Oncol*, 2006, 32(3), 353-7.

[37] Mády, K; Sader, R; Hoole, PH; Zimmermann, A; Horch, HH. Speech evaluation and swallowing ability after intra-oral cancer. *Clin Linguist Phon*, 2003, 17(4-5), 411-20.

[38] Yanai, C; Kikutani, T; Adachi, M; Thoren, H; Suzuki, M; Iizuka, T. Functional outcome after total and subtotal glossectomy with free flap reconstruction. *Head Neck*, 2008, 30(7), 909-18.

[39] Carvalho-Teles, V; Pegoraro-Krook, MI; Lauris, JRP. Speech evaluation with and without palatal obturator in patients submitted to maxillectomy. *J. Appl. Oral Sci.*, 2006, 14(6), 421-426.

In: Speech Disorders: Causes, Treatment and Social Effects ISBN: 978-1-60876-213-2
Editor: Alan E. Harrison, pp. 237-248

Chapter 11

AUDIENCE EFFECTS ON STUTTERING: A JAPANESE CASE STUDY

Jun Yamada and Takanobu Homma
Hiroshima University, Hiroshima, Japan

ABSTRACT

This case report investigated audience/no-audience effects on stuttering, speech rate, and fundamental frequency (F_0) by analyzing the oral reading performance of an adult Japanese male stutterer in an A_1-B_1-A_2-B_2 paradigm, where A represents an audience phase and B a no-audience phase. The subject read a passage five times in each phase. The audience/no-audience effects on the three variables were found significant. The plausibility of higher F_0 as an indicator and 'precursor' of stuttering, in conjunction with the relation of anxiety to stuttering and F_0, is discussed. The possibility is also suggested that oral reading practice in a no-audience condition may be used as treatment for stuttering.

1. INTRODUCTION

Several studies have demonstrated that stutterers' speech is generally much more fluent when stutterers are alone than when they have an audience (Bergmann, 1987; Bloodstein, 1995; Hahn, 1940; Johnson, 1955; Porter, 1937; Yamada & Homma, 2007). We can draw at least two implications from these findings: (1) a major cause of stuttering is anxiety evoked in the presence of an audience (but cf. Messenger, Onslow, Packman, & Menzies, 2004) and (2) the true speech competence of stutterers, which is nearly normal, best manifests itself in the absence of an audience.

To learn more about these implications for clinical and research purposes, we investigated the oral reading performance of an adult Japanese stutterer in an A_1-B_1-A_2-B_2 paradigm, where A represents an audience-present phase and B a no-audience phase. The subject read the same passage five times in each phase, and we measured his reading performance in terms of stuttering frequency, speech rate, and fundamental frequency (F_0).

On the basis of the findings from previous studies, we expected that the subject's reading performance would be much better in the no-audience condition, Phase B, displaying fewer stuttering events and faster speech rates.

Regarding fundamental frequency (F_0), we attempted to demonstrate that F_0 values tend to be lower in a no-audience condition than in an audience condition. It was more than half a century ago when Glasner and Dahl (1952), examining stuttering people, stated that "It has been interesting to observe that as improvement is noted, there is a definite drop in pitch level. The lowering of pitch seems to be one of the first indications of a lessening of tension" (p. 1113). But the relations between anxiety level, stuttering, and F_0 have not been well established in the literature (Atkinson, 1978; Bergmann, 1986; Hall & Yairi, 1992; Sacco & Metz, 1989; Scherer, 1979; Schmitt & Cooper, 1978; Yamada & Homma, 2007).

We also asked a question as to whether there is an adaptation effect (Bloodstein, 1995) in each phase, i.e., whether performance improves as the subject reads the same passage five times.

2. METHOD

2.1. Subject

The subject was the second author (T. H.) of this study, a 31-year-old Japanese male speaker, who also served as a subject in our preliminary study (Yamada & Homma, 2007). His stuttering, assessed as mild to moderate, appeared at the age of two. At the time of testing, he was a doctoral candidate who was doing research on stuttering in children.

2.2. Test Material

The reading passage was taken from a book for the general public written by Umesao (1988, p. 146), a Japanese naturalist. The text consisted of 117 *phonological words* and 476 syllables. A phonological word was defined as a constituent which consists of a content word and optionally following postpositions, e.g., "ima-de-wa," where "ima (now)" is a noun, "de" and "wa" are postpositions. (We will hereafter refer to a phonological word simply as a word.) Although the level of readability was unknown, our judgment was that it is at a high school level.

2.3. Procedure

The experiment used an A_1-B_1-A_2-B_2 design where Phase A represents an audience condition and Phase B a no-audience condition. The experimenter, the first author (J. Y.), a 55-year-old professor, with whom the subject was familiar, served as the only listener present. This condition was considered to be one of the situations which provoke only a small amount anxiety in the subject, but as reported below, it turned out that such was not the case.

The experiment was conducted in a small, relatively quiet room of the university which the subject used almost on a daily basis. The subject was seated at a small table opposite the experimenter. On the table were a Sony dynamic microphone F-V620, a Sony cassette-recorder TCM-1390, and a sheet of paper on which the reading material was printed.

Before the first trial of the audience condition, Phase A_1, the subject read silently the test passage until he was ready to read it orally. (No silent reading session was needed in the subsequent trials.) The experimenter then pressed the record button of the tape-recorder, and the first trial started. After the first trial was finished, a short break was given. In this manner, the subject orally read the passage five times in the first audience condition, Phase A_1. The experimenter then left the room, and the subject attempted five trials in the first no-audience condition, Phase B_1. On the first trial in this condition, the subject pressed the record button by himself, but he soon found himself somewhat tensed in doing so. He thus decided to keep the tape running after the second trial. He also thought that he would need a longer break to make himself more relaxed, and had longer breaks between the subsequent trials. On completing the fifth reading, he called the experimenter, and trials in the second audience condition, Phase A_2, began basically in the same manner as in Phase A_1. After completing five trials in this condition, the final five trials were given in the second no-audience condition, Phase B_2, in a similar fashion.

2.4. Dependent Variables

The subject's oral reading performance in each condition was analyzed in terms of stuttering frequency, speech rate, and mean F_0 maximum value for words. Stuttering frequency was determined by the present authors, who independently assessed stuttered words listening to audiotape. Reliability was computed by dividing twice the stuttered words agreed upon by the total stuttered words identified by the two observers. The mean of the reliability coefficients for the 20 trials was 0.90 (SD = 0.05). Only the stuttering events agreed upon, i.e., clear cases, were used for main analysis.

Speech rate was defined in two ways. The first was the total reading time taken to read the passage. The second was mean duration for *fluent* words. This second measurement was considered necessary to ascertain whether slower speech rate, if indicated by total reading time, is largely due to higher stuttering frequency. A fluent word was defined as a word which neither of the authors identified as stuttered across the whole 20 reading trials. Of the 117 words in the test passage, 33 (28%) were fluent words, and the reading times for 660 such fluent words (33 words × 20 trials) were measured to the nearest millisecond using an Animo SUGI speech analyzer (Version 1.0.7.8).

The first author measured F_0 max values for a total of 2,340 words (117 words × 20 trials) using the same speech analyzer. To confirm the reliability of the measures, he quasi-randomly selected 10% of the total words and measured them again with an interval of more than one month. The correlation between the two measures was .998, df = 232, $p < .0001$, and the mean difference was .01 Hz.

Table 1. Mean of stuttering frequency, total reading time in sec, mean duration for fluent words in msec, and mean F_0 in Hz in each trial

Trials	1	2	3	4	5	Mean
The first audience condition, Phase A_1						
Stuttering frequency	36	46	42	50	40	42.8
Total reading time in sec	224	211	230	229	292	237
Duration for fluent words in msec	646	653	677	682	671	665
Mean F_0	150	152	151	155	153	152
The first no-audience condition, Phase B_1						
Stuttering frequency	27	17	11	17	25	19.4
Total reading time in sec	259	154	144	154	192	181
Duration for fluent words in msec	656	641	640	620	663	638
Mean F_0	144	147	148	148	150	147
The second audience condition, Phase A_2						
Stuttering frequency	42	26	34	41	25	33.6
Total reading time in sec	259	191	202	299	179	226
Duration for fluent words in msec	646	639	638	636	620	636
Mean F_0	150	147	149	147	145	148
The second no-audience condition, Phase B_2						
Stuttering frequency	18	25	29	19	27	23.6
Total reading time in sec	155	163	272	163	209	192
Duration for fluent words in msec	601	634	631	644	632	626
Mean F_0	145	148	150	149	152	149

3. RESULTS

The main results for stuttering frequency (number of stuttering events), two speech rates, i.e., total reading time (sec) and mean durations of fluent words (msec), the mean F_0 max value (Hz) for each trial in each condition are presented in Table 1. In the following three sub-sections, a 2×2 ANOVA with repeated measures on the two factors, audience (audience and no-audience conditions, i.e., Phases A and B) and order (1st two phases and 2nd two phases), was performed using mean measurements for five trials in each phase as units for analysis.

3.1. Stuttering Frequency

The mean stuttering frequency was 42.8 ($SD = 5.4$), 19.4 ($SD = 6.5$), 33.6 ($SD = 8.2$), and 23.6 ($SD = 4.9$) in the first audience (A_1), first no-audience (B_1), second audience (A_2), and second no-audience (B_2), respectively. The effect of audience was significant, $F(1, 4) = 25.67$, $p < .01$, but neither the effect of order nor the interaction between audience and order was significant, $F(1, 4) = 1.34$, *n.s.*, and $F(1, 4) = 2.90$, $p > .1$, respectively. Paired comparisons indicated that the mean (42.8) in the first audience (A_1) condition was significantly higher than those (19.4 and 23.6) in the first and second no-audience (B_1 and B_2) conditions, $t(4) = 4.94, p < .01$, and $t(4) = 6.04, p < .01$, respectively, and that the mean (33.6) in the second audience (A_2) condition was significantly higher than that (19.4) in the first no-audience (B_1) condition, $t(4) = 3.20, p < .05$. These results showed that the subject stuttered significantly less often in the no-audience conditions than in the audience conditions. The mean (42.8) in the first audience (A_1) condition tended to be higher than that (33.6) in the second audience (A_2) condition, $t(4) = 2.05, p < .11$, suggesting a positive effect of the preceding no-audience (B_1) condition on the following audience (A_2) condition. The difference between the first and second no-audience (B_1 and B_2) conditions (19.4 and 23.6), and the difference between the second audience and second no-audience (A_2 and B_2) conditions (33.6 and 23.6) were not significant, $t(4) = 1.00$, and $t(4) = 1.84$, respectively. In summary, the results indicate (1) that, with less audience-associated anxiety in the no-audience (B_1 and B_2) conditions, the subject's oral reading performance was markedly improved and (2) that the preceding no-audience (B_1) condition tended to improve the subject's performance in the following audience (A_2) condition.

3.2. Speech Rate

The mean total reading time was 237 sec ($SD = 31.6$), 181 sec ($SD = 47.5$), 226 sec ($SD = 51.1$), and 192 sec ($SD = 49.3$) in the first audience (A_1), first no-audience (B_1), second audience (A_2), and second no-audience (B_2) conditions, respectively. The effect of audience was significant, $F(1, 4) = 7.76, p < .05$, but neither the effect of order nor the interaction between audience and order was significant, $F(1, 4) < 1$. Paired comparisons indicated that the mean (237 sec) in the first audience (A_1) condition was significantly longer than that (181 sec) in the first no-audience (B_1) condition, $t(4) = 2.36, p < .05$, and tended to be longer than that (192 sec) in the second no-audience (B_2) condition, $t(4) = 2.00, p < .06$. The other differences were not significant.

The mean duration for fluent words ($N = 33$) was 665 msec ($SD = 16$), 638 msec ($SD = 17$), 636 msec ($SD = 10$), and 626 msec ($SD = 16$) in the first audience (A_1), first no-audience (B_1), second audience (A_2), and second no-audience (B_2) conditions, respectively. The pattern of results here was different from that for total reading time. Both the effect of audience and the effect of order were significant, $F(1, 4) = 8.05, p < .05$, and, $F(1, 4) = 16.11, p < .02$, but the interaction between audience and order was not, $F(1, 4) < 1$. Paired comparisons indicated that the mean (665 msec) in the first audience (A_1) condition was significantly longer than that (638 msec) in the first no-audience (B_1) condition, $t(4) = 2.36, p < .05$, and tended to be longer than that (626 msec) in the second no-audience (B_2) condition, $t(4) = 2.00, p < .06$. The mean (665 msec) in the first audience (A_1) condition was significantly longer than that (636 msec) in the second audience (A_2) condition, $t(4) = 3.05, p < .05$, and that (626 msec) in the second no-audience (B_2) condition, $t(4) = 7.69, p < .01$, but the other differences were not significant.

Table 2. Correlations between stuttering frequency, total reading time in sec, mean duration for fluent words in msec, and mean F_0 in Hz, for 20 trials (df= 18)

	SFr	TRT	DFW	MF_0
Stuttering frequency (SFr)	1			
Total reading time (TRT)	.73**	1		
Duration for fluent words (DFW)	.61*	.44	1	
Mean F_0 (MF_0)	.63*	.33	.67**	1

*$p < .01$, **$p < .001$.

This latter finding suggests that speech rate for fluent words may not be correlated with overall speech rate for the text. Indeed, as presented in Table 2, the correlation between mean duration for fluent words and total reading time, $r(18) = .44$, failed to reach the 5% level. The correlation between mean duration for fluent words and stuttering frequency, however, was significant, $r(18) = .61, p < .01$.

3.3. Fundamental Frequency

The mean F_0 max value was 152 Hz (SD = 1.8), 147 Hz (SD = 2.2), 148 Hz (SD = 2.0), and 149 Hz (SD = 2.6) in the first audience (A_1), first no-audience (B_1), second audience (A_2), and second no-audience (B_2) conditions, respectively. Neither the effect of audience nor the effect of order reached significance, $F(1, 4) = 2.52$, $p > .1$, and $F(1, 4) = 5.12$, $p < .09$, but their interaction was significant, $F(1, 4) = 15.13$, $p < .02$. Paired comparisons showed that the mean (152 Hz) in the first audience (A_1) condition was significantly higher than the mean (147 Hz) in the first non-audience (B_1) condition, the mean (148 Hz) in the second audience (A_2) condition, and the mean (149 Hz) in the second no-audience (B_2) condition, $t(4) = 7.07$, $p < .01$, $t(4) = 3.14$, $p < .05$, and $t(4) = 3.88$, $p < .05$, respectively. Interestingly, although the difference was small, the mean (147 Hz) in the first no-audience (B_1) condition was significantly lower than that (149 Hz) in the second no-audience (B_2) condition, $t(4) = 5.72$, $p < .01$.

This pattern of results resembles those for stuttering frequency and mean duration for fluent words. As shown in Table 2, the correlation between stuttering frequency and F_0 was .63, $p < .01$, and that between mean duration for fluent words and F_0 was .67, $p < .001$.

3.4. Some More Exploratory Analysis of the Relation between Stuttering and F_0

It was worth exploring more about the relationship between stuttering and F_0. First, a point-biserial correlation between stuttering events (0 or 1) and F_0 values (df = 115) was carried out for each of the 20 trials. The mean for 20 correlation coefficients for the 20 trials was .29 (SD = .07), $p < .01$, ranging from .13 to .40. The correlations were significant for 18 out of the 20 trials, indicating that F_0 values were higher for stuttered words than for non-stuttered words. These findings, however, may be misleading because stuttering is more likely to occur at the beginning part of a sentence than toward the end, and because F_0 values are generally higher in sentence-initial position and decline toward the end of a sentence.

There would be at least two more ways to examine the relation between stuttering and F_0. The first is to compare F_0 for the stuttered and nonstuttered cases for the same words. We selected words which were stuttered 30% (6 trials) to 70% (14 trials) of the time in the 20 trials. There were 15 such words, and we compared mean F_0 values for their stuttered and nonstuttered cases. The mean was 156 Hz ($SD = 12$) for the stuttered group and 151 Hz ($SD = 12$) for the nonstuttered group, the difference being highly significant, $t(14) = 5.31$, $p < .001$. That is, F_0 was a mean of 5 Hz higher when the word was stuttered than when the same word was not stuttered.

The second way to reveal the relation between stuttering and F_0 is to compare F_0 values for stuttered words in a trial with a higher mean F_0 value on the one hand, and F_0 values for the same stuttered words in a trial with a lower mean F_0 value on the other. If we hypothesize that relatively higher F_0 values are associated with relatively more severely stuttered words, and further, if stuttered words are more severely stuttered in a trial with a higher mean F_0 value than in a trial with a lower mean F_0 value, then we would expect that F_0 values for stuttered words which appeared in a trial with a higher mean F_0 value would be higher than F_0 values for the same stuttered words which appeared in a trial with a lower mean F_0 value. To verify this hypothesis, we compared F_0 values for the same 10 stuttered words between the third trial of the first no-audience (B_1) condition, which exhibited the lowest mean F_0 condition, and the fourth trial of the first audience (A_1) condition, which exhibited the highest mean F_0 condition. (Note that one word which was stuttered in the former condition was not stuttered in the latter condition so that the number of the same words selected was not 11 but 10.) The result was what we expected. The mean for the former was significantly lower than that for the latter, 157 Hz ($SD = 14$) and 169 Hz ($SD = 19$), respectively, $t(9) = 5.36$, $p < .001$.

Given the findings above, we further asked a complementary question: what is the relationship between *nonstuttering* and F_0? A question we asked was whether F_0 values for the nonstuttered words which immediately precede stuttered words are higher than F_0 values for those which immediately precede nonstuttered words. Falck, Lawler, and Yonovitz (1985) gave a repeated-readings task to English-speaking stutterers ($N = 7$), and reported that the mean F_0 value tended to be *lower* for utterances prior to the moments of stuttering (pre-stuttered utterances) than that of identical utterances which were fluently produced (pre-nonstuttered utterances). Their finding was not consistent with our intuition, and thus we addressed the question of whether the same is true with a Japanese case. For our study, the question was whether nonstuttered words which immediately preceded stuttered words exhibit *lower* F_0 values than those which immediately precede nonstuttered words. We selected nine target words out of the 15 words which were stuttered 30% (6 trials) to 70% (14 trials) of the time in the 20 trials. Four words were excluded from the 15 words because they were in sentence-initial and/or pre-pause position, and two were excluded because less than five cases out of the 20 were nonstuttered.

Results showed that the mean F_0 was 152 Hz ($SD = 19.6$) for the pre-stuttered words and also 152 Hz ($SD = 19.9$) for the pre-nonstuttered words, $t(8) < 1$. Inspection of F_0 values for individual words, however, revealed that three nonstuttered words exhibited relatively large differences ($d > 5$ Hz) between the pre-stuttered and pre-nonstuttered conditions. Actually, a significant difference was observed for two of the words, one yielding 161 Hz ($SD = 4.2$) and 156 Hz ($SD = 3.9$), $t(17) = 2.45$, $p < .05$, and the other 164 Hz ($SD = 5.5$) and 157 Hz (SD

=6.7), $t(16) = 2.45$, $p < .05$, in the pre-stuttered condition and in the pre-nonstuttered condition, respectively. The remaining word exhibited the opposite direction, but failed to reach significance, 163 Hz ($SD = 13.0$) and 170 Hz ($SD = 5.2$), $N = 20$, $t(12) = 1.6$, $p > .1$. Overall, these results were not consistent with Falck *et al.*'s finding.

Likewise, F_0 values for the nonstuttered words which immediately follow stuttered words were compared with F_0 values for those which immediately follow fluent words. There were 11 words which were appropriate for analysis, with the remaining four words excluded because they appeared in post-pause position and/or because the number of nonstuttered words was too small. The mean F_0 was 155 Hz ($SD = 15.3$) for the post-stuttered words and 154 Hz ($SD = 13.6$) for the post-nonstuttered words, $t(10) < 1$. There was one word for which the mean F_0 was significantly *lower* in the post-stuttered condition than in the post-nonstuttered condition, i.e., 124 Hz ($SD = 7.8$) and 131 Hz ($SD = 2.9$), $N = 19$, $t(13) = 2.47$, $p < .05$.

In sum, F_0 is closely associated with stuttering, but F_0 values of stuttered words are unlikely to affect those of the immediately preceding or following nonstuttered words.

3.5. The Adaptation Effect

By inspection of Table 1, no apparent adaptation trend may be observed for any of the four variables (stuttering frequency, total reading time, duration for nonstuttered words, and F_0) in each phase. The speech rate for nonstuttered words appears to become much faster from the first audience (A_1) condition to the first no-audience (B_1) condition, and F_0 also seems to become lower in a similar manner.

4. Discussion

This study observed several interesting results, and perhaps the most important ones involve these two: (1) audience/no-audience effects on stuttering frequency and speech rate in an A_1-B_1-A_2-B_2 paradigm, and (2) a possible relationship between anxiety, stuttering, and fundamental frequency F_0.

4.1. Stuttering Frequency and Speech Rate

The association between anxiety and stuttering has been well documented for older children, adolescents, and adults (e.g., Bloodstein, 1995; Ezrati-Vinacour & Levin, 2004; Davis, Shisca, & Howell, 2006; Johnson, 1955; but cf. Miller & Watson, 1992), but regarding the causal direction, Messenger et al. (2004) pointed out the possibility that "social anxiety is an effect of stuttering" (p. 207). The present study indicates that such is not likely to be the case; rather, stuttering is an effect of social anxiety, i.e., an effect of the presence of an audience. In addition to this basic finding, we will here discuss three intriguing yet under-researched characteristics of the audience/non-audience effects: audience type, fluctuations of performance, and the possibility for treatment.

The first is that even the presence of a 'friendly' listener causes a great deal of stuttering, thus the absence of the listener markedly decreasing frequency of stuttering. To our knowledge, no previous study except for our pilot study (Yamada & Homma, 2007) has showen such a large effect of such a listener as an audience. In the present study, the number of stutterings was on average reduced to less than one half in the first no-audience (B_1) condition, as compared to the first audience (A_1) condition. This finding indicates that the present friendly listener failed to create a care-free, less anxiety-evoking situation. This failure then raises a question as to what criteria involving age, sex, trait, and others must be met to be a truly friendly, least-anxiety-inducing, ideal audience. In future research we would need to examine the effects of different types of audience including virtual audience (e.g., Anderson, Zimand, Hodges et al. 2005; Brundage, Graap, Gibbons et al. 2006) and construct an audience-associated anxiety scale where the most demanding or threatening audience would be placed in the rightmost position, and a no-audience condition in the leftmost position. For clinical and research purposes, we would also need to examine more about the effects of the leftmost position on stuttering, for fluctuations in stuttering frequency were unexpectedly great even in such a seemingly relaxed situation.

These great fluctuations in the no-audience condition are taken as the second characteristic of the no-audience effect. Such fluctuations suggest that, even with no audience present, there occur some subtle external and/or internal stimuli which make him anxious, tense, or upset, resulting in more frequent stuttering events. As mentioned in the Method section, the subject felt uneasy when he pressed the record button in the first no-audience (B_1) condition. Also in the second no-audience (B_2) condition, he heard a chime ringing and footsteps outside of the room which he thought were disturbing his reading performance. Anecdotal stories abound about similar events and situations; for example, according to Bloodstein (1995), some stutterers say that "they may stutter if they hear a footstep down the hall, or if they talk 'as though' to a listener, or even if they think, 'If somebody were listening to me I would be stuttering'" (pp. 303-2).

What is the ideal no-audience condition like? Under an ideal condition, can stuttering frequency be kept at nearly zero? This latter question may probably be answered affirmatively, but the reality is that it is extremely difficult to have such an ideal condition. Anxiety-inducing events easily come and go, badly affecting a subject's oral reading performance on a moment-by-moment basis. The finding that the performance was somewhat poorer in the second no-audience (B_2) condition than in the first no-audience (B_1) condition, should be attributed to more occurrences of external/internal stimuli such as a ringing chime.

The third characteristic of the audience/no-audience effect is the tendency of the subject's performance to improve in the second audience (A_2) condition, as compared to that in the first audience (A_1) condition. This tendency is, although not very large, encouraging. We emphasize that the subject exhibited nearly normal oral reading performance in anxiety-free situations, which represents his true competence. Thus, the critical question is how good performance in a no-audience condition can be transferred to audience-present situations. Specifically, how can we remove potential anxiety-causing stimuli in audience-present situations which precipitate him into stuttering. Aside from inherent difficulty identifying such anxiety-causing stimuli, one possibility would be for the subject to have a longer reading practice in a no-audience condition until he/she gains full confidence in the performance.

With regard to speech rate, we only note one point. That is that speech rate measured in terms of total reading time is qualitatively different from speech rate measured by mean duration for fluent words. This conclusion is suggested from the results that there was no significant correlation between them (Table 2), and that total reading time fluctuates more greatly from trial to trial than does mean duration for fluent words (Table 1). Overall fluency would be better represented by total reading time than by mean duration for fluent words. The higher correlation between stuttering and total time than between stuttering and mean duration for fluent words (Table 2) is taken as supporting evidence for that.

4.2. The Relation between Stuttering and F_0

Although the relationship between stuttering and F_0 has remained indeterminate in previous studies (Atkinson, 1978; Bergmann, 1986; Hall & Yairi, 1992; Sacco & Metz, 1989; Scherer, 1979; Schmitt & Cooper, 1978), the present results are clear-cut. As shown in Table 2, stuttering frequency significantly correlates with F_0. What remains to be done is to interpret the result. While the simple correlation between stuttering and F_0 allows several interpretations, we take it as suggesting that both stuttering and F_0 are an indicator of level of anxiety. The finding that mean F_0 became lower after the first audience (A_1) condition is consistent with the notion that the higher state anxiety is ameliorated after this first audience condition. In retrospect, the subject thinks that this seems to have been the case.

The relation between anxiety and stuttering and F_0 was not straightforward, however. Stuttering and F_0 may differentially reflect level of anxiety. We will discuss the relation by considering two levels of effect: a global (or across-conditions) level where generalized state anxiety evoked by the experimental situation may be represented, and a local (or within-condition) level where specific state anxiety arising from particular kinds of stimuli may be represented. At a global level, a rough rule is that for F_0 to be lower than 150 Hz is necessary (though not sufficient) for stuttering frequency to be fewer than 30 per trial (Table 1). There was one exception to this rule (the fifth trial in the second no-audience (B_2) condition, where the number of stutterings was 27 although the mean F_0 was 152 Hz. (Why this exception was observed is unknown. That the trial was the last one of the experiment might have something to do with it.) On the other hand, there were two trials (the third and fourth trials in the second no-audience (B_2) condition) in which F_0 values were 149 Hz and 147 Hz whereas stuttering frequency was 34 and 41, respectively. For these trials, the effects exerting their influence at a local level might have caused more stutterings. For example, the words which the subject stuttered in the preceding audience condition might have become feared words, which in turn induced state anxiety and caused stutterings. Apart from some exceptions, therefore, at a global level, anxiety may first manifest itself as higher F_0 and then as stuttering. In other words, higher F_0 may be a 'precursor' to stuttering rather than the other way around.

At a local level, on the other hand, F_0 is likely to be higher when the word is stuttered than when it is not stuttered. It was noted, however, that there are little or no anticipatory and carry-over effects in the immediate vicinity of stuttered words. This implies that on a local level the rising or falling of F_0 is instantaneous, probably because anxiety appears or disappears instantaneously on that level.

4.3. Further Questions

Several more questions are raised and we will briefly mention three of them. First, this was a case study, where the subject was the second author and the experimenter was the first author. Given this rather rare condition, the generality of the present findings remains unknown, and to what extent the present findings are generalized to other stutterers is a challenge.

Second, can we use an A_1-B_1-A_2-B_2 paradigm for purposes of treatment for stuttering? The answer seems to be in the affirmative. For example, substantial practice in Phase B_1 may well result in good performance in the subsequent situation at least at a global level. Unfortunately, we failed to elicit the best oral reading performance that displays virtually no stuttering in the no-audience condition.

Finally, we conducted no psycholinguistic analysis in this study, and we ask whether such analysis in an A_1-B_1-A_2-B_2 paradigm may shed new light on treatment for individual stutterers. For example, feared and/or difficult sounds, if any, may profitably be compared between the audience and no-audience conditions. In the best trial in this study (the third trial of the first no-audience (B_1) condition, for example, the subject produced 11 stutterings, where only five types of consonants, /s/, /t/, /ʃ/, /k/, and /d/, which may be identified as feared and/or difficult consonants, appeared. On the other hand, in a trial where many more stutterings were yielded, nearly all Japanese consonants were observed. What hierarchy of feared and/or difficult consonants exists remains another interesting question.

Acknowledgments

This study was supported in part by a Japan Ministry of Education, Science, and Technology Grant (No. 18530517). The authors are grateful to Joe Lauer for his comments about an earlier draft of this paper.

References

Anderson, P. L., Zimand, E., Hodges, L. F., & Rothbaum, B. O. (2005). Cognitive behavioral therapy for public-speaking anxiety using virtual reality for exposure. *Depression and Anxiety*, *22*, 156-158.

Atkinson, J. E. (1978). Correlation analysis of the physiological factors controlling fundamental voice frequency. *Journal of Acoustical Society of America*, *63*, 211-222.

Bergmann, G. (1986). Studies in stuttering as a prosodic disturbance. *Journal of Speech and Hearing Research*, *29*, 290-300.

Bloodstein, O. (1995). *A handbook on stuttering*. New York: Chapman & Hall.

Brundage, S. B., Graap, K., Gibbons, K. F., et al. (2006). Frequency of stuttering during challenging and supportive virtual reality job interviews. *Journal of Fluency Disorders*, *31*, 325-339.

Erzrati-Vinacour, R. & Levin, I. (2004). The relationship between anxiety and stuttering: A multidimensional approach. *Journal of Fluency Disorders*, *29*, 135-148.

Falck, F. J., Lawler, P. S. & Yonovitz, A. (1985). Effects of stuttering on fundamental frequency. *Journal of Fluency Disorders, 10*, 123-135.

Glasner, P. J. & Dahl, M. F. (1952). Stuttering – a prophylactic program for its control. *American Journal of Public Health, 42*, 1111-1115.

Hahn, E. F. (1940). A study of the relationship between the social complexity of the oral situation and the severity of stuttering. *Journal of Speech Disorders, 5*, 5-14.

Hall, K. D. & Yairi, E. (1992). Fundamental frequency, jitter, and shimmer in preschoolers who stutter. *Journal of Speech and Hearing Research, 35*, 1002-1008.

Healey, E. C. & Gutkin, B. (1984). Analysis of stutterers' voice onset time and fundamental frequency contours during fluency. *Journal of Speech and Hearing Research, 27*, 219-225.

Homzie, M. J. & Lindsay, J. S. (1984). Language and the young stutterer: A new look at old theories and findings. *Brain and Language, 22*, 232-252.

Johnson, W. (1955). *Stuttering in children and adults: Thirty years of research at the University of Iowa*. Minneapolis: University of Minnesota Press.

Messenger, M. Onslow, M., Packman, A. & Menzies, R. (2004). Social anxiety in stuttering: measuring negative social expectancies. *Journal of Fluency Disorders, 29*, 201-212.

Miller, S. & Watson, B. (1992). The relationship between communication attitude, anxiety, and depression in stutterers and non-stutterers. *Journal of Speech and Hearing Research, 35*, 789-798.

Porter, H. V. K. (1939). Studies in the psychology of stuttering, XIV. Stuttering phenomenon in relation to size and personnel of audience. *Journal of Speech Disorders, 4*, 323-333.

Sacco, P. R. & Metz, D. E. (1989). Comparison of period-by-period fundamental frequency of stutterers and nonstutterers over repeated utterances. *Journal of Speech and Hearing Research, 32*, 439-444.

Scherer, K. R. (1979). Personality markers in speech. In Scherer, K. R. & Giles, H. (eds.). *Social markers in speech*. Cambridge: CUP, pp. 147-209.

Schmitt, L. S. & Cooper, E. B. (1978). Fundamental frequencies in the oral reading behavior in stuttering and nonstuttering children. *Journal of Communication Disorders, 11*, 17-23.

Watson, B. & Alfonso, P. (1987). Physiological bases of acoustic LRT in nonstutterers, mild stutterers, and severe stutterers. *Journal of Speech and Hearing Research, 30*, 434-447.

Umesao, T. (1988). *Nihongo to nihon bunmei* [*The Japanese language and Japanese civilization*]. Tokyo: Kumon Shuppan.

Yamada, J. & Homma, T. (2007). A simple and effective treatment for stuttering: Speech practice without audience. *Medical Hypothesis, 69*, 1196-1199.

In: Speech Disorders: Causes, Treatment and Social Effects ISBN: 978-1-60876-213-2
Editor: Alan E. Harrison, pp. 249-257

Chapter 12

SILENT CHILDREN: UNDERSTANDING AND TREATING SELECTIVE MUTISM

Katharina Manassis

Dr. Manassis is a Staff Psychiatrist, Senior Associate Scientist, and Head of the Anxiety Disorders Program, Department of Psychiatry, Hospital for Sick Children, Toronto, and an Associate Professor of Psychiatry at the University of Toronto.

ABSTRACT

Selective mutism is a poorly understood condition at the interface between speech-language disorders and psychiatric disorders of childhood. Affected children fail to speak in one or more specific situations, impairing their social and academic development, often for years. Previous underestimates of its prevalence may account for the limited research attention it has received. Social anxiety, second language acquisition, developmental delays, auditory processing problems, and subtle language impairments may contribute to selective mutism, but a clear understanding of its etiology remains elusive. Key aspects of assessment include evaluating anxiety, cognition, and language using nonverbal methods and collateral information from parents and schools; obtaining a detailed baseline of communication attempts in various situations; and ruling out the presence of impaired hearing, pervasive developmental disorder, other communication disorders, normal second language acquisition, and mutism secondary to a traumatic event. Intervention has focused largely on behavioral methods to encourage social speech, but adding serotonin-specific medications is often helpful in severe cases, despite some concerns about using these in young children. Teamwork between clinicians, families, and school personnel is essential for treatment success. Further studies to elucidate the etiology of selective mutism and its optimal treatment are needed.

INTRODUCTION

Most papers on selective mutism begin with a definition of the disorder and a comment on its rarity, a clue to how little we know about this perplexing condition of childhood. Children who speak without apparent difficulty with familiar people in familiar circumstances yet are completely silent in other settings (one description of selective mutism) are prone to being misunderstood. Early descriptions of these children often said more about the biases of the observers than about the children themselves. "Elective mutism", the original term for this condition, implied that the child was voluntarily choosing (or "electing") not to speak. The term "selective mutism", used in current diagnostic systems (1), was meant to correct this misperception by linking mutism to selective environments.

A further disadvantage these children face is that they do not clearly fall within the territory of any one profession. Often identified at school (2), they may be referred to special education consultants, family doctors, speech-language pathologists, child psychologists, child psychiatrists or other professionals. Each discipline is likely to have a different perspective on the problem, and consequently a different treatment approach. Rarely do these professionals communicate and pool their expertise for the child's benefit (3). Moreover, selective mutism appears to be an "orphan" in the DSM diagnostic system, as it is not considered an anxiety disorder, nor does it belong to any other large category of disorders (1).

Finally, the infrequency of selective mutism may limit the resources made available to help these children, and the research attention they receive. Recent prevalence estimates are somewhat higher than those previously reported (about 0.7% (2)), but the condition is still considered rare compared to other psychiatric conditions of childhood or (depending on one's perspective) other speech and language disorders of childhood. Nevertheless, this prevalence suggests that at any given time one would expect to find at least one selectively mute child in every elementary school of average size. Girls are more frequently affected than boys (4, 5), onset is typically in preschool or early elementary grades (4), and children who attend schools where they are taught in a language other than their native tongue are at increased risk of selective mutism (6, 7).

In this chapter, what is known and (perhaps more importantly) what is not known about the possible causes and treatment of selective mutism is briefly reviewed. Further research in these areas is crucial to improve the developmental trajectories of affected children. Selectively mute children often show significant social and academic impairments (4, 8). On long term follow-up, many show increased psychiatric problems relative to controls, especially anxiety disorders, even if their social speech improves (8, 9). Developing a clearer understanding of selective mutism and more effective treatments could reduce this unfortunate morbidity.

ETIOLOGY

Social anxiety, auditory processing problems, impaired motor development, speech/language impairments, and being a non-native speaker have all been implicated as risk factors for selective mutism (6, 7, 10-16). Many children with selective mutism are found to have more than one of these factors, but it is unclear how they interact to produce the condition. Similarly, the genetic basis of selective mutism has not yet been studied. The frequent presence of social anxiety in other family members (11), however, and the phenotypic similarity between selective mutism and behavioral inhibition (a highly heritable temperament trait linked longitudinally to social phobia)(17, 18) suggest that genetics of selective mutism (especially in relation to social anxiety), may be a fruitful area of research. Reasons for the gender difference in the prevalence of selective mutism and the possibility of etiologic subgroups also merit further study. Areas for further study regarding the etiology of selective mutism are listed in Table 1.

Table 1. Areas for Further Study in Selective Mutism

Aspect of the Condition	Area for Further Study
Etiology	Genetics
	Relationships between risk factors
	Presence/nature of subgroups
	Reason(s) for female preponderance
Treatment	Preventive interventions (e.g. in ESL or other high risk groups)
	Optimal psychosocial intervention (behavioral or multimodal, individual or group, location—clinic, school, home, combination)
	Criteria for adding SSRI
	Modification in relation to various child characteristics (e.g., age, cognitive level, duration of mutism)
	Optimal role of family in treatment
	Optimal roles of various professional disciplines
Prognosis	Long term speech outcome
	Long term psychiatric outcome
	Long term functional outcome

Social anxiety is the risk factor most consistently linked to selective mutism. It frequently co-occurs with selective mutism (10, 12), is predictive of severity of selective mutism (16), and is prevalent in family members of children with selective mutism (11). Despite the strength of the link between selective mutism and social anxiety, however, children with selective mutism do not report more social anxiety than children with anxiety disorders of childhood (16). Thus, selective mutism cannot merely be considered an extreme form of social anxiety.

Developmental problems of many different types have been associated with selective mutism (13-16). Of these, auditory processing, motor development, and speech/language development have been studied systematically. Arie and colleagues (13) found reduced auditory efferent activity and auditory-verbal memory in children with selective mutism relative to normal controls. Kristensen and colleagues (14, 15) have consistently linked motor deficits to selective mutism, and found that controlling for motor development can eliminate apparent cognitive differences between selectively mute and normal children. Manassis and colleagues (16) found impairments of language in selectively mute children in comparison to children with anxiety disorders and to normal controls, even when they were tested in the home environment.

Finally, recent immigration and attending school where instruction is not in one's native language have been linked to selective mutism (6, 7). Self-consciousness about minor speech irregularities (for example, speaking with an accent) is thought to contribute to selective mutism in this case. Toppelberg and colleagues (19) have emphasized, however, that temporary mutism can be part of normal second language acquisition, so the diagnosis should be reserved for cases where the child is clearly proficient in the second language.

Two separate research groups have now suggested etiologic subgroups within selective mutism (7, 20). Elizur and Perednik (7) studied an Israeli sample and found two groups of selectively mute children: one of native speakers with high rates of developmental delays; one of non-native speakers with high levels of social anxiety. More recently, Cohan and colleagues (20) used a latent profile analysis of parent reports on various child characteristics to identify three groups: one of anxious and mildly oppositional children; one of anxious and communication delayed children; and one of children who were exclusively anxious.

Taking all of these findings into account, one possible etiologic understanding of selective mutism is shown in Figure 1. Of course, other models may also account for these findings and empirical evaluation is needed, but it may provide a helpful framework for beginning to understand the selectively mute child's predicament, and how selective mutism may become entrenched. As shown in the figure, a variety of factors alone or in combination can result in the child perceiving his or her speech as odd. In the case of auditory processing problems, this may be due to a misperception of personal speech. In the case of the other three factors listed (speech-language abnormality, motor abnormality, non-native speaker), the child's speech may actually have some unusual features. When the perception of odd personal speech occurs in the context of social anxiety and/or inhibited temperament, speech anxiety is likely to result in certain environments.

Some children with speech anxiety may respond to environmental pressure or encouragement to speak and thus *not* become selectively mute. Others, however, may find themselves in environments which inadvertently reinforce lack of speech. For example, selectively mute children often have classmates that speak on their behalf, reducing the child's anxiety and allowing for socialization in the absence of social speech. Selective mutism is an adaptive coping strategy in this environment. Alternatively, some children may have rigid, inflexible temperament styles (usually perceived by others as oppositional behavior) that allow the "habit" of avoiding social speech to become entrenched. Then, once selective mutism becomes a consistently used coping strategy for reducing speech anxiety, it can become resistant to change.

TREATMENT

Given the limited etiologic understanding of selective mutism, treatment has been largely symptomatic, using behavioral interventions to gradually promote speech in various social environments (21-25). Areas for further study regarding the treatment of selective mutism are listed in Table 1.

Before beginning treatment, however, careful assessment of psychiatric comorbidities, possible contributory factors, and baseline social communication is advisable to determine additional interventions needed and measure progress over time. Most historical information must be obtained from parents and teachers, as selectively mute children are often silent in clinic settings. Anxiety disorders are the most common psychiatric comorbidity and may contribute to social and academic impairment (4, 12, 16). Disorders which must be ruled out include hearing impairments, communication disorders, pervasive developmental disorders, schizophrenia and other psychotic disorders, and traumatic mutism (1). Mutism following a traumatic event is typically global (i.e., occurring in all environments) rather than selective, and onset is often abrupt and unrelated to the school year (26). Selective mutism, by contrast, usually occurs in children with a history of social reticence and onset often occurs near the beginning of a school year (1).

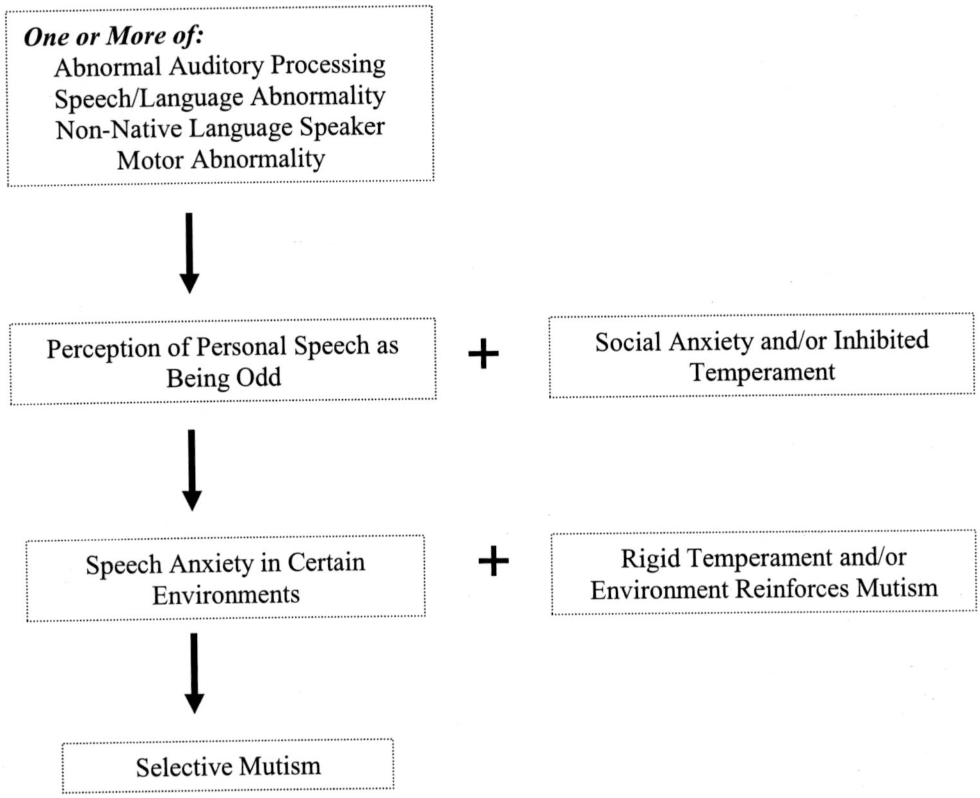

Figure 1. One Possible Etiologic Understanding of Selective Mutism

A careful developmental assessment to address the potential etiologic factors previously described is important, and can be challenging in non-verbal children. However, standardized receptive language tests can often be done by having the child point to responses, and expressive language can be evaluated using audio-taped speech with familiar people in the home environment (see 27, 28). Confirming normal nonverbal IQ (using tests involving pointing) is also important, as children with global intellectual delays sometimes present with selective mutism. A baseline of speech in various environments can be evaluated using the recently standardized Selective Mutism Questionnaire (SMQ) for parents (29). It has good internal consistency, and reliably discriminates children with selective mutism from those with other anxiety disorders.

Despite the emphasis on behavioral intervention in the literature, the only randomized controlled trials of treatment for selective mutism focus on medication, specifically selective serotonin reuptake inhibitors (one with fluoxetine; one with sertraline)(30, 31). There has been more clinical experience with fluoxetine than other medications, so it is often considered the initial medication of choice. Families may be reluctant to consider medication, given the young age of many selectively mute children and recent warnings about suicidal thoughts in youngsters treated with these medications (32). Large meta-analyses suggest a favorable risk-benefit ratio in childhood anxiety disorders though (32), which provides some reassurance given the similarity between selectively mute and anxious children. Careful monitoring of beneficial and adverse medication effects is indicated nonetheless. On balance, most authors advocate reserving medication for severe or refractory cases (3). Unfortunately, there is little agreement as to what constitutes a severe or refractory case.

Several large retrospective studies have demonstrated positive outcomes for behavioral interventions or so-called 'multi-modal interventions' (behavioral intervention with additional family-related, school-related, or other intervention(s)) (21, 23). Key behavioral techniques include shaping, desensitization, stimulus fading and self-modeling. Shaping is the positive reinforcement of speech approximations such as gestures, mouthing, and whispering. In severe cases, every communication attempt, even eye contact, may have to be reinforced initially. Positive reinforcement must be tailored to the child's temperament though, as some selectively mute children are embarrassed by overly exuberant praise resulting in treatment setbacks. Desensitization pairs the child's use of relaxation techniques with a hierarchy of increasingly difficult speech situations. Stimulus fading consists of gradually increasing the number of people and places where the child speaks, while gradually fading out the presence of a reassuring person such as a parent. Self-modeling involves exposing the child to audiotapes or videotapes of himself or herself speaking, edited so the child appears to be speaking in settings where he or she is typically mute.

Not all selectively mute children respond to all techniques, so some trial and error may be needed. Also, social skills training may need to be added in children whose social skills have not developed normally due to selective mutism, or have deteriorated with lack of use (12). Older selectively mute children may benefit from cognitive techniques aimed at anxiety-reduction, in combination with behavioral strategies (22). Thus, some individualization may be needed, which may account in part for the lack of a single "gold standard" psychosocial intervention.

Multimodal interventions address not only child variability but also variability in families, schools, and other systems around the child. Family psychopathology was found to be a significant moderator of outcome in a behavioral intervention study by Sluckin and colleagues (21), supporting this idea. If parents are anxious, for example, modeling of appropriate social behavior, assertively advocating on the selectively mute child's behalf, and instilling confidence in the child are all likely to be difficult. On the other hand, ongoing parent-school partnerships can promote progress in selective mutism and are the mainstay of many multimodal treatments (25). Parent support groups are also important, as families can become demoralized when treatment is ineffective or progresses slowly. Many interventions must be adapted to local education systems, health systems, and community expectations. For example, preventive interventions are more likely to be helpful in education systems where there is preschool attendance by most or all of the population (3). By contrast, interventions that focus on therapists assume a health system that allows most or all of the population to readily access to such professionals. Given the often protracted course of selective mutism (9), a patient but persistent approach by a team of professionals working with the child and family may be needed.

The optimal type of psychosocial intervention for selective mutism and its preferred location (clinic, school, home, combination) remains to be established, as does the best role for the family and for various professional disciplines in treatment. Preventive interventions, group interventions, and interventions tailored to specific child characteristics are all currently being evaluated. As summarized in Table 1, many aspects of treatment require further evaluation. Nevertheless, there is some agreement among professionals as to the long-term goal for children with selective mutism: to improve their ability to speak in social situations, to reduce their suffering from concurrent emotional disorders, and to return them to a more normative developmental course that results in healthy adult functioning (3).

CONCLUSION

Selective mutism is a debilitating disorder with many identified risk factors, but no single clear cause. A preponderance of studies confirms a role for social anxiety, but not all socially anxious children display selective mutism (1, 16). Etiologic subgroups may exist within selective mutism, but remain to be clearly distinguished. Assessment must be done to determine comorbid conditions (commonly, anxiety disorders of childhood) and possible contributory factors (for example, speech/language delay, motor delay, cognitive delay). Due to the nature of selective mutism, clinicians must often rely on nonverbal assessment tools and information obtained from parents and teachers.

Treatment is provided by various professionals, often depending on availability, and is more likely to succeed if these communicate and work as a team (25). It is based largely on behavioral principles, but no "gold standard" intervention exists. Of all treatments evaluated, only selective serotonin reuptake inhibitors have been subjected to randomized controlled trials, but these must be used with caution in young children. Optimal involvement of families and school personnel in the child's treatment, adaptation of treatment to various child characteristics, and preventative interventions remain to be elucidated. Further research is needed to clarify the etiology of selective mutism and treatment(s) which will improve the long-term functioning of affected children, not merely increase their social speech.

REFERENCES

[1] American Psychiatric Association. (1994). Diagnostic and Statistical Manual of Mental Disorders, 4th Edition (DSM-IV). Washington, DC: American Psychiatric Association.

[2] Bergman, R. L., Piacentini, J. & McCracken, J. T. (2002). Prevalence and description of selective mutism in a school-based sample. *Journal of the American Academy of Child and Adolescent Psychiatry*, *41,* 938-946.

[3] Keen, D., Fonseca, S. J. & Wintgens, A. (2008). Selective Mutism: A consensus based care pathway of good practice. *Archive of Diseases of the Child*, *93,* 838-844.

[4] Steinhausen, H. C. & Juzi, C. (1996). Elective mutism: an analysis of 100 cases. *Journal of the American Academy of Child and Adolescent Psychiatry*, *35,* 606-614.

[5] 5. Kristensen, H. (2002). Non-specific markers of neurodevelopmental disorder/delay in selective mutism: a case-control study. *European Child and Adolescent Psychiatry*, *11,* 71-78.

[6] Bradley, S. & Sloman, L. (1975). Elective mutism in immigrant families. *Journal of the American Academy of Child and Adolescent Psychiatry*, *14,* 510-514.

[7] Elizur, Y. & Perednik, R. (2003). Prevalence and description of selective mutism in immigrant and nonimmigrant families: a controlled study. *Journal of the American Academy of Child and Adolescent Psychiatry*, *42,* 1451-1459.

[8] Remschmidt, H., Poller, M., Herpertz-Dahlmann, B., Henninghausen, K. & Gutenbrunner, C. (2001). A follow-up study of 45 patients with elective mutism. *European Archives of Psychiatry and Clinical Neuroscience, 251,* 284-296.

[9] Steinhausen, H. C., Wachter, M., Laimback, K. & Metzke, C. W. (2006). A long-term outcome study of selective mutism in childhood. *Journal of Child Psychology and Psychiatry, 47,* 751-756.

[10] Melfsen, S., Walitza, S. & Warnke, A. (2006). The extent of social anxiety in combination with mental disorders. *European Child and Adolescent Psychiatry, 15,* 111-117.

[11] Chavira, D. A., Shipon-Blum, E., Hitchcock, C., Cohan, S. & Stein, M. B. (2007). Selective mutism and social anxiety disorder: all in the family? *Journal of the American Academy of Child and Adolescent Psychiatry, 46,* 1464-1472.

[12] Cunningham, C. E., McHolm, A., Boyle, M. H. & Patel, S. (2004). Behavioral and emotional adjustment, family functioning, academic performance, and social relationships in children with selective mutism. *Journal of Child Psychology and Psychiatry, 45,* 1363-1372.

[13] Arie, M., Henkin, Y., Lamy, D., Tetin-Schneider, S., Apter, A., Sadeh, A. & Bar-Haim, Y. (2007). Reduced auditory processing capacity during vocalization in children with Selective Mutism. *Biological Psychiatry, 61,* 419-421.

[14] Kristensen, H. (2000). Selective mutism and comorbidity with developmental disorder/delay, anxiety disorder, and elimination disorder. *Journal of the American Academy of Child and Adolescent Psychiatry, 39,* 249-256.

[15] Kristensen, H. & Oerbeck, B. (2006). Is selective mutism associated with deficits in memory span and visual memory? An exploratory case-control study. *Depression and Anxiety, 23,* 71-76.

[16] Manassis, K., Tannock, R., McInnes, A., Garland, E. J., Clark, S. & Minde, K. (2007). The sounds of silence: Language, cognition and anxiety in selective mutism. *Journal of the American Academy of Child and Adolescent Psychiatry, 46,* 1187-1195.

[17] Biederman, J., Hirshfeld, D. R., Rosenbaum, J. F., Hacrot, C., Friedman, D., Snidman, N., Kagan, J. & Faraone, S. V. (2001). Further evidence of association between behavioral inhibition and social phobia in children. *American Journal of Psychiatry, 158*, 1673-1679.

[18] Kagan, J., Reznick, J. S. & Snidman, N. (1987). The physiology and psychology of behavioral inhibition in children. *Child Development, 58,* 1459-1473.

[19] Toppelberg, C. O., Tabors, P., Coggins, A., Lum, K. & Burger, C. (2005). Differential diagnosis of selective mutism in bilingual children. *Journal of the American Academy of Child and Adolescent Psychiatry, 44,* 592-595.

[20] Cohan, S. L., Chavira, D. A., Shipon-Blum, E., Hitchcock, C., Roesch, S. C. & Stein, M. B. (2008). Refining the classification of children with selective mutism: a latent profile analysis. *Journal of Clinical Child and Adolescent Psychology, 37*, 770-784.

[21] Sluckin, A., Foreman, N. & Herbert, N. (1991). Behavioural treatment programs and selectivity of speaking at follow-up in a sample of 25 selective mutes. *Australian Psychologist, 26,* 132-137.

[22] Fung, D., Manassis, K., Kenny, A. & Fiksenbaum, L. (2002). Web-based CBT for selective mutism. *Journal of the American Academy of Child and Adolescent Psychiatry, 41,* 112-113.

[23] Krohn, D. D., Weckstein, S. M. & Wright, H. L. (1992). A study of the effectiveness of a specific treatment for elective mutism. *Journal of the American Academy of Child and Adolescent Psychiatry*, *31,* 711-718.

[24] Sharkey, L., McNicholas, F., Barry, E., Begley, M. & Ahern, S. (2008). Group therapy for selective mutism – A parents' and children's treatment group. *Journal of Behavior Therapy and Experimental Psychiatry*, *39,* 538-545.

[25] McHolm, A., Cunningham, C. & Vanier, M. (2005). *Helping Your Child with Selective Mutism: Practical Steps to Overcome a Fear of Speaking*. California: New Harbinger Publications Inc.

[26] Thorpe, L. U., Keegan, D. L. & Veeman, G. A. (1985). Conversion mutism: case report and discussion. *Canadian Journal of Psychiatry*, *30*, 71-73.

[27] McInnes, A. & Manassis, K. (2005). When Silence Is Not Golden: An Integrated Approach to Selective Mutism. *Seminars in Speech and Language*, *26,* 201-210.

[28] Manassis, K., Fung, D., Tannock, R., Sloman, L., Fiksenbaum, L. & McInnes, A. (2003). Characterizing Selective Mutism: Is it More than Social Anxiety? *Depression and Anxiety*, *18,* 153-161.

[29] Bergman, R. L., Keller, M. L., Piacentini, J. & Bergman, A. J. (2008). The development and psychometric properties of the selective mutism questionnaire. *Journal of Clinical Child and Adolescent Psychology*, *37,* 456-464.

[30] Black, B. & Uhde, T. (1994). Treatment of elective mutism with fluoxetine: A double blind placebo-controlled study. *Journal of the American Academy of Child and Adolescent Psychiatry*, *33,* 1000-1006.

[31] Carlson, J. S., Kratochwill, T. R. & Johnston, H. F. (1999). Sertraline treatment of five children diagnosed with selective mutism: a single case research trial. *Journal of Child and Adolescent Psychopharmacology*, 9, 293-306.

[32] Bridge, J. A., Iyengar, S., Salary, C. B., Barbe, R. P., Birmaher, B., Pincus, H. A., Ren, L. & Brent, D. A. (2007). Clinical response and risk for reported suicidal ideation and suicide attempts in pediatric antidepressant treatment. *Journal of the American Medical Association*, *297,* 1683-1696.

In: Speech Disorders: Causes, Treatment and Social Effects ISBN: 978-1-60876-213-2
Editor: Alan E. Harrison, pp. 259-274

Chapter 13

ORIGINS OF THE MUSCLES OF THE HUMAN TONGUE

Hideto Saigusa
Nippon Medical School, Tokyo, Japan

INTRODUCTION

The tongue of the human being is the muscular mass which takes a seat in the mandibular bone and occupies the oral floor. The musculature of the human tongue is consisted of both four extrinsic lingual muscles and four intrinsic tongue muscles. The extrinsic lingual muscles are attached to the structures outside of the tongue including the jaw, the styloid process, and the hyoid bone, and end in the tongue. The intrinsic lingual muscles are contained entirely within the tongue. It had been considered that the gross position of the tongue body might be accomplished by the contraction of the extrinsic lingual muscles, while the intrinsic lingual muscles might determine the shape of the surface of the tongue. In practice, the extrinsic lingual muscles or the intrinsic muscles work not only respectively, but also together to accomplish more fine and efficiently movement of the tongue, i.e., articulatory movement and masticatiory movement. Before considering the musculature of the human tongue, let us see the history and origins the tongue muscles.

Would you associate with the movement of the tongue in the nature including the human being? The chameleon has a well extended tongue to catch the insects. The snake takes his tongue in and out in trickles in order to smell the game. A salamander uses his tongue as not only a feeding apparatus, but also respiratory organ by mucous pappilae on the surface of the tongue with richly arterial feeding. The puppy sips the water in the dish with his lovely tongue, while he puts out his tongue with overflowing saliva to control his body temperature. The anteater and woodpecker use their long and slender tongues to get their dainty dishes. In the human society, the philosopher might consider the tongue as the organ to express one's emotion or spirit. A language teacher thinks over how tongues of her students should be positioned or moved to produce adequate speech sound. A girl who disputes her friend just now puts out her tongue to her friend. A boy who loses the goal in the soccer game clicks his tongue with the click sound /tut/. A man wondering in a desert all day long desires to make his tongue damp with a cup of water. Thus, it could be considered that the tongue contributes many complex functions including gathering foods, mastication, swallowing, tasting, respiration, smelling, control of body temperature, speech production, expression, and so on. However, it had been believed that all the tongue muscles derived from myotomes originating in occipital somites and differentiated in situ. [1] And it had been explained that the neuro-motor control of the tongue musculature could be accomplished by only the hypoglossal nerve that was derived from somatic motor neurons. Considering the unique and important complex capabilities of the tongue, we could not conclude that the hypoglossus nerve might carry out the neuro-motor control of all the tongue muscles. It could be considered that all the muscles of the human being might be derived from not only somatic muscles that were innervated by somatic motor neurons and were associated with adjustment of the organism to its external environment as the outer tube of the body, but also branchial muscles that were innervated by branchial nerve fibers and were associated with food gathering, breathing, nutrition, digestion, secretion, circulation as the anterior inner tube of the body. That is to say, the muscles of the human tongue should be reflected the origins and history of the vertebrates.

What is the Prototype of the Tongue?

When we would like to understand "true" significance of the origin of an organ or muscle, it is most important to know what the prototype of an organ or muscles is. Unfortunately, we could not see to go down in the history of an organ or a muscle for the beginning of a living thing. However, we could see the history of an organ or muscles by the approach of comparative anatomy. Romer[2] described as following; "the structural modifications witnessed are concerned with functional changes undergone by the vertebrates – changes correlated with the varied environments and modes of life found in the course of their long and eventful history". In that way, before considering the musculature of the human tongue, we will see the prototype of the tongue muscles of the vertebrate of the lower order, including cyclostomes (lamprey) and the chondrichthyes (shark).

The tongue of the Lamprey: We could see the prototype of the tongue in the bottom of the oral cavity of the lamprey. Lampreys belong to the cyclostomes, so called jawless vertebrates. An adult lamprey has a round mouth like a sucker with fine spines like teeth in the inner side of a mouth (Fig. 1a). A lamprey's tongue is a cartilaginous tongue (tongue cartilage) with fine spines and is moved forth to back (Fig. 1b). Sucking with fine spine of a mouth to the prey, with the tongue cartilage lampreys rasp away the flesh of the prey and transport the flesh and blood to the pharyngeal cavity. The mechanism to move the tongue cartilage could be accomplished by different originated two muscles. One is the somatic muscle running from the tail of the lamprey, visceral longitudinal muscles (rectus column muecles), and the other is the branchial muscle innervated from the motor fibers of the first branchial nerve which corresponded to the trigeminal nerve (Fig. 2). The former muscle could retract the inferior side of the tongue cartilage, and the superior structure of the tongue cartilage was moved anteriorly. The later muscle could retract the superior side of the tongue cartilage, and the superior structure of the tongue cartilage could be drawn to the pharyngeal cavity. That is to say, in lampreys, the movements of the prototype of the tongue, the tongue cartilage, were accomplished by both the somatic and the first branchial muscles. The other branchial muscles and nerves under the second branchial arch to the seventh branchial arch are stayed in the pharyngeal tube and do not contribute the movement of the tongue of the lamprey. By the way, the second branchial nerve is corresponded to the facial nerve, the third branchial nerve is corresponded the glossopharyngeal nerve, and the fourth to seventh branchial nerves are corresponded to the vagus nerve.

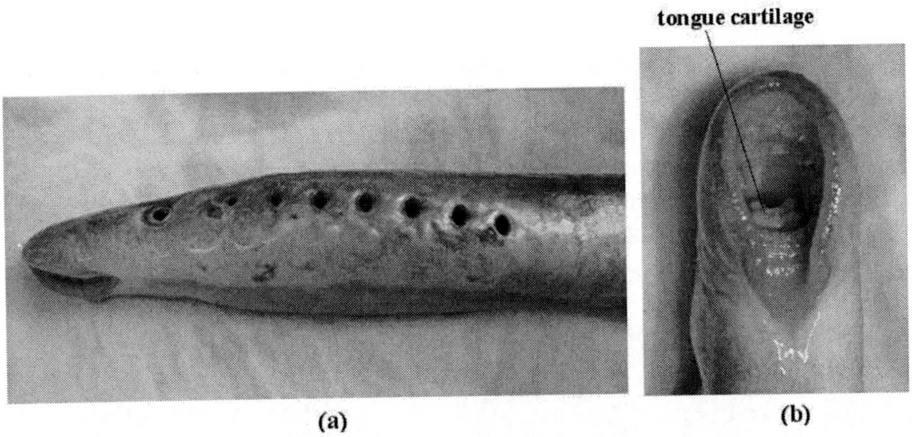

Figure 1. Morphology of the head of the Article Lamprey (*Lampetra Japonica*). (a)Lateral view of the head: one pair of eyes and seven pairs of gill slits without jaws. (b) The tongue cartilage which is moved forth to back is shown in jawless oral cavity with fine spines.

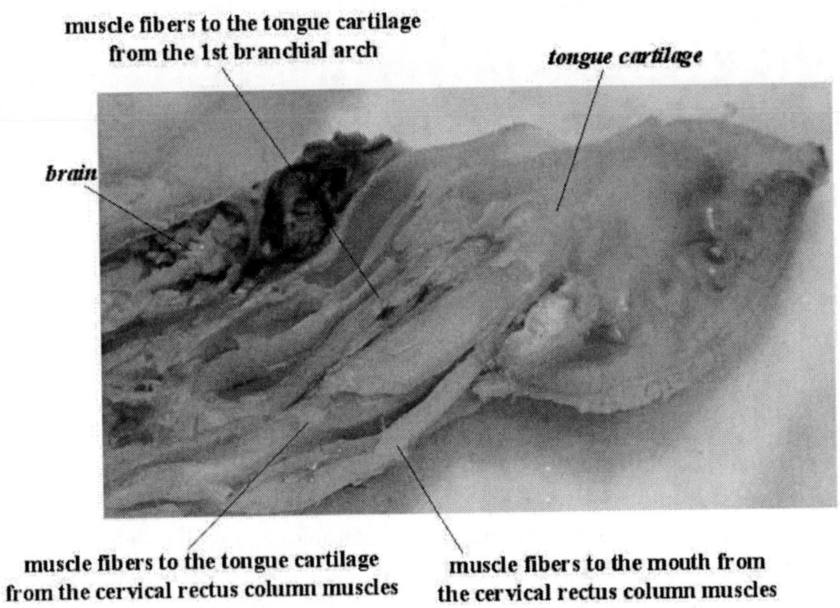

Figure 2. Mid-Sagittal section of the head of the Article Lamprey shows the tongue cartilage is stayed in the jawless oral cavity. The tongue cartilage is supported by the muscle fibers from both the 1st branchial arch and the cervical rectus column muscle.

The Tongue of the Shark

Sharks belong to the chondrichthyes, so called cartilaginous fishes. They have well-formed strong jaws and have survived from the Paleozoic in the sea. A shark has sharp and serrated tooth in the inner surface of the jaws and strong jaw closing muscles derived from the first branchial muscles with assisting by the muscles of the second branchial muscles (Fig. 3a). The rectus column muscles to the mouth and the lower jaw are surrounded with both the first and second branchial muscles. The surface of the tongue is flattened and hard with submucous cartilage (Fig. 3b). The cervical rectus column muscles reach to the jaw and the submucous cartilage of the tongue. The branchial clefts are connected with the both sides of the tongue in continue to the pharyngeal cavity (Fig. 4.). Nerve fiber analysis of the third branchial nerve revealed that the third branchial nerve, which corresponded to the glossopharyngeal nerve, supplies to not only submucosal area of the tongue, but also the muscle fibers of the posterior portion of the tongue (Fig. 5).

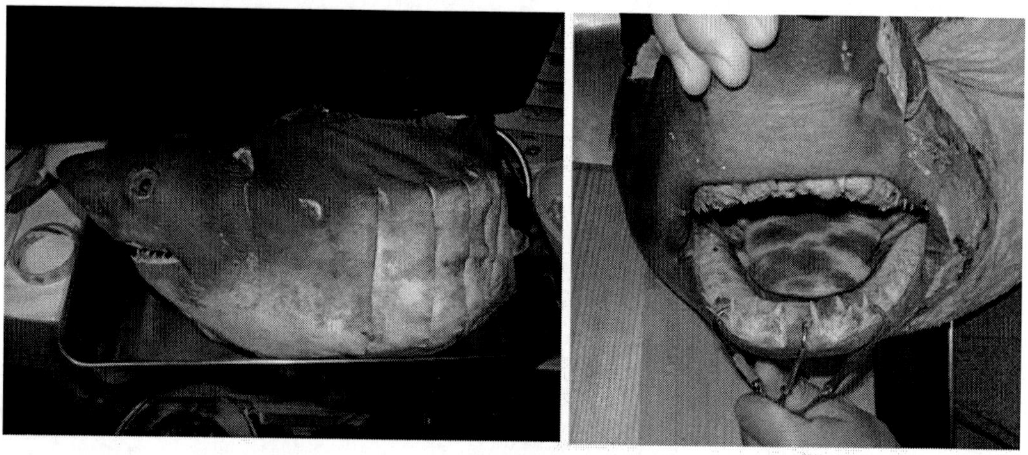

(a) (b)

Figure 3. Morphology of the head of the Salmaon Shark (*Lamna ditropis*) (a) Lateral view of the head: strong jaws with sharp tooth and five gill slits. (b) The hard tongue is stayed in the oral floor and continues to the pharynx with gill slits.

And past literatures about the tongue of the other vertebrate also indicated some significant descriptions. Marcus [3] reported that the tongue of a primeval fish (polypterus), which belong to the Actinopterygii with the lung, was composed of smooth muscle. Portman [4] described that the primordium of a bird's tongue, which had a hard and immobile tongue in the bills, had only motor fiber of the trigeminal nerve without sensory fiber. Hatta [5] described from the embryological studies of tachydromoides, which belong to the Reptiles, the tongue of tschydromoides was derived from the endoderm with the pharyngeal wall.

From those anatomical findings, the muscles of the tongue have the three different origins, the muscles derived from the first branchial arch which were supplied by the trigeminal nerve, the muscles derived from the somatic muscle which supplied by occipital somatic nerve, i.e., the hypoglossal nerve, and the muscles derived from the third branchial arch which supplied by the glossopharyngeal nerve. Thus, it could be considered that the tongue contributes various important roles, including nutrition, breathing, speech production, expression, and so on.

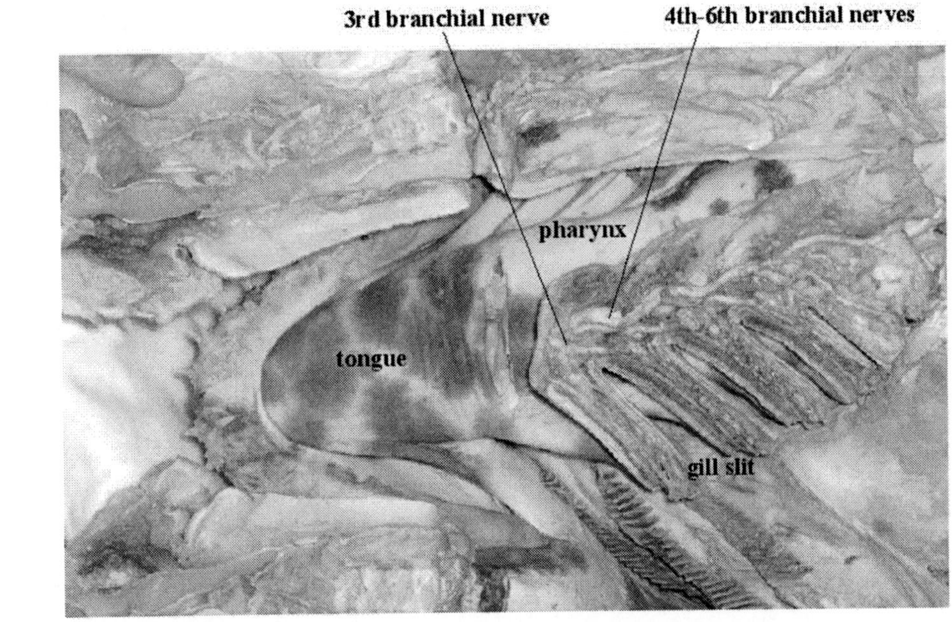

Figure 4. After splitting the upper jaw and the head of the Salmaon shark, the tongue is seen in the oral cavity, and continues to the pharyngeal cavity with gill slits bilaterally.

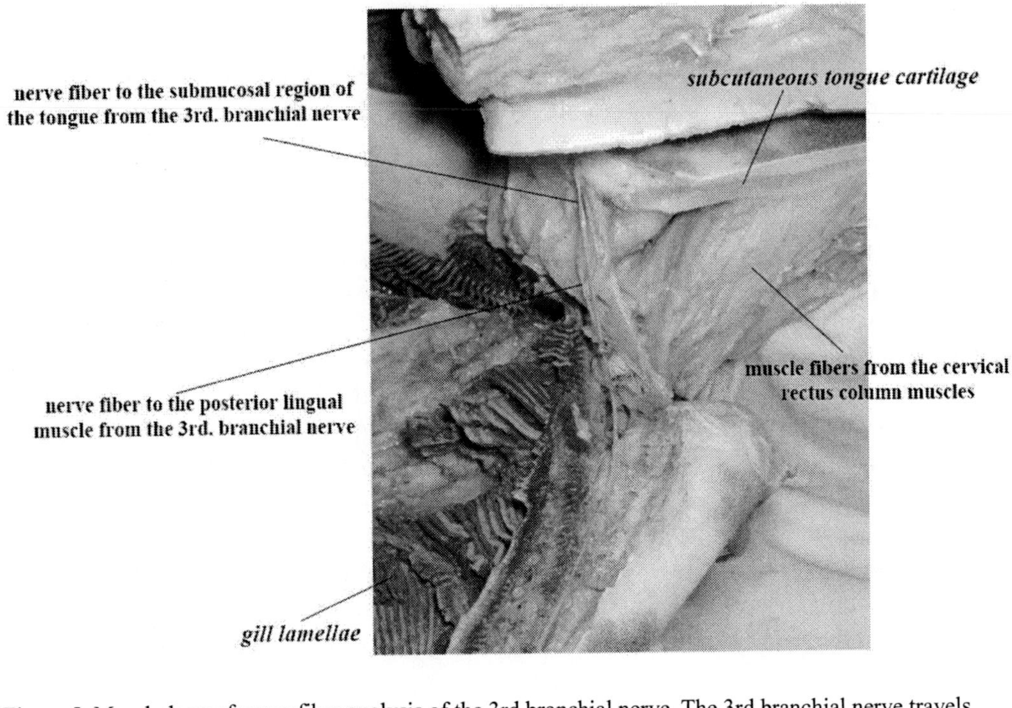

Figure 5. Morphology of nerve fiber analysis of the 3rd branchial nerve. The 3rd branchial nerve travels along the branchial artery and branches to both the submucosal region of the tongue and the posterior part of the lingual muscle.

WHERE THE MUSCLES OF THE HUMAN TONGUE ORIGINATED FROM?

The human tongue is consist of four extrinsic lingual muscles including the genioglossus, styloglossus, hyoglossus, and palatoglossus muscles, and four intrinsic lingual muscles including the superior longitudinal, inferior longitudinal, transverse, and vertical lingual muscles. Gross anatomical findings revealed that neural supplies for the genioglossus, styloglossus, hyoglossus muscles are innervated by the hypoglossal nerve. The origin of a muscle can always be traced, because the nerve supply is derived from its somite or branchial arch. [1, 4] Thus, we can consider that the genioglossus, styloglossus, and hyoglossus muscles are derived from the occipital somites. However, the neuro-motor controls of the four intrinsic lingual muscles and the other extrinsic muscle, i.e., the palatoglossus muscle had not been clarified yet. The reason why the neuro-motor control and neural supply of each muscle of the tongue had not been investigated in detail is due to its complicated structure of the tongue that the intrinsic and the extrinsic tongue muscles crossed each other in the tongue. In spite of complicated muscle structure of the human tongue, it has not been reported about the abnormal fiber arrangement of the musculature of the tongue except cases with aglossia. Thus, it should be considered that each tongue muscle could have its origin and differentiated along its identity. Now we could see the four intrinsic lingual muscles and remaining the extrinsic lingual muscle, the palatoglossus muscle, as revealed by serial section methods and nerve fiber analysis for the lingual and the glossopharyngeal nerves.

Transverse Lingual Muscle and Palatoglossus Muscle

Horizontal serial section of the human tongue revealed the morphological and functional close relationship between the superior pharyngeal constrictor muscle and the transverse lingual muscle as following (Fig. 6).[6] Near the dorsum of the tongue, the muscle fibers of the superior pharyngeal constrictor muscle reached the lateral edge of the tongue, but did not join the tongue musculature. The number of muscle fibers reaching the tongue body increased toward the base of the tongue. The fibers of the superior pharyngeal constrictor muscle become connected to the thick fibers of the transverse lingual muscle at the base of the tongue. Simultaneous contraction on both of the transverse lingual and the superior pharyngeal constrictor muscles could cause constriction of the mid-pharyngeal cavity and allow retrusive movement of the tongue (Fig. 7). The functional relationship could contribute to produce the low vowel /a/ and cause the pharyngeal peristaltic movement starting at the base of the tongue (Fig. 8).[7] Nerve fiber analysis of the glossopharyngeal nerve of a human adult subject revealed that the motor-branch of the glossopharyngeal nerve branched to the styloglopharyngeal muscle and coursed inferoanteriorly, and gave off supplies to the palatopharyngeal, the ringed muscle fibers of the superior pharyngeal constrictor muscle connecting with the transeverse lingual muscle at the base of the tongue, and the palatoglossus muscle (Fig. 9). These findings indicated that the transeverse lingual and the palatoglossus muscles originated from the third branchial muscles and differentiated in the tongue.

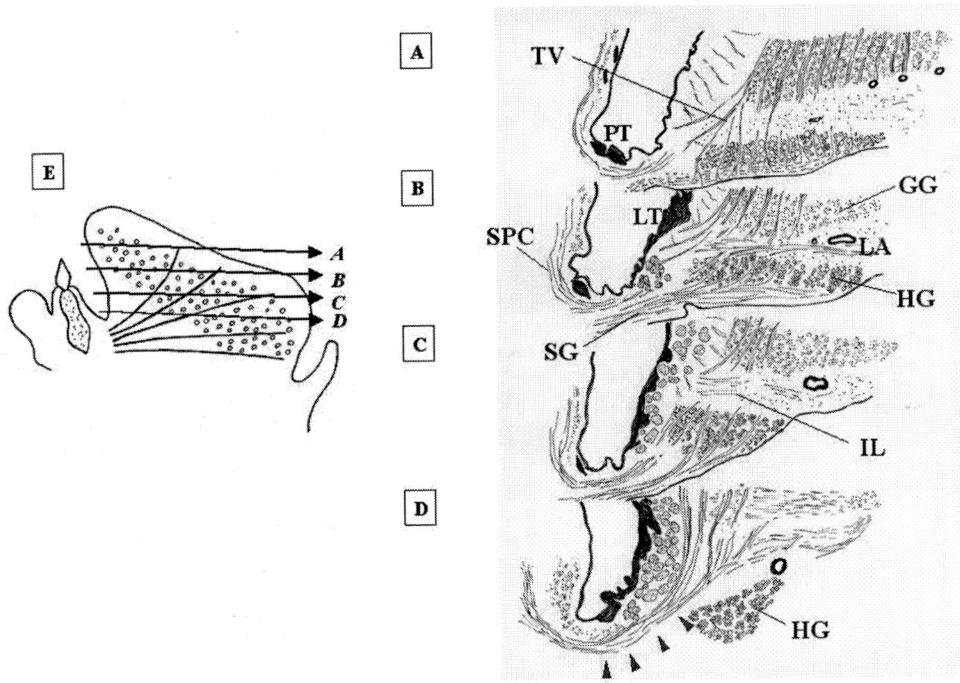

Figure 6. Diagram showing tongue musculature and the midpharyngeal wall in horizontal sections. A-D: Locations of four typical serial sections in the tongue. E: Illustrates (A) through (D).The fibers of the superior pharyngeal constrictor muscle become connected to the thick fibers of the transverse lingual muscle at the base of the tongue (red △). GG, genioglossus muscle; HG, hyoglossus muscle; IL, inferior longitudinal lingual muscle; LA, lingual artery; LT, lingual tonsil; PT, palatal tonsil; SPC, superior pharyngeal constrictor muscle; SG, stylogloossus muscle; TV, transverse lingual muscle.

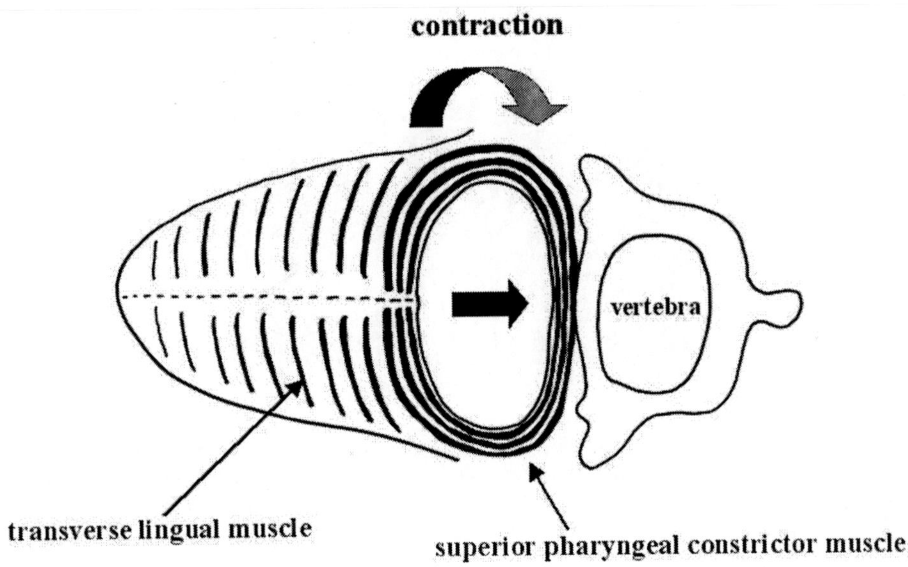

Figure 7. Diagram showing the fiber arrangement of the transverse lingual muscle and its close relationship to the superior pharyngeal constrictor muscle. The contraction of these muscles contributes the retrusive movement of the tongue with constriction of the midpharyngeal cavity at the level of the base of the tongue.

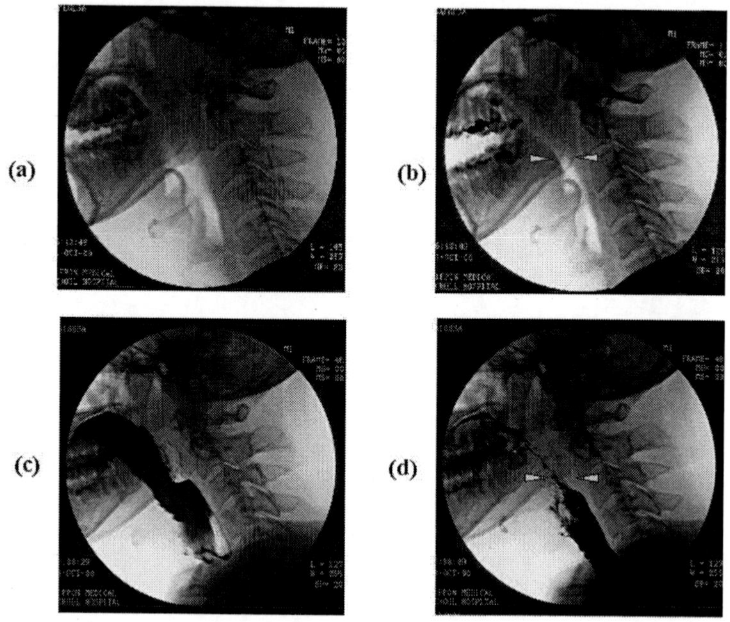

Figure 8. Lateral X-ray imaging of the head and neck. During the production of high vowel /i/ (a), the tongue protrudes with enlargement of the midpharybegeal cavity. Whereas, during the production of low vowel /a/ (b), the tongue retrudes with constriction of the posterior pharyngeal wall at the base of the tongue (yellow △). During swallowing, the tongue moves anteriorly and toward the hard palate (c). Subsequently, the retrusive movement of the tongue forced the bolus of food into the pharyngeal cavity with pharyngeal peristaltic movement starting at the base of the tongue (yellow △) (d).

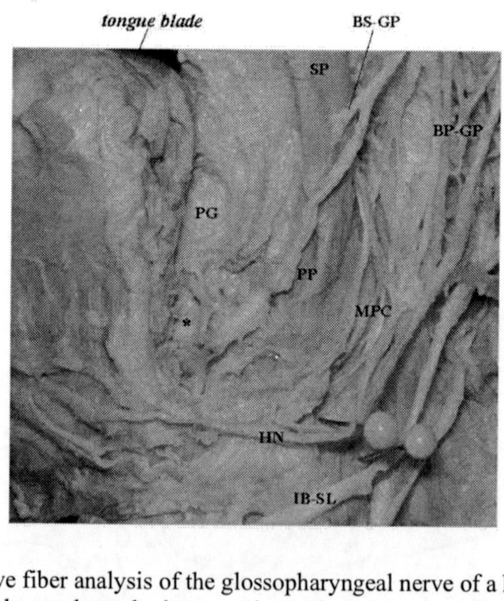

Figure 9. Morphology of nerve fiber analysis of the glossopharyngeal nerve of a human adult subject. The glossopharyngeal nerve branches to the stylopharyngeal muscle and travels inferoanteriorly, and gave off its supplies to the palatopharyngeal muscle, the ringed muscle fibers consisted of both the superior pharyngeal constrictor and the transverse lingual muscles at the base of the tongue (∗), and the palatoglossus muscle. BP-GP, branches of the glossopharyngeal nerve to the pharyngeal plexus; BS-GP, branch of the glossopharyngeal nerve to the stylopharyngeal muscle; HN, hypoglossal nerve; IB-SL, inner branch of the superior laryngeal nerve; MPC, middle pharyngeal constrictor muscle; PG, palatoglossus muscle; PP, palatopharyngeal muscle; SP, stylopharyngeal muscle.

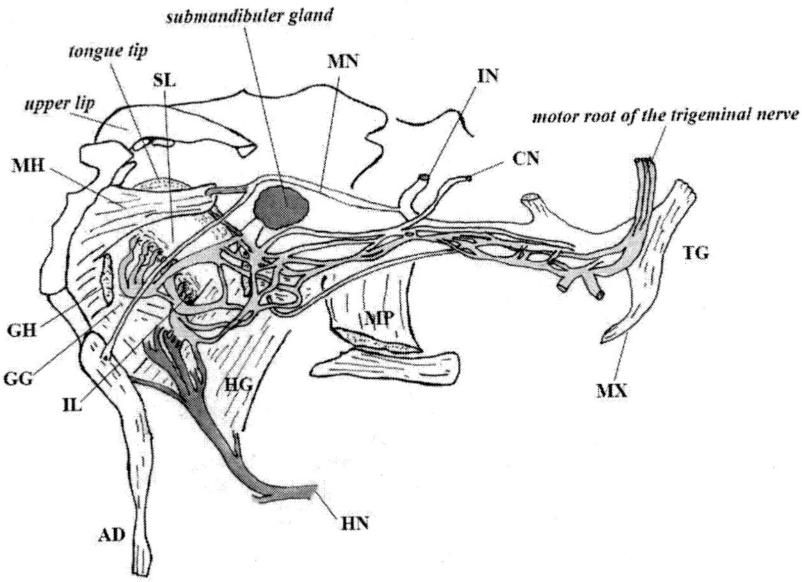

Figure 10. Morphology of nerve fiber analysis of the lingual nerve of a human subject. Motor root of the trigeminal nerve (yellow) gives off its supply to the lingual nerve near the region where the motor root branches to the medial and the lateral pterygoid nerves. The motor fiber travels into the lingual nerve and enters to the muscle layer consisting of the superior and the inferior longitudinal lingual muscles as branches to these muscles. Exra-lingual connections between the lingual and the hypoglossal nerves (orange) are seen. AD, anterior belly of the digastric muscle; CN, chorda tympani; GG, genioglossus muscle; GH, geniohyoid muscle; HG, hyoglossus muscle; HN, hypoglossal nerve; IL, inferior longitudinal lingual muscle; IN, inferior alveolar nerve; LN, lingual nerve; MH, mylohyoid muscle; MN, mylohyoid nerve; MP, medial pterygoid muscle; MX, maxillary nerve; SL, superior longitudinal lingual muscle; TG, trigeminal ganglion.

Superior and Inferior Longitudinal Lingual Muscles

Nerve fiber analysis of the lingual nerve from the trigeminal ganglion to the tongue musculature could reveal that the motor-root of the trigeminal nerve gave off its supply to the lingual nerve and traveled into the lingual nerve (Fig. 10), and branched to the superior and the inferior longitudinal lingual muscles (Fig. 11). [8] Coronal serial sections of the human tongue (Fig. 12) show that the inferior and the superior longitudinal lingual muscles joined each other and surrounded the whole tongue and combined with the sub-mucosal connective tissue closely in the anterior portion of the tongue like the facial muscles. And the lingual nerve entered with the lingual artery into the posterior portion between the genioglossus muscle and the inferior longitudinal lingual muscle, and gave off supplies to the musculature consisting of the inferior and the superior longitudinal lingual muscles. Whereas, the hypoglossal nerve supplied to the genioglossus muscle. These findings indicated that the inferior and the superior longitudinal lingual muscles originated from the first branchial muscles and differentiated in the tongue. The fibers of the superior longitudinal lingual muscle course from the base of the tongue to the anterior portion of the tongue, but scarcely in the tongue tip, on the other side the fibers of the inferior longitudinal lingual muscle course from the tongue tip to the posterior portion of the tongue, but not reaching to the base of the tongue. The slipping fiber arrangements between the superior and the inferior longitudinal lingual muscles might be useful to control the movement of the tongue tip.

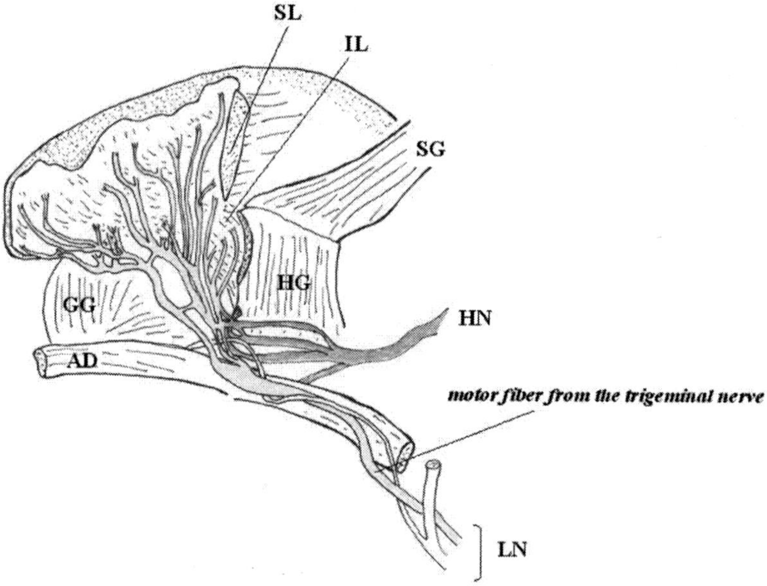

Figure 11. Peripheral morphology of the lingual nerve. Motor fibers (yellow) derived from the motor root of the trigeminal nerve travel into the lingual nerve and give off its supplies to the inferior and the superior longitudinal lingual muscles, and reach the sub-mucosal layer of the tongue. And the motor fibers connect the hypoglossal nerve (orange) before branching the inferior and the superior longitudinal lingual muscles.AD, anterior belly of the digastric muscle; GG, genioglossus muscle; HG, hyoglossus muscle; HN, hypoglossal nerve; IL, inferior longitudinal lingual muscle; LN, lingual nerve; SL, superior longitudinal lingual muscle; SG, styloglossus muscle.

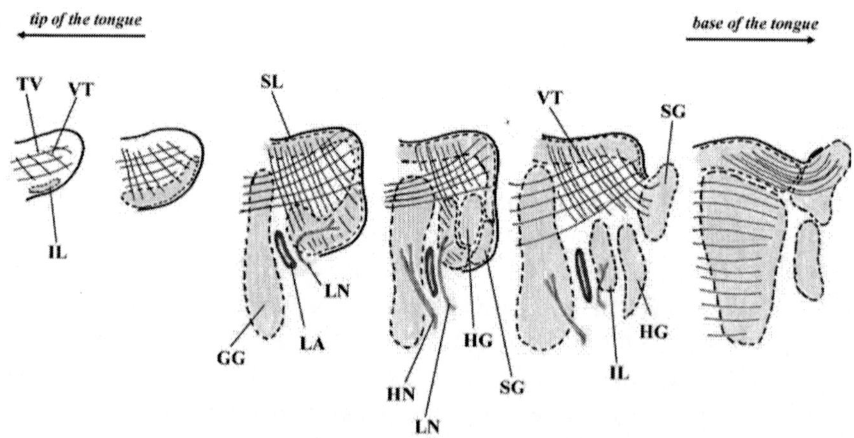

Figure 12. Diagram showing the fiber arrangements of the superior longitudinal and the inferior longitudinal, and the vertical lingual muscles and their relationship with the lingual artery, the hypoglossal nerve, the lingual nerve, and the extrinsic lingual muscles. Fibers of the superior longitudinal lingual muscle become connected with the fibers of the inferior longitudinal lingual muscle at the level of the anterior portion of the tongue. The lingual artery divides the genioglossus muscle from the inferior longitudinal lingual muscle with the hypoglossal nerve (inner side) and the lingual nerve (outer side). Fibers of the vertical lingual muscle become connected with the fibers of the styloglossus muscle at the level of the posterior portion of the tongue. GG, genioglossus muscle; HG, hyoglossus muscle; HN, hypoglossal nerve; IL, inferior longitudinal lingual muscle; LA, lingua artery; LN, lingual nerve; SG, styloglossus muscle; SL, superior longitudinal lingual muscle, TV, transverse lingual muscle; VT, vertical lingual muscle.

Vertical Lingual Muscle

Coronal serial section of the human tongue could also reveal the morphological and functional close relationship between the styloglossus muscle and the vertical lingual muscle as following. [9] In the tip of the tongue, the fibers of the vertical lingual muscle course diagonally from the superior surface of the tip of the tongue to the inferior surface and intersect with the fibers of inferior longitudinal lingual and the transverse lingual muscles. In the anterior part of the tongue body, the fibers of the vertical lingual muscle course diagonally from the superior surface of the body of the tongue to the inferior surface outside of the genioglossus muscle. And fibers of the vertical lingual muscle do not intersect with fibers of the genioglossus muscle, but with the superior longitudinal, transverse, and the inferior longitudinal lingual muscles. In the mid portion of the tongue body, fibers of the vertical lingual muscle course outside of the genioglossus muscle diagonally from the superior surface of the body of the tongue to the inferior longitudinal lingual muscle and near the styloglossus muscle but not reach the mucosal layer of the inferior surface of the body of the tongue. In the posterior portion of the tongue body, the fibers of the vertical lingual muscle coursed diagonally from the superior surface of the dorsum of the tongue and join with fibers of the styloglossus muscle. Simultaneous contraction of both the vertical lingual muscle and the styloglossus muscle could accomplish the postero-superior movement of the whole dorsum of the tongue with the depressive movement of the tip of the tongue (Fig. 13). This functional relationship might contribute to product the high back vowel /u/ which was produced acoustically by two distinct cavities including the pharyngeal cavity and the oral cavity. These findings suggested that the vertical lingual muscle originated or differentiated along with the styloglossus muscle innervated by the hypoglossal nerve.

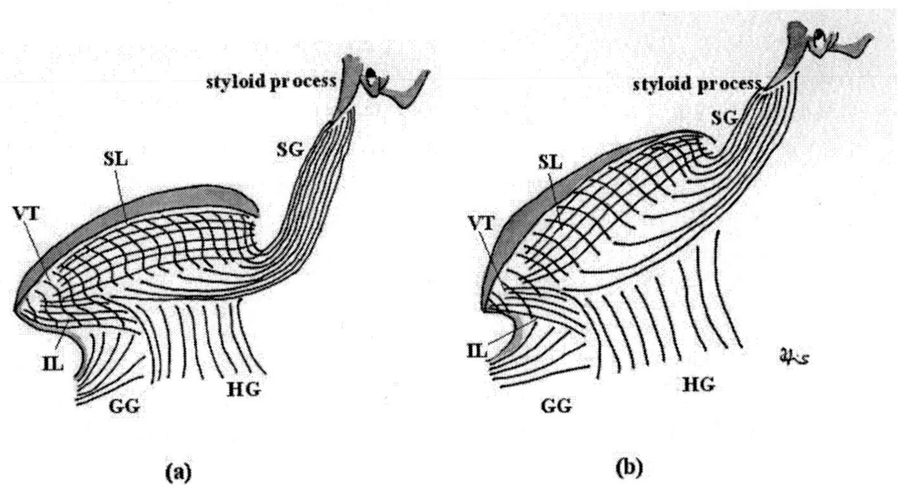

Figure 13. Diagram showing the fiber arrangement of the vertical lingual muscle and its close relationship to the styloglossus muscle (a). The contraction of these muscles contributes the posterosuperior movement of the tongue blade with depression of the tongue tip simultaneously (b). GG, genioglossus muscle; HG, hyoglossus muscle; IL, inferior longitudinal lingual muscle; SG, styloglossus muscle, SL, superior longitudinal lingual muscle; VT, vertical lingual muscle.

Now, we can understand origins and neuro-motor control of the each tongue muscles as Table 1.

Table 1. Origins of the muscles of a human tongue

Muscles		Innervation	Origin of the muscle
Intrinsic lingual muscles	Superior longitudinal lingual	trigeminal	1st branchial arch
	Inferior longitudinal lingual	trigeminal	1st branchial arch
	Transverse lingual	glossopharyngeal	3rd branchial arch
	Vertical lingual	hypoglossal (?)	occipital somites
Extrinsic lingual muscles	Genioglossus	hypoglossal	occipital somites
	Styloglossus	hypoglossal	occipital somites
	Hyoglossus	hypoglossal	occipital somites
	Palatoglossus	glossopharyngeal	3rd branchial arch

A New Theory of the Origination for the Human Tongue

From those anatomical findings, we could consider that all the tongue muscle is not derived from myoblasts originating in occipital somites, but each tongue muscle has its own origin and differentiated with its own history along its own identity. Now, we would like to present a new theory of origination of the human tongue as following.

First, the tongue sprouts near front of or in the area of the first branchial arch with pushing up by the cervical rectus column muscles (visceral longitudinal muscles) which are innervated by somatic efferent motor nerves and course from the bottom of the body to the mouth longitudinally (Fig. 14). Thus, the prototype of the tongue is consisted of both the first branchial muscle and the cervical rectus column muscle. After that, the cartilages of the first branchial arch (Meckel's cartilage) form primitive jaws, and the cartilages of the second branchial arch (Reichert's cartilage) support primitive jaws as the hyomandibular cartilages. With the changes of the first and second branchial cartilages, muscle fibers of the first branchial muscles except muscle fibers consisting of the prototype of the tongue and muscle fibers of the second branchial muscles break out the pharyngeal cavity to the outside of the head and neck. The former muscles differentiate to the masticatory muscles and the latter differentiate to the facial muscles and the cervical subcutaneous muscles. Next, the cervical rectus column muscle pushes up the muscle layer of the third branchial muscle and takes in the third branchial muscle as a tongue muscle (Fig, 15.). After disappearance of the cartilaginous jaws, the bony jaws are made by membranous ossification and some parts of cartilaginous jaws differentiate the occicle bones, i.e., the malleus and the incus. Also almost parts of the second branchial cartilage disappear or differentiate the upper structure of the hyoid bone, the styloid process, and the stapes. With disappearance or differentiating the first and the second branchial cartilages, adhesive regions of the cervical rectum column muscles to the solid structure of the head and neck might change the mandibular bone, the hyoid bone, and styloid process. As results, the muscles originated from the first branchial arch differentiate the superior and the inferior longitudinal lingual muscles, the muscles originated from the third branchial arch differentiate the transverse lingual and the palatoglossus muscles, the muscle derived from the cervical rectus column muscles differentiate the genioglossus, hyoglossus, and styloglossus muscle. And the styloglossus muscle branches muscle fibers into the tongue as the vertical lingual muscles (Fig. 16). These concepts for the musculature of the human tongue might contribute to create more useful or significant approaches for the patients with dysarthria or swallowing disorders.

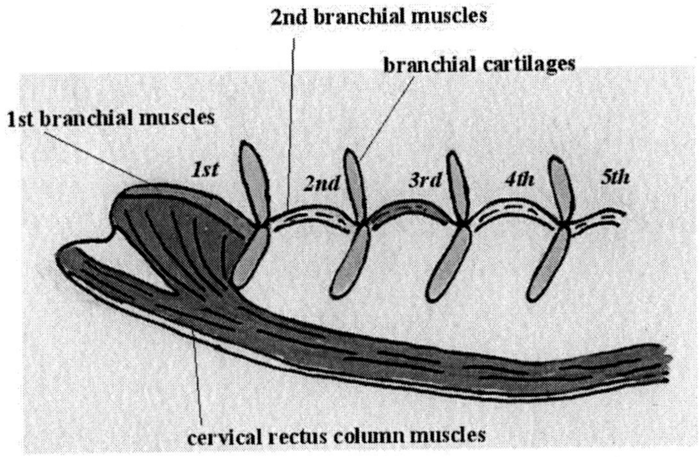

Figure 14. The tongue sprouts near front of or in the area of the first branchial arch with pushing up by the cervical rectus column muscles. The prototype of the tongue is consisted of muscle fibers of both the first branchial muscle (blue) and the cervical rectus column muscles (orange).

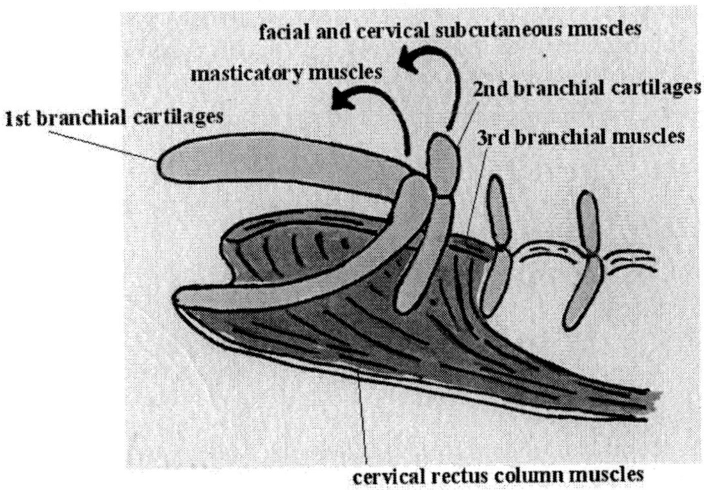

Figure 15. After forming the primitive jaws and their supporting structures with cartilages of the first and second branchial arches, muscle fibers of the first branchial muscles except muscle fibers consisting of the prototype of the tongue (blue), and muscle fibers of the second branchial muscles break out the pharyngeal cavity to the outside of the head and neck. Muscle fibers from the first branchial arch differentiate the masticatory muscles, and muscle fibers from the second branchial arch differentiate the facial and the cervical subcutaneous muscles. Then, the cervical rectus column muscle pushes up the muscle layer of the third branchial muscle (green) and takes in muscle fibers of the third branchial arch as a tongue muscle.

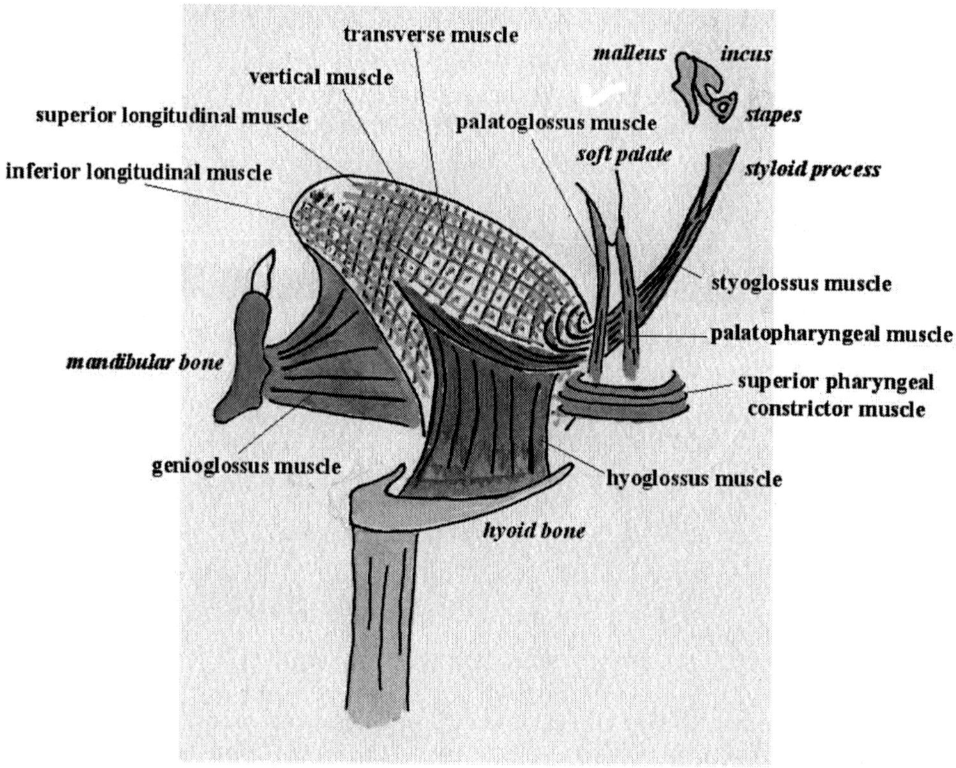

Figure 16. The musculature of the human tongue. Muscles fibers originated from the first branchial arch (blue) differentiate the superior and the inferior longitudinal lingual muscles, muscle fibers originated from the third branchial arch (green) differentiate the transverse lingual and the palatoglossus muscles, muscle fibers derived from the cervical rectus column muscles (orange) differentiate the genioglossus, hyoglossus, and styloglossus muscle. And the styloglossus muscle branches muscle fibers into the tongue as the vertical lingual muscle.

REFERENCES

[1] Sadler TW (2000): *Langman's medical embryology*. 8th edn. Lippincott Williams &Willkins, Baltimore.

[2] Romer AS (1970): *The vertebrate body*. 4th Edn. W.B.Saunders, Philadelphia.

[3] Marcus H (1934): Zur stammesgeschichte der Zunge? *Ueber Muskulatur in der polypteruszunge*. Anat Anz 77.

[4] Portman A (1969): *Einführung in die vergleichende morphogie der wirbeltiere*. Schwabe & Co, Basel.

[5] Hatta S (1931): Comparative embryology. 1st Edn. Tohe Shoin, Tokyo.

[6] Saigusa H, Yamashita K, Tanuma K, Saigusa M, Niimi S (2004): Morphological studies for retrusive movement of the human adult tongue. *Clin Anat* 17:92-98.

[7] Kokawa T, Saigusa H, Aino I, Matsuoka C, Nakamura T, Tanuma K, Yamashita K, Niimi S (2005): Physiological studies of retrusive movements of the human tongue. *J of Voice* 20:414-422.

[8] Saigusa H, Tanuma K, Yamashita K, Saigusa M, Niimi S (2006): Nerve fiber analysis for the lingual nerve of the human adult subjects. *Surg Radiol Anat* 28:59-65.

[9] Saigusa H, Aino I, Tanuma K, Yamashita K, Saigusa M, Niimi S (2009): Morphological Study related to the Jaw-Tongue Reflux in Human Adults. *J of Voice* (in press).

In: Speech Disorders: Causes, Treatment and Social Effects ISBN: 978-1-60876-213-2
Editor: Alan E. Harrison, pp. 275-287

Chapter 14

EFFECTIVENESS OF SPEECH RATE-CONVERSION SOFTWARE FOR PATIENTS WITH DYSARTHRIA

Masaki Nishio[1], Yasuhiro Tanaka[2], Chikako Sakakibara[3] and Naoko Abe[4]

[1]Department of Speech, Language and Hearing Sciences, Niigata University of Health and Welfare, 1398, Shimami-cho, Kita-ku, Niigata, 950-3198, Japan

[2]Graduate School of Health and Welfare, Niigata University of Health and Welfare 1398, Shimami-cho, Kita-ku, Niigata, 950-3198, Japan

[3]Department of Rehabilitation, Uno Hospital, 1-10, Nakaokazaki-cho, Okazaki, 444-0921, Japan

[4]Department of Rehabilitation, Kaetsu Hospital; 1-23, Nakazawa-cho, Akiha-Ku, Niigata, 956-0831, Japan

ABSTRACT

The effectiveness of using speech rate-conversion software by artificially decreasing sound waveforms without changing the pitch was studied in 62 individuals with dysarthria. Besides having patients read a standard common passage entitled "The North Wind and the Sun" aloud, they had casual conversations on a different occasion. Both reading and conversations were recorded on a digital audiocassette recorder in a sound-treated studio. Using speech rate-conversion software, the two types of speech samples (reading and speaking) were played back under 5 rate-delay conditions (100, 150, 200, 250, and 300% slower than the original recording) for evaluation of intelligibility and naturalness by 3 speech and language pathologists. With regard to both intelligibility and naturalness, a significant difference was observed among the 5 rate-delay conditions regardless of the type and severity of dysarthria. A 200% delay in rate delivered the greatest improvement in intelligibility; conversely, any rate-delay less or more than 200% resulted in slight deterioration. In addition, a 150% rate-delay in speech yielded the greatest improvement in naturalness, while any delay less or more than 150% resulted in a significant deteriorating tendency. These findings suggest that reducing verbal speed within the range of 150 - 200% may be useful in the clinical management of dysarthria.

Keywords: dysarthria, speech rate-conversion software, intelligibility, naturalness

INTRODUCTION

It is widely known that slowing the rate of speech can improve intelligibility in individuals with dysarthria (Yorkston, Beukelman, Strand, and Bell, 1999; Duffy, 2005; Nishio, 2007). In the clinical setting, different rate-control techniques such as alphabet board supplementation (Beukelman and Yorkston, 1977; Hunter, Pring, and Martine, 1991; Beliveau, Hodge, and Hagler, 1995; Dowden, 1997; Hustad and Beukelman, 2001, 2002; Hustad and Garcia, 2002; Beukelman, Fager, Ullman, Hanson, and Logemann, 2002; Nishio and Niimi, 2005), pacing board (Helm, 1979; Pilon, Mcintosh, and Thaut, 1998; Nishio, Tanaka, Abe, Shimano, and Yamaji, 2007), rhythmic cueing (Yorkston and Beukelman, 1981; Yorkston, Hammen, Beukelman, and Traynor, 1990), delayed auditory feedback (DAF) (Hanson and Metter, 1980; Downie, Low, and Lindsay, 1981; Hanson, Gerratt, and Ward, 1983; Dobbs, Bowes, Henley, Charlett, O'Neill, Dickins, Nicholson, and Dobbs, 1993; Dagenais, Southwood, and Lee, 1998) and visual feedback (Berry and Goshorn, 1983) have been used to slow the speech of individuals with dysarthria to improve intelligibility and/or naturalness in speech.

On the other hand, artificially converting and editing speech by acoustic techniques, where the speech rate is modified using speech rate-conversion software (Nakamura, Seiyama, Ikezawa, Takagi, and Miyasaki, 1994; Watanabe, 1996), has recently been developed. Much attention has been focused on the useful time-domain harmonic scaling (TDHS) method (Malar, 1979), where the speech rate is modified by extending the sound waveform against time without altering the pitch. As such, multiple modified and improved versions of the TDHS method have been developed to date.

The innovated software programs and related devices, which were originally developed for the enhancement of linguistic education/training, have also been extensively employed in the elderly with hearing impairment to improve their speech perception ability. Although unreported to date, these software and devices may be useful in the prosthetic management of dysarthria in clinical treatment on the whole. Of cases worthy of using these innovations are patients who find difficulty in speech training; these recently innovated software and devices may in fact serve as useful alternatives along with voice amplifiers and relevant devices.

In this chapter, we elucidated the effects of speech rate-conversion software on speech intelligibility and naturalness of Japanese patients with dysarthria. The following issues were addressed accordingly:

1. The relationships of speech rate-delay and intelligibility and naturalness in individuals with dysarthria were investigated, and optimal speech rate-delay conditions for the respective speech features were established.
2. The efficacy of speech rate-conversion software in relation with the type of dysarthria was elucidated.
3. The effect of dysarthria severity on the efficacy of speech rate-conversion software was also investigated.

METHODS

Subjects

A total of 62 individuals with dysarthria (male: 42; female: 20; mean age: 60.0 years; SD=14.4) participated in the investigation. The mean ages of males and females were 62.5 (SD=12.0) and 54.8 (SD=17.8) years, respectively. In tandem with the objectives of the present chapter, the distributions of dysarthria were categorized according to the etiological factors (Table 1) and dysarthria types (Table 2) . Based on an extensively employed and commonly accepted standard classification system in the field of speech pathology (Darley, Aronson, and Brown, 1975), dysarthria was categorized accordingly (Table 2). A defect in the unilateral upper motor neurons (UUMN), which is often quoted in current studies, was also included as a type of dysarthria (Table 2). Patients were categorically enrolled in the investigation according to the following criteria:

1. Adult-onset dysarthria,
2. Dysarthria without other speech or language disorders,
3. Dysarthria without history of either speech disorder prior to disease onset,
4. Dysarthria without tracheostomy.

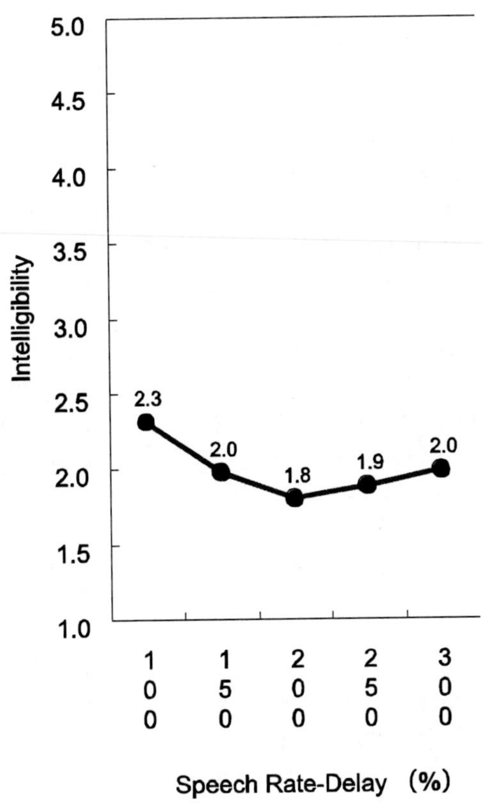

Figure 1. Intelligibility scores at the respective rate-delay conditions in 62 patients with dysarthria showed highest improvement in speech intelligibility levels at 200% rate-delay in speech. Rate-delays of less or more than 200% produced reversed tendencies in intelligibility levels.

Recording Procedures

The speech samples employed to measure speech intelligibility and naturalness included reading of a standard passage aloud entitled "The North Wind and the Sun" in Japanese (reading), and casual question-response conversations on seven items with a speech pathologist (speaking). Patients were each asked to read a passage once at his/her own pace with habitual and comfortable pitch, volume/loudness, and rate. All speech samples were recorded on a digital audio-cassette recorder （Sony TCD-D10） with a sampling rate of 44.1 kHz in a sound-treated studio. The vocal input receptacle of a microphone (Shure, SM48) was placed and positioned directly opposite (180°) to the mouth of patients with a constant mouth-to-microphone distance of 15 cm.

Speech Intelligibility and Speech Naturalness

The speech samples (reading and speaking) were reproduced with their speech rate delayed using time-warping (i.e. speech rate-conversion software) equipped with optional auditory feedback tools of the Computerized Speech Lab (CSL-Model: 4400, KayPentax). The present device was capable of reproducing and delaying speech rate input by 300% via either conduction through the connecting cord or through the microphone per se. During playback, the articulation time (i.e. time-intervals where speech segments are reproduced) and pause-time (i.e. silent periods in the speech waveforms) were identified, and were extended accordingly under different rate-delay conditions.

Using above-mentioned speech rate-conversion software, the two speech samples (reading and speaking) were all played back under 5 rate-delay conditions (100, 150, 200, 250 and 300%), and the intelligibility and naturalness were evaluated by three 'blind' listeners based on a 9-grade rating scale (Table 3). At 100% speech rate-delay, the speech speed was reduced by 1 fold or in other words the speech rate remained unchanged. At 150 and 300%, the rates were respectively reduced by 1.5 and 3 fold, and so on.

The listeners were asked to rate the patient's speech intelligibility perceptually using the 9-grade rating scale, where the speech intelligibility level was scored according to severity in understanding the speech content. A highest score of 5 was given to speech not understandable at all, a lowest score of 1 was given to speech fairly understandable, and so on (Table 3). This rating system was developed by Taguchi (1966), revised by Itoh (1992), and has been extensively applied in speech and linguistic studies in Japan since 1992. Furthermore, the reliability of this 9-grade rating scale has previously been confirmed by Nishio and Niimi (2001).

Speech performance with regard to naturalness was perceptually rated with a 5-point severity-rating scale as follows: extremely natural (1; without any unnatural elements); fairly natural (2; with slight unnatural elements); natural (3; natural with negligible unnatural elements); unnatural (4; with certain unnatural elements); and extremely unnatural (5; without any natural element). This severity scale developed by Nishio has its reliability confirmed in 2004.

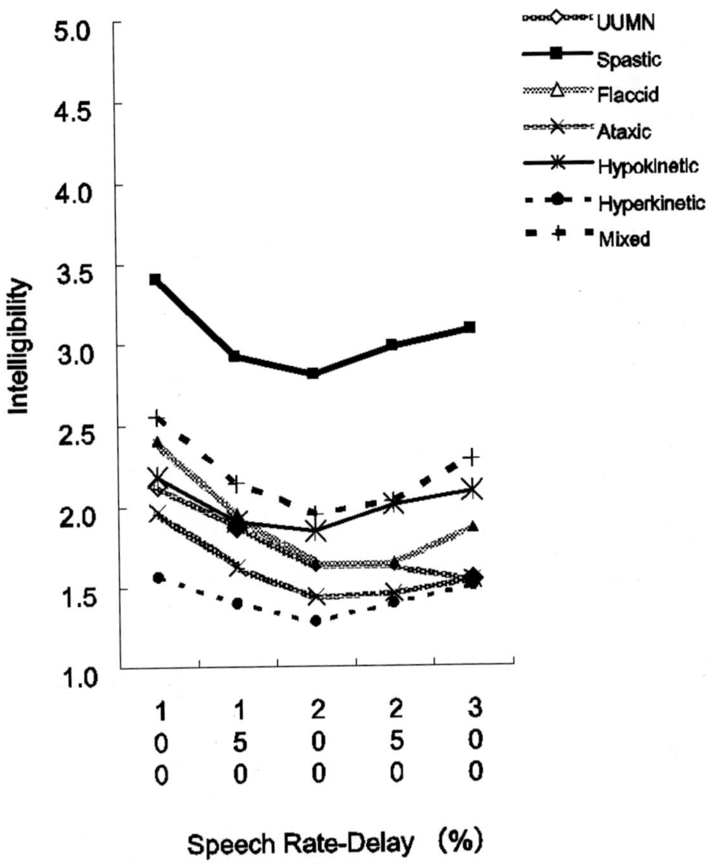

Figure 2. Intelligibility scores of the different types of dysarthria under various speech rate-delay conditions. Except for the unilateral upper motor neuron (UUMN) type, all other types (spastic, flaccid, ataxic, hypokinetic, hyperkinetic and mixed) indicated highest improvement in intelligibility levels at 200% rate-delay in speech. Rate-delays of less or more than 200% for all types (except UUMN) registered reversed effects in intelligibility levels, indicating that speech comprehension was best attained at 200% rate-delay in speech of dysarthria patients.

Table 1. Distribution of etiologies

Etiological factors	Cases (n)
Cerebrovascular disease	23
Spinocerebellar degeneration	12
Amyotrophic lateral sclerosis	9
Parkinson's disease	9
Neuropathy	2
Encephalitis	2
Others (one for each etiology) Myasthenia gravis, Dystonia, Myoclonus, Shy-Drager Syndrome, Brain injury	
Total	62

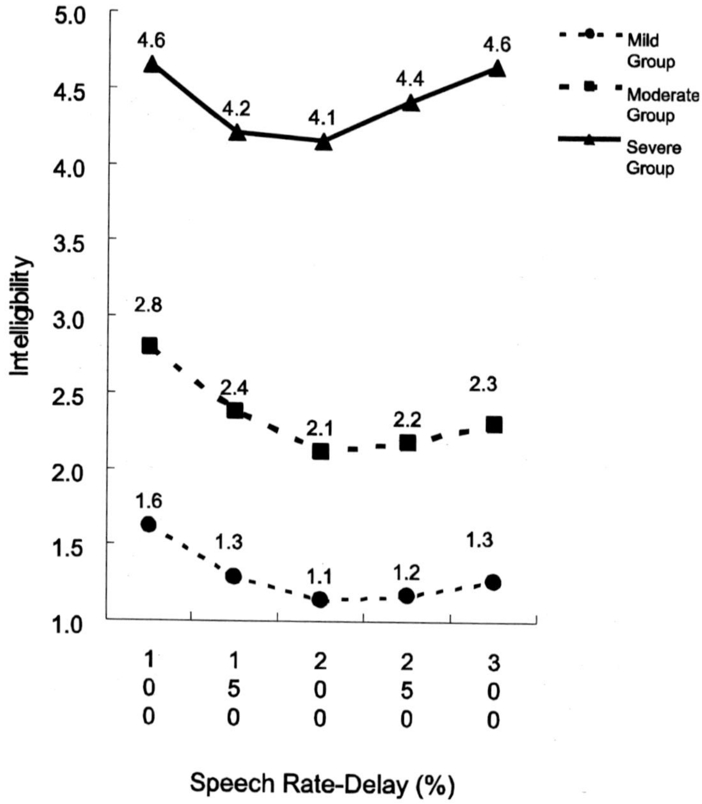

Figure 3. The relationships between the 3 severity (mild, moderate and severe) groups and the rate-delay conditions portrayed the highest improvement in intelligibility level at 200% rate-delay in speech for all groups.

Scoring by the Listeners

Three speech and language pathologists assessed the listening aspect and rated both the intelligibility levels and naturalness consistently for each speech sample (played back under 5 rate-delay conditions in speech). A mean score was computed for each speech sample by averaging the rating scores of the three listeners.

Severity Level

The intelligibility scores on severity of dysarthria of patients were homogenously graded into 3 groups with 3 different intelligibility levels (Table 3): mild (<2.3), moderate (<3.7) and severe (>3.7), where the higher the speech intelligibility scores, the more severe was the pathological state. In our findings, 36 (male: 20; female: 16; mean age: 59.0 years, SD=16.4), 17 (male: 15; female: 2; mean age: 61.6 years, SD=11.0) and 9 (male: 7; female: 2; mean age: 61.4 with SD=12.4) patients were distributed in the mild, moderate and severe dysarthria groups, respectively. Significant differences in age between any of 2 of the 3 groups were not established with one-way analysis variance assay.

Table 2. Distribution according to dysarthria types

Dysarthria type	Cases (n)
Flaccid	7
Spastic	11
Ataxic	19
Hypokinetic	9
Hyperkinetic	3
Mixed	9
UUMN*	4
Total	62

*: UUMN=unilateral upper motor neuron.

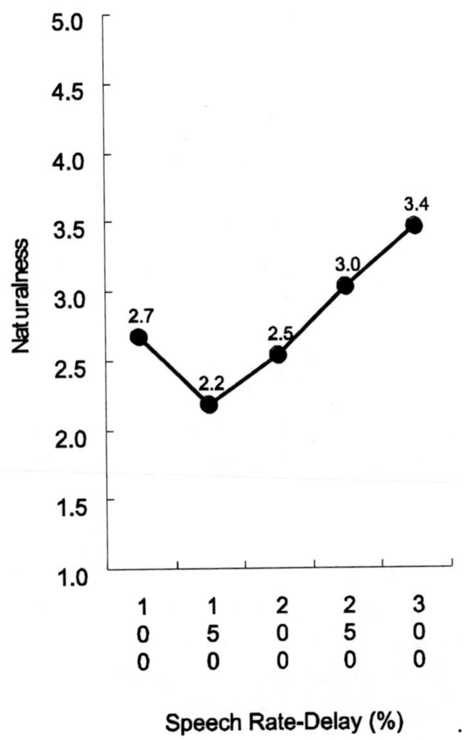

Figure 4. On comparing the 5 rate-delay conditions in 62 cases with dysarthria, the naturalness levels established the highest improvement at 150% rate-delay in speech, while naturalness portrayed a distinct decreasing tendency under rate-delays of less or more than 150%.

Method Reliability

With regard to the evaluated intelligibility levels and naturalness by the 3 listeners, the 5 rate-delay conditions (100, 150, 200, 250 and 300% delay in speech speed) provided Kendall's coefficient of concordance and yielded extremely high levels of W=0.95 with significant differences ($p<0.001$) in intelligibility and naturalness.

Table 3. Rating scale for speech intelligibility

Scores	Comprehensive levels of speech
1	Speech is fairly understandable
1.5	Between levels 1 and 2
2	Speech is understandable in large part, but with some difficulty
2.5	Between levels 2 and 3
3	Speech is understandable if the listener knows the content spoken
3.5	Between levels 3 and 4
4	Speech is understandable in small part
4.5	Between levels 4 and 5
5	Speech is not understandable at all

RESULTS

Speech Intelligibility

The relationships between speech intelligibility and 5 different rate-delay conditions in 62 cases of dysarthria (Figure 1) indicated the peak improvement in speech intelligibility was achieved at 200% rate-delay in speech. Delay rates less than or more than 200% portrayed a reversed tendency, where speech intelligibility would be reduced accordingly. Significant improvements ($p<0.001$) in speech intelligibility were established with the 5 different rate-delay conditions when verified with the Kruskal-Wallis test.

From data on the speech intelligibility levels of the different types of dysarthria evaluated under 5 different rate-delay conditions (Figure 2), the levels registered the highest improvement at 200% delay in speech rate in 6 of 7 listed types of dysarthria (exception: UUMN). Delay rates less than or more than 200% indicated a reversed tendency; i.e. improvements of the speech intelligibility were reduced. When verified with the Friedman's two-way analysis of variance, significant differences ($p<0.001$) were established. Although ataxic dysarthria was the only type that showed significant improvement ($p<0.05$) in speech intelligibility, other types did not indicate any significant difference when compared with the 5 rate-delay conditions using the Kruskal-Wallis test.

In a fashion similar to dysarthria types (Figure 2), the relationships between the severity groups and the rate-delay conditions (Figure 3) portrayed a similar tendency in intelligibility levels with rate-delay condition; viz., the highest improvements of intelligibility levels were established in all (mild, moderate and severe) groups at 200% delay in speech rate/speed. In a manner similar to intelligibility levels and rate-delay conditions of the different dysarthria types (Figure 2), a significant difference ($p<0.01$) was established when verified with the Friedman's two-way analysis of variance. In group comparisons under the 5 rate-delay conditions using the Krustal-Wallis test; although a significant difference ($p<0.001$) in intelligibility scores was established between the mild and moderate groups, significant difference was not verified with the severe group.

Speech Naturalness

On comparing the 5 rate-delay conditions in 62 cases with dysarthria, the naturalness levels achieved highest improvements at 150% rate-delay in speech, while naturalness portrayed a distinct decreasing tendency under a rate-delay of less or more than 150%. Comparisons with the Kruskal-Wallis test indicated significant differences ($p<0.001$) in speech naturalness under the 5 rate-delay conditions (Figure 4).

In correlating the dysarthria types with speech naturalness under the 5 different rate-delay conditions, all types established improvements in speech naturalness levels at 150% rate-delay in speech (Figure 5). The naturalness levels of all dysarthria types indicated a markedly reversed (i.e. decreased) tendency when the rate-delay was less or more than 150%. On comparison with the Friedman's two-way analysis variance, significant differences ($p<0.001$) were noted. Although the ataxic ($p<0.001$), hypokinetic ($P<0.05$), mixed ($p<0.05$) and UUMN ($p<0.05$) types established significant differences, the flaccid, spastic and hyperkinetic types indicated insignificant tendencies when the respective types were each compared under the 5 rate-delay conditions using the Kruskal-Wallis test.

On correlating naturalness with the severity groups under the 5 rate-delay conditions in speech, peak improvements of naturalness were established at 150% rate-delay condition while any rate-delay lower or higher than 150% would markedly reduced the naturalness levels (Figure 6). When verified by the two-way analysis variance test, significant differences ($p<0.01$) were noted. Although the mild and severe groups indicated significant differences ($p<0.001$) under the 5 rate-delay conditions, comparisons with the severe group did not show any significant difference when verified with the Kruskal-Willis test (Figure 6).

DISCUSSION

From the present results, speech intelligibility and naturalness reflected the highest comprehensive levels at 200% and 150% rate-delay conditions in speech, respectively. As such, in cases where speech rate-conversion software was employed in the clinical treatment of dysarthria, the most effective management would be established within the range of 150 - 200% rate-delay conditions in speech. Intelligibility levels would instead be exacerbated if the rate-delay were either less or more than 200%, disproving the simple proportional relationship that intelligibility levels would improve with increases in the rate-delay condition (i.e. lower speech rate) when applying present speech rate-conversion software. .

Improvement in speech intelligibility increased with speech rate-delay in the present investigation may be attributed to: 1) elevation of speech perception ability related with segmental information via an increase in the articulation time; and 2) a delayed speech rate facilitated comprehension on the listener side by providing more time for processing acoustic signals. Furthermore, the rationales for the decrease in speech intelligibility with rate-delay of more than 200% include: 1) prevalence of noise incorporating intermittent consonants such as plosive, affricate and fricative sounds; 2) perception on the listener side of elevated noise components (produced by abnormal articulatory movement due to time-delay; 3) probable degradation of segmental information structuring the connected speech.

These findings advocate that not only the adjuvant effect of using speech rate-conversion software in clinical treatment of dysarthria (incorporation with various currently employed techniques used in the speech training) was constructive, but the use of said software to merely delay the speech rate may also indirectly elevate the value-added communication ability in some dysarthric speakers who find medical (internal medicine) problems with certain devices routinely used for speech-training

Hitherto, naturalness displays a decreasing tendency with delay in speech rate (Yorkston, Beukelman, Strand, and Bell, 1999; Nishio, 2007). In the present chapter, a 150% rate-delay in speech improved naturalness compared with either 100% or >150% rate-delays, regardless of the type and severity of dysarthria. The rationales for the improvement in naturalness with 150% rate-delay in speech may include: 1) a reduction of hoarseness (especially rough hoarseness) with rate-delay in speech; 2) an elevated speech-perception ability of segmental information on the listener side due to probable attenuation in articulatory distortion. The distinct exacerbations in naturalness with increases in rate-delays exceeding 150% may be attributable to: 1) perceptional extension of abnormality in prosody with delay in the speech rate; 2) degradation of suprasegmental information and/or prosodic features such as rhythm, stress and intonation accompanying delay in the speech rate; and 3) factors related to voice-synthesizing components in speech.

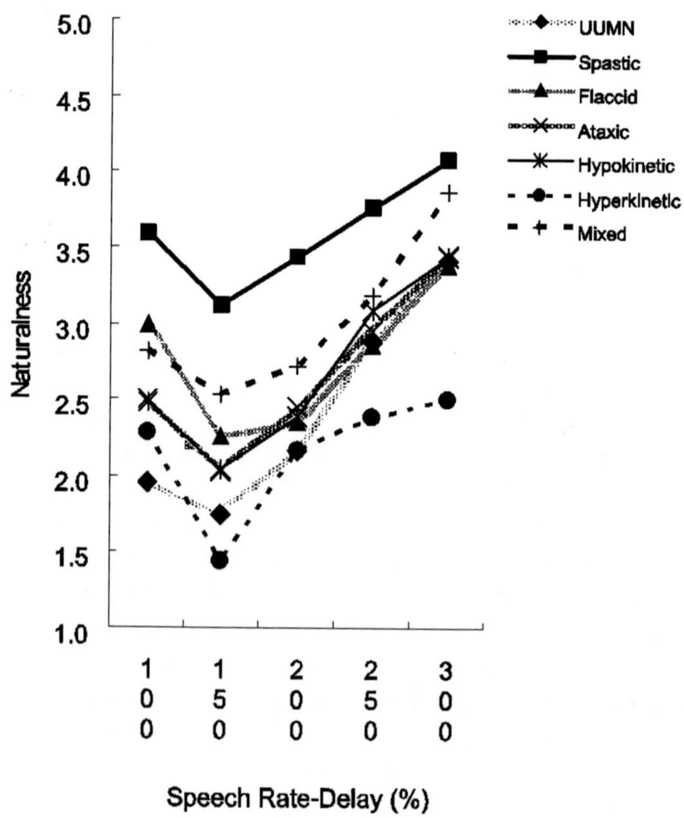

Figure 5. All types of dysarthria established the highest improvement in speech naturalness levels at 150% rate-delay conditions; however the naturalness levels indicated a markedly reversed (i.e. decreased) tendency when the rate-delay was less or more than 150%.

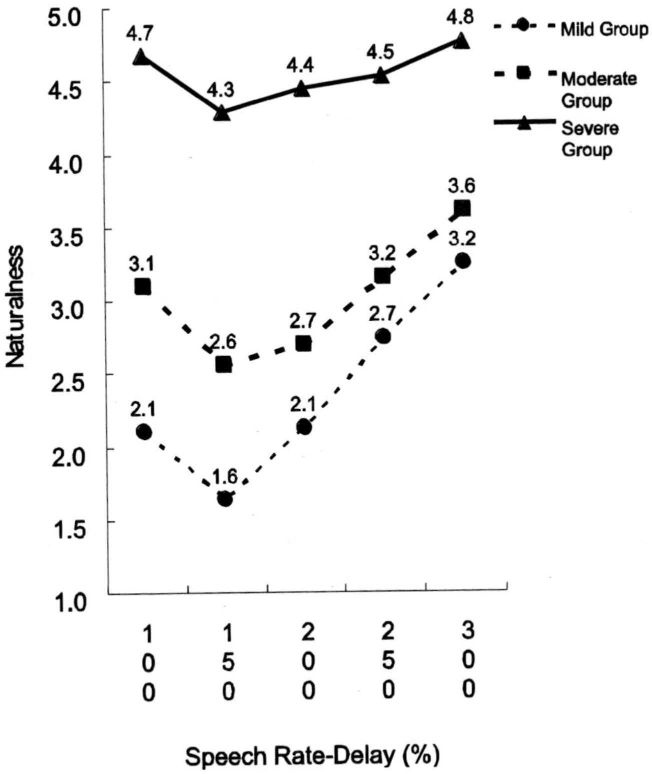

Figure 6. On correlating naturalness with the severity groups under the 5 rate-delay conditions in speech; peak improvement in naturalness was establsihed at 150% rate-delay in speech, while any delay lower or higher than 150% would markedly reduced the naturalness levels.

The results of using speech rate-conversion software in the present chapter are probably different from those clinical outcomes obtained in behavioral management approaches of speech rate control. In behavioral management of speech rate control; when the speech rate of patients with dysarthria is deliberately delayed, the following events occur: 1) coordination is enhanced through interactions of various speech components; and 2) actualization with emphasis on speech intelligibility through interactions of various speech subsystems attributable to delay in articulatory movement (Yorkston, Beukelman, Strand, and Bell, 1999; Nishio, 2007).

In summary, speech intelligibility and/or speech perception ability on the listener side can be potentially improved when the speech rate of patients with dysarthria is subjected to conditioning training with complementary use of speech rate-conversion software.

References

Beliveau, C., Hodge, M. & Hagler, P. (1995). Effect of supplemental linguistic cues on the intelligibility of severely dysarthric speakers. *Augmentative and Alternative Communication*, *11*, 176-186.

Berry, W. R. & Goshorn, E. L. (1983). Immediate visual feedback in the treatment of ataxic dysarthria: a case study. In Berry WR (Ed.) *Clinical Dysarthria* (pp.253-256). San Diego, California: College-Hill Press.

Beukelman, D. R. & Yorkston, K. M. (1977). A communication system for the severely dysarthric speaker with an intact language system. *Journal of Speech and Hearing Disorders*, *42*, 265-270.

Beukelman, D. R., Fager, S., Ullman, C., Hanson, E. & Logemann, J. A. (2002). The impact of speech supplementation and clear speech on the intelligibility and speaking rate of speakers with traumatic brain injury. *Journal of Medical Speech-Language Pathology*, *10*, 237-242.

Dagenais, P. A., Southwood, M. H. & Lee, T. L. (1998). Rate reduction method for improving speech intelligibility of dysarhric speakers with parkinson's disease. *Journal of Medical Speech-Language Pathology*, *3*, 143-157.

Darley, F., Aronson, A. & Brown, J. (1975). Motor Speech Disorders. Saunders . Philadelphia: W. B. Saunders Company.

Dobbs, R. J., Bowes, S. G., Henley, M., Charlett, A., O'Neill, C. J. A., Dickins, J., Nicholson, P. W. & Dobbs, S. M. (1993). Assessment of the bradyphenia of parkinsonism: A novel use of delayed auditory feedback. *Acta neurologica Scandinavica, 87*, 262-267.

Dowden, P. A. (1997). Augmentative and alternative communicative decision making for children with severely unintelligible speech. A*ugmentative and Alternative Communication*. *13*, 48-58.

Downie, A. W., Low, J. M. & Lindsay, D. D. (1981). Speech disorders in parkinsonism: Usefulness of delayed auditory feedback in selected cases. *British Journal of Disorders of Communication*, *16*, 135-139.

Duffy, J. R. (2005): Motor speech disorders: substrates, differential diagnosis, and management (2nd edition), St Louis: Mosby.

Hanson, W. R. & Metter, E. J. (1980). DAF as instrumental treatment for dysarthria in progressive supranuclear palsy: a case report. *Journal of Speech and Hearing Disorders*, *45*, 268-276.

Hanson, D. G., Gerratt, B. R. & Ward, P. H. (1983). Glottographic measurement of vocal dysfunction : a preliminary report. *The Annals of otology, rhinology, and laryngology*, *92*, 413-420.

Hunter, L., Pring, T. & Martine, S. (1991). The use of strategies to increase speech intelligibility in cerebral palsy: an experimental evaluation. *British Journal of Disorders of Communication*, *26*, 163-174.

Hustad, K. C. & Beukelman, D. R. (2001). Effects of linguistic cues and stimulus cohesion on intelligibility of severely dysarthric speech. *Journal of Speech and Hearing Research*, *44*, 497-510.

Hustad, K. C. & Beukelman, D. (2002). Listener comprehension of severely dysarthric speech: effects of linguistic cues and stimulus cohesion. *Journal of Speech and Hearing Research*, *45*, 545-558.

Hustad, K. C. & Garcia, J. M. (2002). The influences of alphabet supplementation, iconic gestures, and predictive messages on intelligibility of a speaker with cerebral palsy. *Journal of Medical Speech-Language Pathology*, *10*, 279-285.

Itoh, M. (1992). Single-word intelligibility test for evaluating speech of adult with articulation disorders. *Jpn J Logop Phoniatr*, *33*, 227-236.

Malar, S. (1979). Time-domain algorithms for harmonic bandwidth reduction & time scaling of speech signals. *IEEE, Trans. Acoust., Speech, Signal Processing*, ASSP-27, 2.

Nakamura, A., Seiyama, N., Ikezawa, R., Takagi, T. & Miyasaki, E. (1994). Real time voice speed converting system without small impairment. *The Journal of the Acoustical Society of Japan*, *50*, 509-520.

Nishio M. & Niimi, S. (2001). Speech intelligibility in dysarthric speakers. *The Japan Journal of Logopedics and Phoniatrics, 42*, 9-16.

Nishio, M. (2004). Assessment of motor speech for dysarthria. Tokyo: Interuna Publishers.

Nishio, M. & Niimi, S. (2005). Effects of initial letter cueing on intelligibility of Japanese speakers with dysarthria. *Journal of Multilingual Communication Disorders*, *3*, 183-193.

Nishio, M. (2007). Standard textbook of dysarthria. Tokyo: Ishiyaku Publisher.

Nishio, M., Tanaka, Y., Abe, N., Shimano, A. & Yamaji, H. (2007). Efficacy of speech therapy for dysarthria. *The Japan Journal of Logopedics and Phoniatrics*, *48*, 215-224.

Pilon, M. A., Mcintosh, K. W. & Thaut, M. H. (1998). Auditory vs visual speech timing cues as external rate control to enhance verbal intelligibility in mixed spastic ataxic dysarthric speakers: a pilot study. *Brain Injury*, *12*, 793-803.

Taguchi, T. (1966). Introduction to logopedics. Tokyo: Igaku Shoin Publisher.

Watanabe, W. (1996). A study on the effect of slower speech rate produced by the speech rate converter. *Nippon Jibiinkoka Gakkai kaiho*, *99*, 445-453.

Yorkston, K. & Beukelman, D. (1981). Ataxic dysarthria: treatment sequences based on intelligibility and prosodic considerations. *Journal of Speech and Hearing Disorders*, *46*, 398-404.

Yorkston, K. M., Hammen, V. L., Beukelman, D. R. & Traynor, C. D. (1990). The effect of rate control on the intelligibility and naturalness of dysarthric speech. *Journal of Speech and Hearing Disorders*, *55*, 550-560.

Yorkston, K. M., Beukelman, D. R., Strand, E. A. & Bell, K. R. (1999). Management of motor speech disorders in children and adults. Austin, Texas: Pro-Ed

In: Speech Disorders: Causes, Treatment and Social Effects ISBN: 978-1-60876-213-2
Editor: Alan E. Harrison, pp. 289-310

Chapter 15

SPEECH PROBLEMS IN DYSLEXIA: EVIDENCE FROM AUDITORY AND VISUAL SPEECH PERCEPTION

Joshua Ramirez and Virginia Mann
University of California, Irvine

ABSTRACT

The persistent reading difficulties of developmental dyslexics are often accompanied by a host of speech processing deficits (Brady *et al.* 1983; Boets *et al.* 2001; Cunningham *et al.*, 2001; Elbro, 1990; Veuillet *et al.*, 2007; Watson & Miller; 1993; Wible *et al.*, 2002). Dyslexics typically have inordinate difficulties in processing noise-degraded speech as opposed to non-speech stimuli despite exhibiting normal audiometric profiles. Furthermore, dyslexics often show relatively poor categorization of phonetically similar but phonologically contrastive speech sounds. However, some speech contrasts such as /d/-/g/ provoke more discriminative difficulty than others such as /b/-/s/ or /b/-/w/. If speech and speech disorders are modular, as suggested by Liberman and Mattingly (1985), the dyslexic pattern of speech problems may not be limited to the auditory domain. Less often reported in the literature is a reduced influence of visual articulatory gestures on dyslexic perception of auditory cues (Ramirez and Mann, 2005). The question posed by the current study is whether or not dyslexic speech processing in the auditory channel is similarly nuanced in the visual channel. To this end, an auditory-visual twist on the standard categorical perception experiment was used to assess dyslexics' and controls' categorization of synthetic speech sounds along /ada/-/aga/ and /aba/-/awa/ continua. Presentation of each acoustic continuum involved a 3-factor design: 1) noise masked vs. clear presentation, 2) with and without a simultaneous video of a speaker, 3) articulating either endpoint of the respective continua. Results show that the dyslexics exhibited less precise, flatter categorical functions for acoustic /ada/ vs. /aga/ in noise; their responses were also less influenced by the introduction of visual cues to /d/ or /g/ than were those of the controls. In contrast, the dyslexics showed more control-like categorization of acoustic /aba/-/awa/ stimuli, as well as greater influences of the corresponding visual cues than controls. This parallel between the visual and auditory speech perception of dyslexics can be described phonologically: dyslexics may find place of articulation contrasts more problematic than manner contrasts. It is possible that poor apprehension or representation of key phonological features may imperil the categorical labeling of minimally contrastive speech stimuli. Discussion considers this account as compared to auditory temporal accounts, general magnocellular dysfunctions, and integrative failures.

INTRODUCTION

During the course of early literacy training, an estimated 5-10% of children find that their otherwise normal academic achievement is marred by inordinately low proficiency in reading and writing (Shaywitz *et al.*, 1990). Although a general consensus has ruled out low motivation, poor intellectual capacity, and lack of social or educational opportunity as causal factors (for review see Snowling, 2000; Vellutino, 1979), there is still far less agreement among the various etiological theories of reading disability regarding the sensorial or perceptual aberrations that actually typify dyslexia. The persistent reading difficulties of these developmental dyslexics are typically accompanied by a host of subtle speech perception deficits. Inordinate difficulties in identifying speech in noise (Brady *et al.* 1983; Boets *et al.* 2001; Cunningham *et al.*, 2001; Veuillet *et al.*, 2007; Watson & Miller; 1993; Wible *et al.*, 2002), and problems with categorical perception (Breier *et al.*, 2004; Bogliotti, *et al.*, 2002; Bogliotti, *et al.*, 2008; De Weirdt, 1988; Elliot & Hammer, 1998; Godfrey *et al.*, 1981; Joanisse *et al.*, 2000; Reed 1989; Serniclaes *et al.*, 2001, 2004; Snowling *et al.*, 1986; Werker & Tees, 1987) have been observed among dyslexics in the face of normal audiometric profiles. These deficits have been and continue to be the subject of extensive study as they offer insights into the sensory acuity (Gaab *et al.,* 2007; Demb *et al.* 1998a; Demb *et al.*, 1998b; Ridder *et al.*, 1997; Stein & Walsh, 1997; Tallal *et al.* 1993; Tallal & Piercy 1973a and b, 1975) and/or phonological processing difficulties (Chiappe *et al.*, 2001; Chiappe *et al.* 2002; de Gelder & Vroomen, 1998; Rosen & Manganari, 2001; Share *et al.*, 2002; Stanovich, 1998; Studdert-Kennedy & Mody, 1995) that have been well documented in the literature on reading disabilities.

It would appear that at the segmental level, these speech perception deficits are nuanced. Typically, reading disabled individuals find it particularly difficult to discriminate stop-consonants from one another (Brandt & Rosen, 1980; De Weirdt, 1988; Elliot et al. 1989; Godfrey et al. 1981; Kraus et al 1996; Leonard & McGregor, 1992; Lieberman *et al.,* 1985; Mody et al. 1997; Sussman, 1993; Tallal & Piercy, 1974; Tallal and Piercy 1975; Tallal and Stark, 1981; Werker & Tees, 1987). However, some stop vs. fricative (Mody *et al.* 1997), and stop vs. glide consonant contrasts (Kraus *et al.*, 1996; Bradlow *et al.* 1999) do not provoke perceptual difficulty.

One possible explanation for these nuances in the dyslexics' acoustic contrast perception is derived from classic rapid temporal processing (RTP) accounts of reading disability (Gaab *et al.,* 2007; Tallal & Piercy, 1974, 1975). RTP accounts of poor reading achievement among dyslexics and developmental dysphasics (referred to as specific language impaired (SLI) in more recent literature) have pointed to a pervasive failure in temporal acuity for processing rapid acoustic events (Farmer & Klein, 1995a, 1995b; Stark & Tallal, 1988; Tallal, 1980; Tallal *et al.*, 1991; Tallal & Stark, 1982). Dyslexics and SLI individuals have exhibited deficits in temporal order judgment (TOJ) and gap detection tasks (McKrosky & Kidder, 1980; Tallal & Piercy, 1973a and 1973b) that employed rapidly presented speech and non-speech stimuli. Performance in these tasks improved with increases in interstimulus intervals (ISI). Tallal and Piercy (1975) have further suggested that reading/learning disabled individuals also have inordinate difficulties in processing the fast-formant transitions of stop-consonant vowel (CV) syllables /ba/, /da/, and /ga/. In line with this account, there is some evidence that extending the brief formant transition durations of syllables like /ba/ and /da/ can help improve SLI subjects' ability to discriminate these syllables (Tallal *et al.* 1993).

In one supporting study, Kraus *et al.* (1996) measured just noticeable differences (JNDs) for two CV continua, /da/-/ga/ and /ba/-/wa/, in a group of learning-disabled (LD) children and controls. Where the shorter first and second formant (F_1 and F_2, respectively) transition durations for /ba/ distinguish it from /wa/'s more gradual transition, /da/ and /ga/ differ spectro-temporally in terms of both the onset and slope of the third formant (F_3) onset frequency. Results showed that the LD group's JNDs were worse for the /da/-/ga/ contrast. Kraus *et al.* (1996) also examined electrophysiological responses that reflect how the dyslexic brain registers an apparent change from the /b/ acoustic category to /w/. They found that the resulting mismatch negativity (MMN) responses to /b/ and /w/ were equally robust for LD and control subjects. The RTP model would, thus, anticipate that reading impaired individuals would not have difficulties in differentiating /ba/ from /wa/ as they are highly contrastive in formant transition duration. It follows that /ba/ and /wa/ offer a natural foil to consonant contrasts like /da/ vs. /ga/ that possess briefer transitions. Furthermore, the RTP model would suggest that increasing the formant transition durations of the /da/ and /ga/ contrast might enhance their distinctiveness.

In extending the F_3 transition durations for a /da/-/ga/ acoustic continuum, Bradlow *et al.* (1999) found that MMN responses of their LD and control groups were much more similar compared to when the F_3 duration was shorter. However, Bradlow *et al.*'s LD children also exhibited inflated discrimination thresholds for the /da/-/ga/ continuum regardless of whether the critical F_3 transition duration was relatively short or long. In the case of perceptual discrimination, transition duration did not matter, despite the fact that the longer transitions gave rise to a more robust neural response than shorter transitions. Bradlow *et al.* thus interpreted their results as suggesting that the locus of impairment may be situated at a higher—possibly phonetic—level of processing.

Mody *et al.*'s (1997) study offers some insight into why the speech perception problems that appear in the dyslexic literature are nuanced. Mody *et al.*'s sample of reading impaired children showed marked deficits in discrimination and TOJ tasks with synthetic /ba/-/da/ stimuli at short ISIs, echoing Tallal and Piercy's (1975) previous observations. However, Mody *et al.*'s subjects were much sharper in their categorization of /ba/-/sa/ and /da/-/ʃa/. These syllable pairs were phonetically more contrastive than /ba/-/da/, differing in manner of articulation as well as in place. Taken together with Bradlow *et al.'s* findings, it is possible that phonetic features are the critical mitigating factors in dyslexic/LD individuals' phonetic contrast perception. As Elbro (1996) and Fowler and Swanson (1998) both make reference to impoverished phonetic representations as a factor in dyslexia, it is possible that imprecise specification of phonetic features can lead to naming problems and problems with phonological awareness and working memory. In their view we might speculate that if manner differences, for some reason, are easier to discern or are more likely to be correctly represented than place differences, then dyslexics would have greater success with manner contrasts like /b/-/w/, /b/-/s/, and /da/-/ʃa/ than with place contrasts like /b/-/d/ or /d/-/g/. Not only would this account for the pattern of phonetic contrasts that dyslexics find most problematic (as catalogued by Bradlow *et al.*, 1999), but it would also be consistent with studies that have found that acoustic cues for manner of articulation are more salient than those for place among both English and non-English speakers (Zhang, 1996). It would also agree with the pattern of consonant confusions that most commonly occur in normal listening conditions and in noise (Miller & Nicely, 1955).

One question we could ask is whether we could expect to see a similar pattern manifest in other channels of speech perception. After all, it has been theorized that speech perception is modular (Liberman, 1985; Whalen & Liberman, 1996): it is not merely an acoustic entity but a visual one as well. The literature has amply acknowledged this. Although visual speech perception is generally less accurate than auditory or bimodal speech perception (Auer, 2002), clearly the discrimination and identification of many speech 'sounds' can be influenced by a video of a talker articulating in synchrony with acoustic cues (Brancazio & Miller, 2005; Massaro & Cohen, 1983; McGurk & MacDonald, 1976; Sumby & Pollack, 1954), and can improve auditory perception even under the most impoverished of listening conditions (Ramirez & Mann, 2005; Summerfield, 1987). Furthermore, it has been demonstrated that some individuals who have been congenitally deaf since birth are more adept than normal hearing, good readers at visual speech-reading (Mohammed *et al.* 2005). This is a particularly intriguing phenomenon in that the intended phonetic structure of a speaker's articulations can sometimes be determined in the absence of clear acoustic-based representations that are typically acquired during the linguistic development of normal listeners. The perception of speech is, thus, hypothesized to be supra-modal in nature (Schmid & Ziegler, 2006), and this prompts us to ask whether dyslexic individuals have problems with the perception of speech information regardless of the sensory channel from which it is drawn.

A phonological account of dyslexic speech processing might anticipate similar patterns of phonetic feature perception deficits in *both* auditory *and* visual speech perception. A strictly auditory RTP account would not. Whether or not variants on that account, such as those that reference magnocellular (m-cell) deficits (Demb *et al.* 1998a; Demb *et al.*, 1998b; Ridder *et al.*, 1997; Stein & Walsh, 1997) would anticipate this pattern is a matter we shall return to in the discussion. For the most part, individual differences in visual speech perception skill have been studied with regard to specific cognitive factors rather than visual ones. For example, a number of studies have suggested that nonverbal IQ is a poor predictor of visual speech-reading skill (e.g. Elphick, 1996; Jeffers & Barley 1971; Mohammed *et al.* 2005). With regard to psycholinguistic factors, the literature offers some evidence that dyslexics do have problems with visual speech perception. de Gelder and Vroomen (1998) have shown that some poor readers' consonant categorizations are generally less influenced by visual articulatory cues that have been synchronized with audio tokens along a /b/-/d/ continuum. Despite failing to show a significant group x visual cue interaction, de Gelder and Vroomen have, nevertheless, demonstrated that poor readers are generally worse than controls in correctly identifying visual cues. The basic trends in de Gelder and Vroomen's data are wholly consistent with a broader phonological account of visual speech perception. However, they are also partly at odds with the results of Hayes *et al.*'s (2003) auditory-visual studies. When given incongruent audio and visual speech cues, Hayes *et al.*'s sample of LD children were overwhelming biased toward reporting the visual components when their corresponding audio tokens were heavily masked by noise. Oddly enough, these LD subjects were also significantly poorer than controls at identifying visual tokens in quiet. More consistent data is offered by Ramirez and Mann (2005). Not only did their sample of dyslexic adults exhibit poor baseline identification of visual tokens, but also the dyslexics' showed little improvement in their ability to identify noise-degraded audio CV tokens despite the introduction of corresponding visual cues. In the same study both age-matched normal readers and adults who suffered from neuropathic hearing loss showed the opposite trend. It should be noted, though, that Ramirez and Mann's (2005) previous study focused on a broad range of natural CV tokens that were not considered with any specific regard to the kinds of consonant contrasts that are most problematic for dyslexics and, therefore, does not allow us to draw conclusions about its bearings on the predictions of a featural account of phonological processing.

For the following experiment, we applied an audio-visual approach to the stimulus contrasts used by Bradlow *et al.* (1996). Based on that study, we can anticipate that, at least in the auditory channel, categorization difficulties would be most apparent in the /d/-/g/ place of articulation contrast, and not in the /b/-/w/ manner contrast. We used a categorical perception paradigm in order to assess the sharpness with which dyslexics categorize the range of audio tokens along acoustic continua for these two contrasts, and also to see if we could replicate the general trends in Bradlow *et al.*'s previous study. As noise is particularly detrimental to dyslexic speech perception (Brady *et al.,* 1983; Breier *et al.,* 2004; Veuillet *et al.,* 2007), we also wanted to examine how well that dissociation in dyslexics' /d/-/g/ and /b/-/w/ perception fares under impoverished listening conditions. Lastly, and most importantly, we wanted to examine the dyslexics' categorization of speech sounds that have been digitally synchronized with visual articulatory cues to the respective endpoints of each continua, and to see if their performance follows the trends apparent in both Bradlow *et al.* and Kraus *et al.*'s (1996) previous studies even though there is visual information about the identity of the stimuli.

The following were hypothesized: 1) Given Bradlow *et al.*'s data, one could expect that dyslexics, on average, will show a sharper categorical function for the /b/-/w/ contrast than for /d/-/g/. 2) The typical sigmoid-shape of the categorical function for both acoustic continua would be distorted by the presence of simultaneous noise, and there should be greater noise induced distortion in the case of dyslexics. This might result in poorer categorization of the acoustic stimuli at the endpoints as well. 3) Subjects on average should tend to be biased towards reporting any accompanying visual speech cues, especially in noise. However, given that place contrasts tend to be more problematic than manner contrasts, 4) in line with a phonological account of dyslexic perceptual impairments, difficulties in processing the audio tokens for the /d/-/g/ contrast should be accompanied by similar difficulties in processing the corresponding visual cues. If noise proves to be an effective masker, the visual cues for either /d/ or /g/ should not consistently bias the dyslexics' categorization of the audio tokens toward either endpoint.

METHODS

A. Participants

Unlike de Gelder and Vroomen, Ramirez and Mann (2005) previously focused on adult dyslexics who had experienced a lifetime of poor reading. Although Scarborough (1984) has shown that childhood reading disabilities share some continuity with adult reading achievement, in keeping with the methods employed by both de Gelder and Vroomen and Tallal and Piercy (1975), the following experiment examined elementary level children instead of adults for whom a lack of reading experience could possibly be used as an account of poor phonological perception. 15 reading impaired children (6 males, 9 females, mean age: 8:4) who were formally diagnosed as dyslexic were recruited from the Prentice School in Santa Ana, CA, a school that thoroughly screens for concomitant deficits of hearing loss, attention, memory, non-verbal intelligence, etc. prior to identifying children as dyslexic in which case they are eligible for enrollment. Likewise, 15 normal reading control subjects (7 males, 8 females, mean age: 8:9) were recruited from the greater Orange County and Los Angeles County areas using advertisements and were matched with the dyslexic subjects on chronological age (with a difference of no more than 7 months between subjects). All subjects served as paid volunteers. Subjects were screened for hearing loss (20 dB or more from 250 to 8000 Hz in both ears) using a software based audiometer. They were also tested for level of reading achievement using the Woodcock (1998) Word ID and Word Attack basic skill cluster subtests, the former testing for subjects' word reading mastery, and the latter, used to gauge pseudoword decoding.

Audiometry tests yielded normal hearing thresholds for controls and dyslexics. However, the dyslexics typically scored at or below the 20th percentile on Word ID (m = 55.3, $s.d.$ = 4.7 vs. m = 69.5, $s.d.$ = 2.9 for controls, $t(14) = 11.85$, $p < .01$) and Word Attack subtests (m = 18.1, $s.d.$ = 3.8 vs. m = 32.1, $s.d.$ = 2.8 for controls, $t(14) = 7.723$, $p < .01$), where the controls scored at or above the 50th percentile on both measures.

B. Design

Two synthetic acoustic speech sound continua were designed: 1) /ada/-/aga/, comprising a spectro-temporal contrast that turns on the onset and consequently the slope of the F_3 formant transitions with a constant duration of 35 msec and 2) /aba/-/awa/, comprising a temporal duration contrast that turns on a 5 to 50 msec variation in the F_1 and F_2 transition duration but keeps the onset spectra constant. In each case, a 10-step continuum was prepared and factorially combined with noise and visual speech cues. The visual cues were videotaped from a full frontal facial view of a male native speaker of English producing the endpoints of each of the continua: /ada/ and /aga/, /aba/ and /awa/. Subjects were presented with either continuum, with or without noise, and either without visual cues, or with cues corresponding to the continuum presented such that the 10 audio tokens in the /ada/-/aga/ continuum were presented to subjects with the visual cue for /ada/ and for /aga/, only; likewise, for the /aba/-/awa/ continuum.

This experimental paradigm is an adaptation of the design used by Massaro and Cohen (1983). To illustrate, for those conditions where the audio tokens were synchronized with visual cues, we presented the entire /ada/-/aga/ acoustic series with a single visual cue: once with the visual cues articulating /ada/ and once with the visual cues articulating /aga/. Given a single visual token, we would be able to see how each visual cue would bias subjects' responses when it either matched or conflicted with the audio tokens. A similar convention applied to the visual cues for /aba/ and /awa/ for their respective acoustic series.

Lastly there was a visual baseline condition for both continua, with tokens of the visual articulatory cues for /ada/, /aga/, /aba/, and /awa/, presented without audio and randomly throughout testing, five times each.

C. Stimuli and Apparatus

A PC Klatt-based formant synthesizer was used to generate synthetic /ada/-/aga/ and /aba/-/awa/ speech sound continua. For both continua, the initial /a/ steady state vowel sound ran for approximately 150 msec, with vowel frequencies set at approximately 750, 1200, and 2300 Hz for F_1, F_2, and F_3, respectively and a fundamental frequency (F_0) initially set at 120 Hz, tapering down to 90 Hz at the end of the vowel. This was followed by 50 msec of silence that was edited into the waveform after synthesis.

For the /ada/-/aga/ continuum, the gap was then followed by a 35 msec formant transition, the spectro-temporal characteristics of which were manipulated as follows: to remain more or less consistent with the stimulus designs used by Cunningham *et al.* (2002), F_3 varied at onset from 2060 Hz (/g/) to 2600 Hz (/d/) in 10 steps of 60 Hz each, while F_1 and F_2 starting frequencies for the consonants were set at 220 and 1700 Hz, respectively; F_0 was set at 120 Hz. For the /aba/-/awa/ continuum, the duration of the first and second formant transition varied from 5 msec (/b/) to 50 msec (/w/) in 10 steps of 5 msec each. Starting frequencies for the consonants were set at 400, 1000, and 2000 Hz for F_1 (rising linearly to about 750 Hz), F_2 (rising linearly to 1250 Hz), and F_3 (rising linearly to 2300 Hz), respectively; F_0 was again set at 120 Hz. Lastly, the consonants in both continua transitioned into a 150 msec vowel sound /a/, again with vowel frequencies set at 750, 1200, and 2300 Hz for F_1, F_2, and F_3, respectively, and with F_0 tapering down to 90 Hz during the final 30 msec.

For both continua, amplitude voicing (AV) was held stable at 75 dB from stimulus onset, dropping off steadily to 45 dB starting at the last 30 msec of playback. Noise masked stimuli were presented at a -9 dB signal-to-noise ratio (SNR). For the noise-masked condition, for the duration of each trial, audio tokens were masked with a digital audio track of speech shaped noise approximating the mean long term spectrum of the four audio tokens. The auditory stimuli were played to subjects using a pair of Maxell HP-NC1 noise-cancelling headphones.

For trials on which visual articulatory cues were provided, the audio tokens were digitally synchronized with video footage of a male speaker pictured from the neck up in 32-bit color, covering roughly 75% of a 600 X 800 pixel window, and situated in front of a neutral white background, illuminated from above by soft white fluorescent lighting. Four types of video clips were used during testing. They showed the male speaker articulating either /ada/, /aga/, /aba/, or /awa/. For each VCV syllable, five versions were videoed and one best exemplar for each consonant category was chosen for testing after a pilot run determined which of the potential visual cues best controlled for inadvertent eye-blinks, head movements, etc. The stimuli were carefully matched for initial vowel and consonant onset and ended with the speaker open mouthed after the production of the second vowel. The duration of each of the video clips was set to 400 msec to compensate for the maximum stimulus duration required for the /aba/-/awa/ acoustic series. The video clips were sampled at 30 fps and presented to subjects in a video window controlled by Voyetra media software. On trials that were not accompanied by visual articulatory cues, the video window presented subjects with an empty black field. The video window was displayed foveally on a high-resolution height adjustable

Dell LCD monitor, at a viewing distance of approximately 40.64 cm. The monitor was connected to a Sony VAIO laptop that was used to control the presentation of stimuli.

D. Procedure

In a testing room, subjects were administered reading and hearing tests by an experimenter. They were subsequently seated in front of a computer monitor and fitted with noise-cancelling headphones. Subjects were then given five practice trials. They were verbally instructed by the experimenter to watch the computer monitor, and to listen for speech sounds over the headphones. They were then instructed to say what they thought the speaker had said for each trial, and the experimenter recorded each response. For each of these practice trials, subjects were provided with feedback regarding the correct response. The stimuli in the practice sessions were representative of the conditions they would experience in the actual experimental trials. Following practice, there were a total of 260 experimental trials. For the actual experiment, presentation of stimuli was blocked by speech sound continuum, the order of which was counterbalanced across subjects. For each block, each step along a 10-step continuum (/ada/-/aga/ vs. /aba/-/awa/) was presented in six different conditions corresponding to 6 factorial combinations of noise level (in quiet vs. with noise) and visual cue condition (no visual cues, vs. with visual cues /ada/ or /aba/ vs. alternative cues /aga/ or /awa/, depending on the continuum presented). Presentation of each stimulus was randomized for subjects. Additionally, 5 trials randomly interspersed in each block presented the visual cues without audio, bringing the total number of trials to 65 stimuli per block. As in Ramirez and Mann's (2005) prior work, stimuli from each continuum was presented twice, and each factorial combination was also presented twice. Subjects were informed before the start of each block as to which continuum they would be presented with. If presented with the /ada/-/aga/ continuum, subjects were asked to report whether the speech sound presented was either /ada/ or /aga/ only, and to take a best guess if they were not sure. They were also told in advance that they would not receive feedback on the experimental trials. Subjects were permitted a brief break after every block, if so desired.

E. Scoring

Subject responses were recorded according to the consonant reported for each VCV stimulus. Though not common, if the subject responded with a consonant not found in the continuum presented—for example, a subject reported /aba/ when given a block of /ada/-/aga/ VCV stimuli—the subject's response was considered an error and not counted in the total number of either /ada/ or /aga/ responses (and likewise for the /aba/-/awa/ continuum).

F. Analysis

For the /ada/-/aga/ continuum, the mean proportion of subjects' /ada/ responses was computed. Likewise, for the /aba/-/awa/ continuum, the mean proportion of /awa/ responses was computed. These values were then used as the dependent measures for two separate repeated measures analyses of variance (ANOVA)—one for each continuum—to assess main effects for Noise (in quiet vs. in noise), Visual Cues (no visual cues vs. with visual cues: /ada/ or /aba/ vs. alternative visual cues: /aga/ or /awa/) and Step (i.e., stimulus position along the 10 step F_3 onset frequency series for /ada/-/aga/, or along the 10 step F_1-F_2 formant transition duration series for /aba/-/awa/). Group (dyslexic vs. control) served as a between subject factor in each repeated measures ANOVA. One-way ANOVAs were used as needed to assess critical group differences per condition.

RESULTS

The /ada/-/aga/ Continuum

Of the 15 dyslexic subjects examined in this study, 13 subjects were included here for analysis and were matched accordingly with normal reading controls by age. Two subjects did not complete testing with the /ada/-/aga/ stimuli due to fatigue and were thus, excluded.

For the /ada/-/aga/ continuum, the main effects for Group and Noise did not reach significance [$F(1, 24) = 0.963$. $p > .05$; $F(1, 24) = 1.73$. $p > .05$, respectively]. However, the main effects for Step [$F(9, 216) = 35.09$, $p < .001$] and Visual Cue [$F(2, 48) = 15.21$, $p < .001$] were significant. There was also a significant three-way interaction, Noise x Step x Group [$F(9, 216) = 3.16$, $p < .001$] and a significant two-way interaction, Visual Cue x Group [$F(2, 48) = 14.778$, $p < .001$].

Figures 1A and 1B plot the mean proportion of subjects' /ada/ responses at each step along the /ada/-/aga/ continuum in quiet and in noise, respectively. Contrary to our initial prediction, in quiet, the controls and dyslexics exhibited very similar categorical functions (see Figure 1A). In noise, however, the dyslexics' /ada/-/aga/ categorical function appears flattened and distorted (see Figure 1B). In order to more closely study the nature of the three-way interaction, group differences in the proportion of /ada/ responses were examined along each stimulus position and at each level of noise. One-way ANOVAs reveal significant group differences in the proportion of /ada/ responses at the three outermost stimulus positions on either side of the continuum in noise ($p < .05$). In noise, the controls were more likely than the dyslexics to identify stimuli from 2060 to 2180 Hz as being categorically /aga/, and likewise, stimuli from 2480 to 2600 Hz as being categorically /ada/. In quiet, group differences in their categorization of the same endpoint stimuli were not significant ($p > .05$).

As Figure 1C shows, both groups exhibited similar categorical functions when visual articulatory cues were synchronized in quiet with the /ada/-/aga/ audio tokens. In noise, however, the endpoints of the dyslexics' /ada/-/aga/ categorical function are not systematically biased towards either /d/ or /g/ responses despite the introduction of visual cues (see Figure 1D). In order to further evaluate the influence of the different visual cues on subjects' categorization of the audio tokens, in a manner similar to de Gelder and Vroomen (1998), we computed a measure of visual influence by subtracting the proportion of /ada/ responses given visual /aga/, from the proportion of /ada/ responses given visual /ada/, averaging across the 10 steps. We assessed this in quiet and in noise. Generally speaking, the larger this value is, the greater the degree of visual influence on subjects' categorization of the audio tokens.

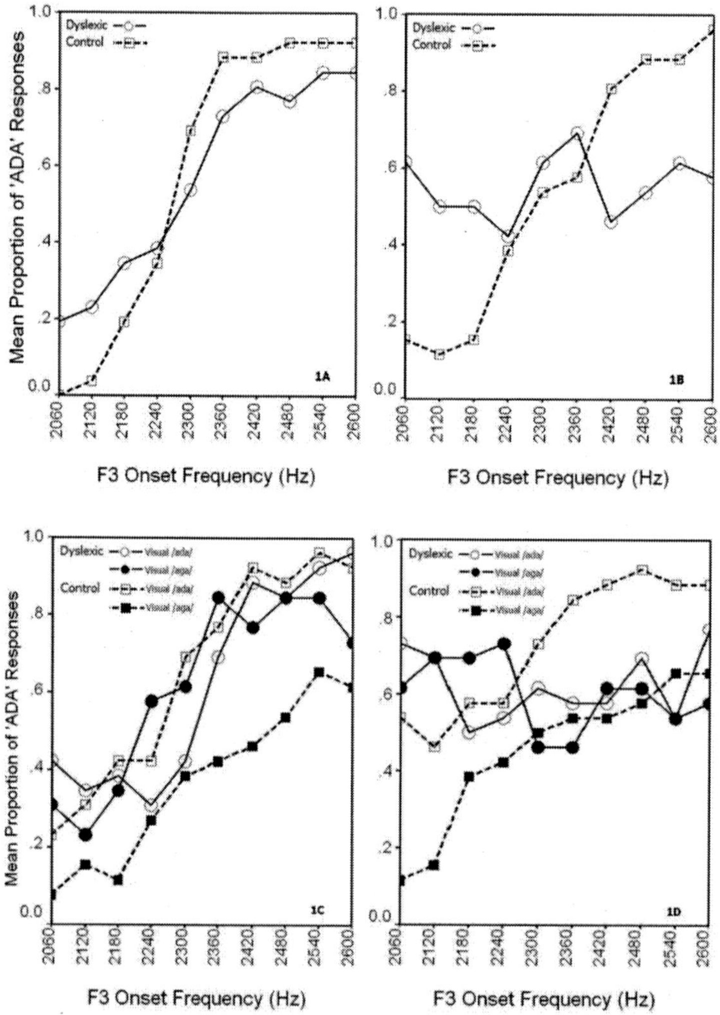

Figures 1. A-D: Subjects' mean proportion of /ada/ responses, plotted across the 10-step /ada/-/aga/ series (1A) in quiet; (1B) in noise; (1C) in quiet with visual cues; and (1D) in noise with visual cues.

The resulting difference values calculated in quiet were significantly larger [$F(1, 24) = 18.86$, $p < .05$] for the controls than for the dyslexics. The same holds true in noise [$F(1, 24) = 6.09$, $p < .05$]. Compared to their performance in quiet, simple effects analyses suggest that the controls generally show an increase in the proportion of /ada/ responses in noise when given visual /ada/ [$F(1, 12) = 9.47$, $p < .05$]. Given visual /aga/, the controls show a slight, but significant increase in the proportion of /ada/ responses in noise [$F(1, 12) = 7.67$, $p < .05$]. Controls were also generally better than the dyslexics in their baseline identification of the /ada/ and /aga/ visual cues, themselves [$F(1, 25) = 24.61$, $p < .05$; $F(1, 25) = 34.98$, $p < .05$, respectively]. On average, given either visual cue, the proportion of /ada/ responses reported by the dyslexics in quiet is not significantly different from that reported in noise [given visual /ada/: $F(1, 12) = .052$, $p > .05$; given visual /aga/: $F(1, 12) = .014$, $p > .05$]. Taken together, it appears that the switch over in the visual cues had stronger consequences on the controls' perception of /d/ vs. /g/ and played a greater role in their categorization of the acoustic stimuli when noise was added. The same cannot be said for the dyslexics.

The /aba/-/awa/ Continuum

Turning to the /aba/-/awa/ continuum, the following analyses included data from 12 of the original 15 dyslexics. Data from three of these subjects was excluded from the analysis since they did not complete testing on the /aba/-/awa/ stimuli due to fatigue. Significant main effects were observed for Visual Cue [$F(2, 44) = 78.74$, $p < .001$], Noise [$F(1, 22) = 10.21$, $p < .05$], Step [$F(9, 198) = 74.50$, $p < .001$], and Group [$F(1, 22) = 12.64$, $p < .05$]. There was a significant three-way Visual Cue x Noise x Group interaction [$F(9, 198) = 2.42$, $p < .05$] as well as two-way interactions, Visual Cue x Noise [$F(2, 44) = 19.96$, $p < .001$] and Visual Cue x Group [$F(2, 44) = 7.04$, $p < .05$].

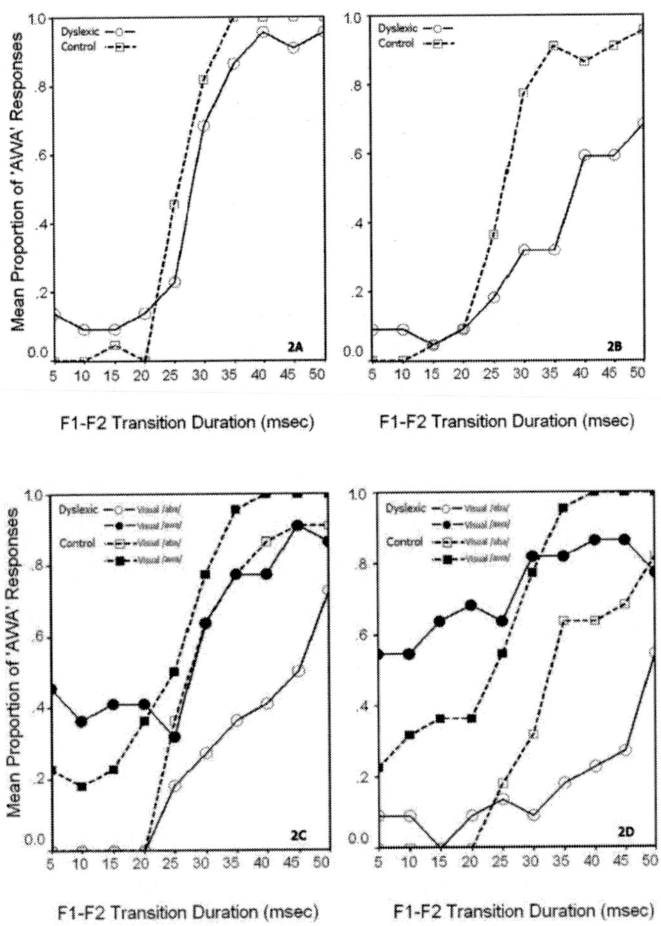

Figures 2. A-D: Subjects' mean proportion of /awa/ responses, plotted across the 10-step /aba/-/awa/ series (2A) in quiet; (2B) in noise; (2C) in quiet with visual cues; and (2D) in noise with visual cues.

Figure 2A shows that the dyslexics and controls exhibited very similar /aba/-/awa/ categorical functions in quiet. One-way ANOVAs comparing the proportion of /awa/ responses across each stimulus position in quiet reveal no significant group differences ($p > .05$). In noise, however, significant group differences ($p < .05$) in the proportion of /awa/ responses were observed at each step from 30 to 50 msec, with the dyslexics showing a more gradual rise in the proportion of /awa/ responses in noise than that exhibited by the controls (see Figure 2B).

In sharp contrast to their performance with the /ada/-/aga/ auditory-visual stimuli, effects of the visual cues on the /aba/-/awa/ continuum are evident in both groups, and are actually stronger for the dyslexics. Again, simple effects analyses were applied to examine how each group differed in terms of their provision of the visual cues in quiet and in noise. As Figure 2D shows, given visual /aba/, the proportion of /awa/ responses in noise was significantly lower than that reported in quiet ([$F(1, 11) = 6.70$, $p < .05$]; compare with Figure 2C) as the F_1 and F_2 transition durations approached 50 msec. Likewise, given visual /awa/, the proportion of /awa/ responses reported by the dyslexics in noise was higher than that reported in quiet [$F(1, 11) = 10.10$, $p < .05$] as the F_1 and F_2 transition durations approached 5 msec. Among the controls, similar effects were observed for visual /aba/ [$F(1, 11) = 7.63$, $p < .05$]. Given visual /awa/, the controls performed very similarly in their categorization of the /aba/-/awa/ stimuli in quiet and in noise [$F(1, 11) = 3.69$, $p > .05$].

To examine the effects of the visual cues on perception more closely, as with the /ada/-/aga/ continuum, we subtracted the proportion of /awa/ responses given visual /aba/, from the proportion of /awa/ responses given visual /awa/, again, averaging across the 10-step series. The resulting difference values calculated for the /aba/ and /awa/ visual cues, both in quiet and in noise, are actually larger for the dyslexics than the controls [$F(1, 22) = 3.09$, $p < .05$; $F(1, 22) = 7.43$, $p < .05$, respectively]. This suggests that, especially in noise, the dyslexics were more biased toward reporting the identity of the visual cues than the controls. These results, coupled with data that shows that, especially in noise, visual /awa/ shifted perception across the continuum more towards /awa/ (and likewise for visual /aba/), suggest that the dyslexics were better at discerning a contrast in the visual articulations for /b/ and /w/ than they were for /d/ vs. /g/. That no group differences were observed in the baseline identification of visual /aba/ and /awa/ [$F(1, 23) = 3.83$, $p > .05$; $F(1, 23) = .002$, $p > .05$, respectively] is in keeping with this assertion.

DISCUSSION

This categorical perception experiment attempted to probe the basis of dyslexics' inordinate difficulties in processing certain speech contrasts. We assessed dyslexics' and age-matched controls' categorization of synthetic vowel-consonant-vowel (VCV) sounds along /ada/-/aga/ and /aba/-/awa/ continua that were factorially combined with noise and visual articulatory cues corresponding to the endpoints of their respective continuum. We interpret our preliminary findings with some caution given 1) the need for a larger N for our sample population and 2) the need to include younger, reading level-matched controls, as is often called for in studies of dyslexic phonological processing to rule out reading experience as a potential confound. That being said, we readily note that our data are wholly consistent with the pattern of contrast perception difficulties heretofore reported in the literature.

As expected from prior studies (Bradlow *et al.*, 1999; Brady *et al.* 1983; Cunningham *et al.,* 2001) the dyslexics showed inordinately poor categorization of /ada/-/aga/ stimuli in noise. We further find that they showed poorer perception of isolated visual cues to this same contrast, and when the auditory and visual cues to /d/-/g/ were played in synchrony, the dyslexics showed little or no discernable bias towards reporting the visual cue that was present, even in noise. As expected from other work (Kraus *et al.* 1996) the dyslexics also showed more success with the /b/-/w/ distinction. In this case, their categorization of the acoustic /aba/-/awa/ stimuli was more significantly affected by noise than that of the controls. Furthermore, the dyslexics and controls were equally accurate in their perception of the isolated visual /aba/ and /awa/ stimuli, and their responses demonstrated a heightened bias for reporting the identity of the visual cues when the /aba/-/awa/ continuum was presented in noise.

As noted in the introduction, individuals who have reading disabilities find it particularly difficult to discriminate consonants that differ on place of articulation, but are generally better at discriminating consonants that contrast on manner of articulation. Our data are in keeping with these trends, extending previous findings about acoustic stimuli under quiet conditions to perception in noise, and to perception of visual speech stimuli. How do other accounts of our data fare? There are three that we shall consider in turn: those couched in terms of auditory-RTP deficits, magnocellular (m-cell) deficits, and integration failures. The first of these is the most straightforward to address. That the dyslexics performed much better with the acoustic /b/-/w/ contrast is not a surprise for proponents of the traditional RTP account. At least in the auditory domain, /b/ and /w/ have been previously used as a control and natural foil for the /d/-/g/ contrast (Bradlow *et al.* 1999; Kraus *et al.* 1996; Tallal & Piercy, 1975) and are not expected to provoke perceptual difficulty. That noise causes the dyslexics in this study more difficulty with both /d/ and /g/, and /b/ and /w/ in this experiment, as it has in other cases (e.g., Brady *et al.*, 1983, Cunningham *et al.*, 2001; Watson & Miller; 1993; Wible *et al.*, 2002) is not anticipated by acoustic accounts in general. Most importantly, these acoustic accounts are not consistent with our findings that dyslexics are significantly poorer than controls in their baseline identification of visual /d/ and /g/ cues and that their perception of noise-masked acoustic stimuli is, generally, less influenced by the introduction of these visual cues.

It is not simply the case that dyslexics fail to use visual cues under just any condition; the results from the /aba/-/awa/ continuum show that dyslexics were particularly biased toward reporting the corresponding visual cues when the audio tokens were masked by noise. In sharp contrast to their performance with the /ada/ and /aga/ visual cues, the dyslexics show an overall increase in the proportion of /awa/ responses across the /aba/-/awa/ continuum when given /awa/ visual cues, and a corresponding decrease in /awa/ responses when given /aba/ visual cues, especially in noise.

Perhaps a more attractive account of the difference between /d/-/g/ and /b/-/w/ in both the acoustic and visual domains would couch the RTP account in terms of multiple modalities, in which case deficits in the processing of /ada/ and /aga/ visual cues merely represent the visual analogue of an auditory deficit. To their credit, researchers who investigate m-cells processes have taken great strides to consolidate the disparate unimodal processing deficits that have been reported in the dyslexic literature. They point to a neural substrate that could explain a unitary sensory dysfunction that affects the processing of dynamic stimuli (for a review, see Ramus *et al.* 2003). Although the auditory system possesses no m-cell pathway of the sort that contributes to vision, it does possess an analogous set of large cells at the level of the medial geniculate nucleus (Livingstone *et al.*, 1991; Galaburda *et al.*, 1994) that encode the frequency and amplitude characteristics of acoustic stimuli.

The literature on m-cell research (Demb *et al.* 1998a; Demb *et al.*, 1998b; Ridder *et al.*, 1997; Stein & Walsh, 1997) has indeed brought forth a wide array of experimental evidence cataloging various anomalies in visual spatial and temporal perception. However, unlike the stimuli used in our study, these involved transient, low contrast, monochromatic stimuli that are normally presented to the visual periphery at near scotopic-level luminance to selectively tap m-cell function for early visual processing of form and motion (for review see Skottun, 1997, 2000; Skottun & Skoyles, 2008; Skoyles & Skottun, 2004). Calling attention to potential links between m-cell processes and visual speech perception, Mohammed *et al.* (2005) reported a correlation between visual speech-reading skill and sensitivity measures of m-cell function (e.g., visual coherent motion sensitivity) among deaf individuals. This relationship, however, was not found to be significant for normal listeners. Mohammed *et al.* (2006) have further shown that dyslexics are poor visual speech readers for a broad class of segmental and sentential stimuli and speculated that speech-reading deficits may be linked to dyslexics' poor m-cell function. From our perspective, however, if poor spatial and temporal acuity are the primary problems in dyslexia, one would expect that the effects of m-cell visual deficits would be far more widespread and not merely limited just to the domain of visual speech-reading. To our knowledge, no clear psychophysical link has been established that clearly demonstrates a relationship between poor m-cell function and deficits in visual speech-reading among dyslexics. We are currently investigating this putative link to complement the results of this auditory-visual categorical perception study. That being said, sensory aberrations that are reflective of m-cell dysfunction appear to be correlates of reading achievement, and thus, may have some potential prognostic value, but that does not necessarily imply that they are proximal factors in reading disability.

Turning finally to problems with auditory-visual integration: these were once a popular account of dyslexia, but they have long since been dismissed in favor of phonological accounts (for reviews, see Benton, 1975; Mann, 2003; Rutter & Yule, 1973). Could a more sophisticated, perceptual variation of these accounts explain our data? Cavé *et al.* (2007) have shown that poor readers exhibit fewer McGurk percepts relative to controls when presented with incongruent auditory and visual speech components. For example, they are less likely than controls to 'see' /g/, while 'hearing' /b/ and then report 'd'. But the problem in proposing that this perceptual difference is due to an integrative failure is one of garbage in—garbage out: one cannot easily untangle the effects of poor phonetic feature extraction stemming from a supra-modal phonological deficit from an acute failure of cross-modal/dynamic integration. McGurk responses (or lack thereof) are ambiguous in that regard, which is why we examined responses to unimodal and bimodal presentations of visual and auditory speech stimuli. The presence of an impairment in unimodal perception, by itself, makes it more plausible to say that a phonological deficit, from the top down, serves as the bottleneck on integration. Furthermore, auditory-visual speech perception may not be a mere ancillary property of general cross-modal integration. Schmid and Ziegler *et al.* (2006), for example, have demonstrated a potential dissociation between bimodal speech and non-speech perception in patients with receptive aphasia and oral apraxia. In a discrimination task, the patients clearly benefited from the bimodal presentation of non-speech bilabial and alveolar articulatory gestures and sounds (e.g., whistles, and clicks). No such advantage was found for bimodally presented speech stimuli. Clearly more study is required in this particular area of speech perception as it would be interesting to see if dyslexics exhibit a similar dissociation in bimodal perception. For now, we note that there has been much more progress in refining the phonological deficit hypothesis and its extension to phonological perception, phonological working memory, and phonological awareness (Mann, 2003; Shaywitz, 2008; Shaywitz *et al.*, 2003, 2005; Stanovich, 1998) than there has been in establishing either integrative or modality-based deficits.

Our primary point is that reference to the units implied by phonological representations–namely phonetic features–can describe the pattern of our results in both the auditory and the visual modes of speech perception. Reference to phonological units, in and of itself, does not offer an explicit stance on why nuances appear in the dyslexics' phonetic feature perception. However, Mody (2003) offered potential insights into the context dependencies of a core phonological deficit by proposing that poor speech perception results from a poor grasp of the subtleties involved in speech production. Poor or imprecise representations of certain core coarticulatory processes that underlie the place features that differentiate speech sounds, or a poor mapping of the underlying speech gestures to phonetic percepts could contribute to potential confusions between phonetically similar but phonologically contrastive speech sounds and, by extension, their visual articulatory counterparts.

It has been suggested that feedback from the articulators can fine-tune the perception of category boundaries (Werker & Tees, 1987) and that dyslexics may use motor-articulatory strategies during phonetic processing of auditory-visual speech to compensate for their difficulties in auditory speech perception. Pekkola *et al.*'s (2006) functional magnetic resonance imaging (fMRI) study revealed heightened activation in response to the viewing of McGurk type stimuli in both Broca's area and left premotor cortex among reading impaired individuals. Interestingly, these areas are highly implicated in speech production and motor coordination. Furthermore, Shaywitz *et al.* (1998) and Pugh *et al.* (2000) have reported that dyslexics showed greater activation in Broca's area relative to controls, whereas controls showed greater activation in Wernicke's area (which is often associated with more receptive phonological processing) on silent reading tasks. This would suggest that dyslexics differentially engage those cortical areas devoted to production to laboriously uncover the articulatory basis of the corresponding sounds in words. The trends in our data, however, suggest that such strategies afford dyslexics varying degrees of success in their on-line processing of the phonetic features of speech. It is possible that critical articulatory representations that underlie auditory-visual speech perception are either lacking, or are less refined, or are otherwise less automatic/accessible for dyslexics. As subtle articulatory disorders have been observed among pre-school children and are prognostic of rhyme and phonological awareness problems (Mann & Foy, 2007), it follows that early intervention training in articulatory awareness may go a long way to help remediate their phonological processing deficits (Wise & Olson, 1995).

CONCLUSION

We describe the pattern of our data with the hypothesis that dyslexics have difficulties in discriminating both sounds and sights that convey differences in place of articulation. Our data are not well described by auditory-RTP accounts which would anticipate intact visual speech perception. Furthermore, our data are problematic for m-cell accounts to the extent that the critical parameters of our visual stimuli do not readily map onto m-cell attributes. Lastly, they are problematic for integrative accounts because unimodal visual discrimination is compromised for consonants that differ in place of articulation. Although it remains to be determined *why* place contrasts are more difficult than manner contrasts, perhaps future work could attempt to conceptually reconcile articulatory-based arguments with the featural accounts of Elbro (1996) and Fowler and Swanson (2004) by critically examining the underlying articulatory gestures/representations that signal key differences in place and manner features. For now, our findings are more confluent with the assertions of a supra-modal phonological processing account of dyslexia by demonstrating that speech processing deficits are similarly nuanced in both the auditory and visual modes of perception. We feel that this avenue of research warrants further study as auditory-visual speech perception is a relatively underutilized avenue of research in dyslexia that could be used to further test the respective propositions of phonological and sensory based accounts of reading disability.

Acknowledgments

The authors wish to thank the staff of the Prentice School in Santa Ana, CA, and in particular, its principal and executive director, Mrs. Carol Clark, for providing access to the dyslexic children in this study. This research was generously supported by fellowship funding by the National Institutes of Health (NIH/NICHD: 5F31HD046411-04).

References

Auer, E. T., Jr. (2002). The influence of the lexicon on speech read word recognition: Contrasting segmental and lexical distinctiveness. *Psychonomic Bulletin and Review*, *9*, 341–347.

Benton, A. (1975). Developmental dyslexia: Neurological aspects. In. W. J. Freelander (Ed.) *Advances in Neurology: Vol. 7*. (pp.1-47). New York: Raven Press.

Brady, S., Shankweiler, D. & Mann, V. A. (1983). Speech perception and memory coding in relation to reading ability, *Journal of Experimental Child Psychology*, *35*, 345–367.

Bradlow, A. R., Kraus, N., Nicol, T. G., McGee, T. J., Cunningham, J., Zecker, S. G. & Carrell, T. D. (1999). Effects of lengthened formant transition duration on discrimination and neural representation of synthetic CV syllables by normal and learning-disabled children. *Journal of the Acoustical Society of America, 106(4)*, 2086-2096.

Brancazio, L. & Miller, J. (2005). Use of visual information in speech perception: Evidence for a visual rate effect both with and without a McGurk effect. *Perception and Psychophysics*, *67(5)*, 759-769.

Brandt, J. & Rosen, J. J. (1980). Auditory phonemic perception in dyslexia: Categorical identification and discrimination of stop consonants. *Brain and Language*, *9*, 324–337.

Breier, J. I., Fletcher, J. M., Denton, C. & Gray, L. C. (2004). Categorical perception of speech stimuli in children at risk for reading difficulty. *Journal of Experimental Child Psychology, 88*, 152–170.

Bogliotti, C., Messaoud-Galusi, S. & Serniclaes, W. (2002). Relations entre la perception catégorielle de la parole et l'apprentissage de la lecture, ("The relationship between the categorical perception of speech and learning to read"). *XXIVèmes Journées d'Etudes sur la Parole*, 197-200.

Bogliotti, C., Serniclaes, W., Messaoud-Galusi, S. & Sprenger-Charolles, L. (2008). Discrimination of speech sounds by children with dyslexia: Comparisons with chronological age and reading level controls. *Journal of Experimental Child Psychology, 101(2)*, 137-155.

Cavé, C., Stroumza, A. & Bastien-Toniazzo, M. (2007). "The McGurk effect in dyslexic and normal-reading children: an experimental study," In proceedings from the International Conference on Auditory-Visual Speech Processing, 2007, paper P02.

Chiappe, P., Chiappe, D. L. & Siegel, L. (2001). Speech perception, lexicality, and reading skill. *Journal of Experimental Child Psychology, 80*, 58-74.

Chiappe, P., Stringer, R., Siegel, L. S. & Stanovich, K. E. (2002). Why the timing deficit hypothesis does not explain reading disability in adults. *Reading and Writing: An Interdisciplinary Journal, 15*, 73-107.

Cunningham, J., Nicol, T., Zecker, S., Bradlow, A. & Kraus, N. (2001). Neurobiologic responses to speech in noise in children with learning problems: deficits and strategies for improvement. *Clinical Neurophysiology, 112*, 758-767.

de Gelder, B. & Vroomen, J. (1998). Impaired speech perception in poor readers: Evidence from hearing and speech reading. *Brain and Language, 64*, 269–281.

De Weirdt, W. (1988). Speech perception and frequency discrimination in good and poor readers. *Applied Psycholinguistics, 9*, 163-183.

Demb, J. B., Boytnon, G. M. & Heeger, J. G. (1998a). Functional magnetic resonance imaging of early visual pathways in dyslexia. *Journal of Neuroscience, 18(17)*, 6939-6951.

Demb, J. B., Boytnon, G. M., Heeger, J. G. & Best, M. (1998b). Psychophysical evidence for a magnocellular pathway deficit in dyslexia. *Vision Research, 38(11)*, 1555-1559.

Elbro, C. (1996). Early linguistic abilities and reading development: A review and a hypothesis. *Reading and Writing: An Interdisciplinary Journal, 8*, 453-485.

Elliot, L. L. & Hammer, M. A. (1988). Longitudinal changes in auditory discrimination in normal children and children with language-learning problems. *Journal of Speech and Hearing Disorders, 53*, 467-474.

Elliott, L. L., Hammer, M. A. & Scholl, M. E. (1989). Fine-grained auditory discrimination in normal children and children with language learning problems. *Journal of Speech and Hearing Research, 32*, 112–119.

Elphick, R. (1996). Issues in comparing the speechreading abilities of hearing-impaired and hearing 15 to 16 year-old pupils. *British Journal of Educational Psychology, 66*, 357-365.

Farmer, M. E. & Klein, R. M. (1995a). The evidence for a temporal processing deficit linked to dyslexia. *Psychonomic Bulletin Review, 2*, 460-493.

Farmer, M. E. & Klein, R. M. (1995b). Dyslexia and temporal processing deficit: a reply to the commentaries. *Psychonomic Bulletin Review, 2*, 515-526.

Fowler, A. E. & Swanson, B. (2004). Relationships of naming skills to reading, memory, and receptive vocabulary: evidence for imprecise phonological representations of words by poor readers. *Annals of Dyslexia, 54(2)*, 247-280.

Gaab, N., Gabrieli, J. D. E., Deutsch, G. K., Tallal, P. & Temple, E. (2007). Neural correlates of rapid auditory processing are disrupted in children with developmental dyslexia and ameliorated with training: An fMRI study. *Restorative Neurology and Neuroscience, 25*, 295-310.

Galaburda, A. M., Menard, M. T. & Rosen, G.D. (1994). Evidence for aberrant auditory anatomy in developmental dyslexia. *Proceedings from the National Academy of Sciences, 91*, 8010-8013.

Godfrey, J. J., Syrdal-Lasky, A. K., Millay, K. & Knox, C. M. (1981). Performance of dyslexic children on speech perception tests. *Journal of Experimental Child Psychology, 32*, 401– 424.

Hayes, E. A., Tiippana, K., Nicol, T. G., Sams, M. & Kraus, N. (2003). Integration of heard and seen speech: a factor in learning disabilities in children. *Neuroscience Letters, 351*, 46-50.

Jeffers, J. & Barley, M. (1971). *Speechreading (Lipreading)*, Springfield, IL: C. C. Thomas.

Joanisse, M. F., Manis, F. R., Keating, P. & Seidenberg, M. S. (2000). Language deficits in dyslexic children: Speech perception, phonology, and morphology. *Journal of Experimental Child Psychology, 77*, 30-60.

Kraus, N., McGee, T. J., Carrell, T. D., Zecker, S. G., Nicol, T. G. & Koch, D. B. (1996). Auditory neurophysiologic responses and discrimination deficits in children with learning problems. *Science, 273*, 971–973.

Leonard, L. B., McGregor, K. K. & Allen, G. D. (1992). Grammatical morphology and speech perception in children with specific language impairment. *Journal of Speech and Hearing Research, 35*, 1076–1085.

Liberman, A. M. & Mattingly, I. G. (1985). The motor theory of speech perception revised. *Cognition, 21,* 1–36.

Lieberman, P., Meskill, R. H., Chatillon, & Schupack, H. (1985). Phonetic speech perception deficits in dyslexia. *Journal of Speech and Hearing Research, 28*, 480-486.

Livingstone, M. S., Rosen, G. D., Drislane, F. W. & Galaburda A. M. (1991). Physiological and anatomical evidence for a magnocellular defect in developmental dyslexia. *Proceeds from the National Academy of Sciences, 88*, 7943-7947.

Mann, V. A. (2003). "Language Processes: Keys to Reading Disability." In H. L. Swanson, K. R. Harris and S. Graham (Eds.) *Handbook of Learning Disabilities* (pp. 213-228). New York: Guilford Press.

Mann, V. & Foy, J. (2007). Speech development patterns and phonological awareness in preschool children. *Annals of Dyslexia, 57*, 51-74.

Massaro, D. W. (1984). Children's perception of visual and auditory speech. *Child Development, 55*, 1777-1778.

Massaro, D. W. (1987). "Categorical partition: A fuzzy-logical model of categorization behavior," in S. Harnad (Ed.) *Categorical Perception: The Groundwork of Cognition*, New York, NY: Cambridge University Press.

Massaro, D. W. & Cohen, M. M. (1983). Evaluation and integration of visual and auditory information in speech perception. *Journal of Experimental Child Psychology, 41*, 751-753.

McCrosky, R. L. & Kidder, H. C. (1980). Auditory fusion among learning disabled, reading disabled, and normal children. *Journal of Learning Disabilities*, *13*, 18–25.

McGurk, H. & MacDonald, J. (1976). Hearing lips and seeing voices. *Nature*, *264*, 746-748.

Miller, G. A. & Nicely, P. (1955). An analysis of perceptual confusions among some English Consonants. *Journal of the Acoustical Society of America*, *27(2)*, 338-352.

Mody, M. (2003). Phonological basis in reading disability: A review and analysis of the evidence. *Reading and Writing: An Interdisciplinary Journal*, *16*, 21-39.

Mody, M. & Studdert-Kennedy, M. & Brady, S. (1997). Speech perception deficits in poor readers: Auditory processing or phonological coding? *Journal of Experimental Child Psychology*, *64*, 199–231.

Mohammed, R., Campbell, R., MacSweeney, M., Barry, F. & Coleman, M. (2006). Speechreading and its association with reading among deaf, hearing and dyslexic individuals. *Clinical Linguistics and Phonetics*, *20(7-8)*, 621-630.

Mohammed, R., Campbell, R., MacSweeney, M., Milne, E., Hansen, P. & Coleman, M. (2005). Speechreading skill and visual movement sensitivity are related in deaf speechreaders. *Perception*, *34*, 205-216.

Pekkola, J., Laasonen, M., Ojanen, V., Autii, T., Ja¨a¨skela¨inen, I. P., Kujala, T. & Sams, M. (2006). Perception of matching and conflicting audiovisual speech in dyslexic and fluent readers: an fMRI study at 3T. *Neuroimaging*, *29*, 797-807.

Pugh, K.R., Mencl, W.E., Jenner, A.R., Katz, L., Frost, S.J., Lee, J.R., Shaywitz, S.E. & Shaywitz, B.A. (2000). Functional neuroimaging studies of reading and reading disability. *Mental Retardation and Development Disabilities Review, 6*, 207–213.

Ramirez, J. & Mann, V. (2005). Using auditory-visual speech to probe the basis of developmental dyslexia and auditory neuropathy. *Journal of the Acoustical Society of America*, *118(2)*, 1122-1133.

Ramus, F., Rosen, S., Dakin, S. C., Day, B. L., Castellote, J. M., White, S. & Firth, U. (2003). Theories of developmental dyslexia: insights from a multiple case study of dyslexic adults. *Brain*, *126(4)*, 841-865.

Ridder, W. H. 3rd, Borsting, E., Cooper, M., McNeel, B., and Huang, E. (1997). Not all dyslexics are equal. *Optometry and Vision Science*, *74*, 99-104.

Reed, M. A. (1989). Speech perception and the discrimination of brief auditory cues in dyslexic children. *Journal of Experimental Child Psychology*, *48*, 270-292.

Rosen S. & Manganari, E. (2001). Is there a relationship between speech and nonspeech auditory processing in children with dyslexia? *Journal of Speech Language and Hearing Research*, *44*, 720-736.

Rutter, M. & Yule, W. (1973). The concept of specific reading retardation. *Journal of Child Psychiatry*, *16*, 181-198.

Scarborough, H. S. (1984). Continuity between childhood dyslexia and adult reading. *British Journal of Psychology*, *75*, 329-348.

Schmid, G. & Ziegler, W. (2006). Audio-visual matching of speech and non-speech of oral gestures in patients with aphasia and apraxia of speech. *Neuropsychologia*, *44*, 546-545.

Serniclaes, W., Sprenger-Charolles, L. Carré, R. & Demonet J. F. (2001). Perceptual discrimination of speech sounds in developmental dyslexia. *Journal of Speech Language and Hearing Research*, *44(2)*, 384-399.

Serniclaes, W., Van Heghe, S., Mousty, P., Carré, R. & Sprenger-Charolles, L. (2004). Allophonic mode of speech perception in dyslexia. *Journal of Experimental Child Psychology*, *87*, 336-361.

Share, D. L., Jorm, A. F., MacLean, R. & Matthews, R. (2002). Temporal processing and reading disability. *Reading and Writing: An Interdisciplinary Journal*, *15*, 151-178.

Shaywitz, S. E. & Shaywitz, B. A. (2003). "Neurobiological indices of dyslexia." In Swanson, H. Lee; Harris, Karen R.; Graham, Steve (Eds.) *Handbook of Learning Disabilities* (pp. 514-531). New York, NY: Guilford Press.

Shaywitz, S. E. & Shaywitz, B. A. (2005). Dyslexia (Specific Reading Disability). *Biological Psychiatry*, *57(11)*, 1301-1309.

Shaywitz, S. (2008). "Why some smart people can't read." In Immordino-Yang, Mary Helen (Eds.) *The Jossey-Bass Reader on the Brain and Learning*. (pp. 242-250). San Francisco, CA: Jossey-Bass.

Skottun, B. C. (1997). The magnocellular deficit theory of dyslexia. *Trends in Neurosciences*, *20*, 397–398.

Skottun, B. C. (2000). On the conflicting support for the magnocellular theory of dyslexia. *Trends in Cognitive Sciences*, *4(6)*, 211-212.

Skottun B. C. & Skoyles J. R. (2008). Dyslexia and rapid visual processing: a commentary. *Journal of Clinical and Experimental Neuropsychology*, *30(6)*, 666-673.

Skoyles, J. & Skottun, B. C. (2004). On the prevalence of magnocellular deficits in the visual system of non-dyslexic individuals. *Brain and Language*, *88*, 79-82.

Snowling, M. J. (2000). *Dyslexia* (2nd ed.). Malden, MA: Blackwell Publishers.

Snowling, M., Goulandris, N., Bowlby, M. & Howell, P. (1986). Segmentation and speech perception in relation to reading skill: A developmental analysis. *Journal of Experimental Child Psychology*, *41*, 489-507.

Stanovich, K. E. (1998). Explaining differences between the dyslexic and the garden-variety poor reader: The phonological-core variable-difference model. *Journal of Educational. Psychology*, *86*, 24-53.

Stark, R. E. & Tallal, P. (1988). *Language, Speech and Reading Disorders in Children: Neurobiological Studies*, San Diego; College Hall Press.

Stein, J. & Walsh, V. (1997). To see but not to read: the magnocellular theory of dyslexia. *Trends in Neurosciences*, *20*, 147–152

Studdert-Kennedy, M. & Mody, M. (1995). Auditory temporal perception deficits in the reading impaired: A critical review of the evidence. *Psychonomic Bulletin Review*, *4*, 508-514.

Sumby, W. & Pollack, I. (1954). Visual contribution to speech intelligibility in noise. *Journal of the Acoustical Society of America*, *26*, 212-215.

Summerfield, Q. (1987). "A comprehensive account of audio-visual speech perception," In B. Dodd and R. Campbell (Eds.) *Hearing by Eye: The Psychology of Lip-Reading,* London: Erlbaum, 3–51.

Sussman, J. E. (1993). Perception of formant transition cues to place of articulation in children with language impairments. *Journal of Speech and Hearing Research, 36*, 1286–1299.

Tallal, P. (1980). Auditory temporal perception, phonics and reading disabilities in children *Brain and Language*, *9*, 182-198.

Tallal, P., Fitch, R. H. & Miller, S., (1993). Neurobiological basis of speech: a case for the preeminence of temporal processing. *Annals of the New York Academy of Sciences, 682*, 27-47.

Tallal, P. & Piercy, M. (1973a). Defects of non-verbal auditory perception in children with developmental aphasia. *Nature, 241*, 468–469.

Tallal, P. & Piercy, M. (1973b). Developmental aphasia: impaired rate of non-verbal processing as a function of sensory modality. *Neuropsychologia, 11*, 389-398.

Tallal, P. & Piercy, M. (1974). Developmental aphasia: Rate of auditory processing and selective impairment of consonant perception. *Neuropsychologia, 12*, 83–93.

Tallal, P. & Piercy, M. (1975). Developmental aphasia: The perception of brief vowels and extended stop consonants. *Neuropsychologia, 13*, 69-74.

Tallal, P., Sainburg, R. L. & Jernigan, T. (1991). The neuropathology of developmental dysphasia: behavioral, morphological, and physiological evidence for a pervasive temporal processing disorder. *Reading And Writing: An Interdisciplinary Journal, 3*, 363-377.

Tallal, P. & Stark, R. E. (1981). Speech acoustic-cue discrimination abilities of normally developing and language-impaired children. *Journal of the Acoustical Society of America, 69*, 568–574.

Tallal, P. & Stark, R. (1982). Perceptual/motor profiles of reading impaired children with or without concomitant oral language deficits. *Annals of Dyslexia, 32*, 163-176.

Veuillet, E., Magnan, A., Ecalle, J., Thai-Van, H. & Collet, L. (2007). Auditory processing disorder in children with reading disabilities: effect of audiovisual training. *Brain, 130*, 2915-2928.

Vellutino, F. R. (1979). *Dyslexia: Theory and Research.* Cambridge, MA: MIT Press.

Watson, B. U. & Miller, T. K. (1993). Auditory perception, phonological processing and reading ability/disability. *Journal of Speech and Hearing Research, 36(4)*, 850–863.

Werker, J. F. & Tees, R. C. (1987). Speech perception in severely disabled and average reading children. *Canadian Journal of Psychology, 41*, 48-61.

Whalen, D. H. & Liberman, A. M. (1996). Limits on phonetic integration in duplex perception. *Perception and Psychophysics, 56*, 857–870.

Wible, B., Nicol, T. & Kraus, N. (2002). Abnormal neural encoding of repeated speech stimuli in noise in children with learning problems. *Clinical Neurophysiology, 113(4)*, 485–494.

Wise, B. W. & Olson, R. K. (1995). Computer-based phonological awareness and reading instruction. *Annals of Dyslexia, 45*, 99–122.

Woodcock, R. W. (1998). *Woodcock Reading Mastery Tests—Revised, Normative Update* (American Guidance Services, Inc., Circle Pines, MN).

Zhang, J. L. (1996). "On the syllable structures of Chinese relating to speech recognition," In proceedings from the Fourth International Conference on Spoken Language, *4*, 2450-2453.

Index

A

B

C

D

E

F

G

H

I

J

K

L

M

N

O

P

Q

R

S

T

U

V

W

Y